Nutrition Almanac

Nutrition Almanac

FIFTH EDITION

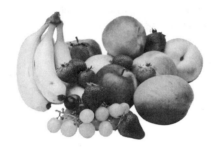

Lavon J. Dunne

McGraw-Hill

New York   Chicago   San Francisco   Lisbon   London   Madrid
Mexico City   Milan   New Delhi   San Juan   Seoul
Singapore   Sydney   Toronto

Library of Congress Cataloging-in-Publication Data

Dunne, Lavon J.
    Nutrition almanac / Lavon J. Dunne.—5th ed.
        p.   cm.
    Includes bibliographical references and index.
    ISBN 0-07-137338-1
    1. Nutrition. 2. Health. 3. Food—Composition—Tables. I. Title.
    RA784.N387   2001
    613.2—dc21

                                                    2001041013

McGraw-Hill

A Division of The McGraw·Hill Companies

1 2 3 4 5 6 7 8 9 0 PBT/PBT 0 9 8 7 6 5 4 3 2 1

ISBN 0-07-137338-1

The sponsoring editor for this book was Mark Licker, the editing supervisor was David E. Fogarty, and the production supervisor was Pamela A. Pelton. It was set in New Caledonia by North Market Street Graphics.

Printed and bound by Phoenix Book Tech.

 This book was printed on recycled, acid-free paper containing a minimum of 50% recycled, de-inked fiber.

McGraw-Hill books are available at special quantity discounts to use as premiums and sales promotions, or for use in corporate training programs. For more information, please write to the Director of Special Sales, Professional Publishing, McGraw-Hill, Two Penn Plaza, New York, NY 10121-2298. Or contact your local bookstore.

First McGraw-Hill paperback edition 1975
Revised McGraw-Hill paperback edition 1979
Second McGraw-Hill paperback edition 1984
Third McGraw-Hill paperback edition 1990
Fourth McGraw-Hill paperback edition 1996
Fifth McGraw-Hill paperback edition 2002

CONTENTS

Preface ix

SECTION I
Nutrients   1

Macronutrients 5
Carbohydrates 5
Fats 7
Protein 9
Micronutrients 10
Vitamins 10
   Vitamin A .10
   B Complex 11
   Thiamine (Vitamin B_1) 11
   Riboflavin (Vitamin B_2) 11
   Niacin (Vitamin B_3) 11
   Pyridoxine (Vitamin B_6) 11
   Vitamin B_{12} 12
   Folic Acid 12
   Pantothenic Acid 12
   Biotin, Choline, Inositol, and PABA 12
   Vitamin C (Ascorbic Acid) 13
   Vitamin D 13
   Vitamin E 13
   Vitamin K 14
Minerals 14
   Calcium 14
   Chromium .14
   Copper 15
   Iodine 15
   Iron 15

   Magnesium .15
   Manganese .15
   Potassium and Sodium 16
   Selenium 16
   Zinc 16
Water 16

SECTION II
Alternative Medicine
and Therapies   19

Aromatherapy .21
Ayurvedic Medicine 23
Bodywork 25
Therapeutic massage 25
Deep Tissue Manipulation 25
Movement Therapies 26
Energy Balancing 26
Reflexology 27
Chinese Medicine 27
Chiropractic 28
Herbal Therapy 28
Homeopathy 31
Mindbody Therapy 32
Meditation 32
Biofeedback 32
Imagery 33
Hypnotherapy .33

SECTION III
Health Conditions   35

Abscess 37

Acne 38

AIDS 40

Allergy 42

Alzheimer's Disease 44

Anemia 45

Arthritis 47

Asthma 50

Atherosclerosis 52

Athlete's Foot 54

Back Pain .54

Bronchitis .56

Bruises 58

Burns 59

Bursitis 61

Cancer 62

Canker Sores 64

Carpal Tunnel Syndrome 65

Chronic Fatigue Syndrome 66

Colds and Flu 67

Constipation 69

Crohn's Disease 71

Cystitis 72

Depression .73

Diabetes 76

Diarrhea 78

Diverticulitis 80

Ear Infection 80

Eczema 81

Epilepsy 83

Eye Problems 84

Cataracts 84

Conjunctivitis 84

Glaucoma .84

Macular Degeneration 84

Night Blindness 85

Fibrocystic Breast Disease 85

Fibromyalgia 86

Gallbladder Disease 87

Gingivitis 88

Gout 89

Headache .91

Heart Attack 93

Heartburn .95

Hemorrhoids 96

Hepatitis 97

Herpes 99

Hypertension—High Blood Pressure . . .100

Infection .102

Insomnia .104

Irritable Bowel Syndrome 106

Kidney Stones 107

Lupus—Systemic Lupus Erythematosus, SLE 108

Menopause 109

Menstrual Problems 111

Multiple Sclerosis 113

Osteoporosis 115

Overweight 116

Pregnancy 118

Premenstrual Syndrome (PMS) 120

Prostate Problems 122

Psoriasis .123

Raynaud's Disease 124

Stress 126

Stroke 128

Ulcers 129

Vaginitis .131

SECTION IV
Foods   133

Food Groups 137

Fruits and Vegetables 137

Legumes .137

Grains 138

Nuts and Seeds 139

Meats and Poultry 139

Seafood 140

Eggs 140

Dairy Products .140

Seaweed 140

Fermented Foods 141

Sweeteners 141

Food Lists 142

Pharmacological Activity 142

Rich Sources of Nutrients 144

Glycemic Index .150

SECTION V
Diet and Food Composition 155

Weights and Measures 157

Recommended Dietary Intake Chart . . .158

Table of Food Composition 162

References 257

Selected Bibliography 263

Index 267

PREFACE

When I began research for the *Nutrition Almanac* in the early seventies, scientific information on health and nutrition was scarce and difficult to find. In recent years, however, there has been a plethora of studies and most are easier to access. The database of the National Library of Medicine, for example, lists over 40,000 articles specifically on alternative medicine.

Alternative therapies focus on the underlying cause. The side effects often experienced from prescription drugs become unneccessary as there are, in many cases, viable and equally effective remedies that are natural and work in tandem with the body. Over 100,000 deaths a year are associated with prescription or over-the-counter drugs; as a contrast, U.S. mortality statistics from 1981 to 1993 registered one death as a result of vitamins and minerals, and since then, several deaths connected to the herb ephedra.

One aspect of wellness that has become clear is the interrelationship between the body, mind, and emotions, a concept that goes beyond the limited vision of allopathic medicine which views the body as functioning like a machine. Studies have shown that a negative attitude can hinder the healing process. Often called the placebo effect, as any physician will acknowledge, it is impossible to determine whether the effect of an intervention, be it a prescription drug or a natural therapy, is due to the medicinal activity and/or its placebo response. A positive outlook often enhances the efficacy of any treatment, including surgery.

The wisest course of action in keeping well and healthy throughout life is prevention, keeping the internal environment inhospitable to disease by reinforcing the body's instrinsic defense mechanisms and controlling the variable risk factors. Food is not only the best alternative medicine, but one of the most effective preventive measures. Scientific studies have proven that elements in food can affect health right down to the cellular level. Supplements are excellent short-term therapy, but for the long run, what we eat will determine our fundamental health status as we age.

Regular exercise, managing stress, and sufficient sleep are the other crucial factors in maintaining a high quality of well-being. Consistently depriving the body of adequate sleep impairs mental and physical biochemical processes. Exercise improves and stimulates the cardiovascular and respiratory systems, increases muscle mass, and decreases body fat. It also affects the symptoms of stress. In a study at the University of New Mexico, more stress hormones and lower levels of endorphins, which are mood enhancing substances, were found circulating in the bodies of sedentary men as opposed to those who exercised.

In this edition, there is an emphasis on the most recent and salient points of the differing aspects of health and nutrition, and on what really works as remedies for many common health conditions. Any questions or comments can be sent to me in care of the publisher.

Lavon J. Dunne

Nutrition Almanac

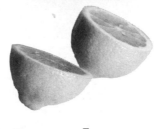

Nutrients

Optimal health and well-being require that carbohydrates, fats, protein, vitamins, minerals, and other micronutrients be supplied to the body in adequate and balanced amounts. These macro- and micronutrients are vital for normal organ development and functioning, for cell reproduction, growth, and maintenance; for high energy and working efficiency; for resistance to infection and disease; and for the ability to repair bodily damage or injury. No nutrient works alone; each is dependent on the presence of others for its best effects.

Although everyone needs the same nutrients, each individual is different in his or her genetic and physiological makeup and therefore individual quantitative nutritional needs differ. Prevention is the wisest strategy in keeping healthy by getting periodic health checks, eating a nutrient-dense diet, exercising on a regular basis, and reducing or managing stress.

The foods eaten by humans are chemically complex. They must be broken down by the body into simpler chemical forms so that they can be absorbed through the intestinal walls and transported by the blood to the cells. There they provide energy and the correct building materials to maintain human life.

Digestion is a series of physical and chemical changes by which food, taken into the body, is broken down in preparation for absorption from the intestinal tract into the bloodstream. These changes take place in the digestive tract, which includes the mouth, pharynx, esophagus, stomach, small intestine, and large intestine.

Beginning in the mouth, chewing breaks large pieces of food into smaller pieces. Food that is masticated well allows for more complete enzymatic action. If left in chunks, food that passes into the stomach and intestine will likely remain undigested as enzymes are only able to work on the surface of these larger particles.

The enzyme that is secreted in the mouth from the salivary glands is ptyalin, which is necessary for the breakdown of carbohydrates. Ptyalin breaks the starch chain into smaller subchains. Certain links of a fibrous nature cannot be broken and their components are left inaccessible to the body. The masticated food mass passes back to the pharynx under voluntary control, but from there on, through the esophagus and into the stomach the process of movement is carried on by *peristalsis,* a slow wavelike motion occurring along the entire digestive tract.

As there are no enzymes released in the stomach for further starch digestion, ptyalin continues to work if an alkaline condition remains. Division into simple sugars occurs later in the small intestine where the pancreas secretes the enzyme amylase.

The stomach has six different sets of glands, and the most important substances they secrete are hydrochloric acid (HCl) and a number of enzymes, including pepsin, which digest protein. These enzymes need an acid environment in order to break the amino acid bonds. The stomach actually begins secreting HCl and other enzymes while protein food is still being chewed, as the body reacts to the sight and taste of the food. The first stages in the digestion of protein can take several hours after which the partially digested food passes into the small intestine where further breakdown of the amino acids takes place as the pancreas secretes the enzyme protease.

Experiments with animals have shown that the stomach has a built-in timetable for gastric secretion. When bread, which contains both carbohydrate and protein, is swallowed, little HCl is released at first while a large amount of pepsin keeps the climate in an alkaline condition and allows ptyalin to continue digesting the starch. Meanwhile, the pepsin begins working on the protein. Once the carbohydrate process is near completion, more gastric juice is released that rapidly accelerates the digestion of the protein. It was also discovered that foods arranged in the stomach remain in the order they are eaten even while the contents are being churned; and liquids consumed while food is in the stomach pass around the food mass and enter the small intestine.

Liquid alone leaves the stomach rather quickly unless it is a thick mixture or puree. Fruits are next, then vegetables, unless eaten with fat or sauces, followed by starches, and then starches mixed with legumes or meats because of the added protein content. Fats take the longest and slow emptying of the stomach if combined with any other food. Stimulants such as coffee, tea, and strong spices can hasten emptying time of the stomach and may also affect digestion by irritating the stomach walls. Certain food additives and excess salt may have the same effect.

Cells in the stomach also secrete mucus. Mucus inhibits the gastric acids from digesting the stomach itself. The mucus constantly flows across the surface of the stomach to maintain the acid and enzyme balance. Too much acid can result in an irritated or ulcerated stomach. Over-abundance of mucus, however, can encourage bacterial growth because gastric acid is necessary to keep the intestinal tract free of bacteria. It is estimated that nearly half of the population may be deficient in HCl, especially among the elderly.

After one to four hours, depending on the combination of foods ingested, peristalsis pushes the food, now in the liquid form of chyme, out of the stomach and into the first part of the small intestine through a valve called the *duodenum*. The pancreas secretes proteolytic enzymes in varying proportions depending on what kind of food is present. If there is any fat, bile, which is produced by the liver from cholesterol, is released from the gallbladder where it has been stored. Bile disperses the fat globules into small droplets so that the pancreatic enzyme lipase can break them down into fatty acids.

If bile contains large amounts of cholesterol, crystals or stones can form in the gallbladder. The crystals obstruct the flow of bile into the small intestine and inhibit fat digestion. Cholesterol levels rise, and if the stones become so large they completely block the bile ducts, pain results. After the bile salts are finished they are transported out of the body through the elimination tract. Quick exit time through bowel action decreases the amount of cholesterol that remains in the body as bile salts. If contents of the bowel move more slowly, the cholesterol can be reabsorbed and recirculated in the system.

Food molecules continue to be broken down as they move along the remaining 20 ft or so of the small intestine, which is lined with millions of fingerlike projections called *villi* that give a furlike appearance. These villi contain microvilli which greatly increase the surface area available for absorption. Nutrients are absorbed by the villi and carried through their tiny blood vessels into the bloodstream. Normally, the villi act as a filter and barrier for undesirable and harmful elements by preventing their absorption. However, this defense mechanism can be compromised and weakened by a number of conditions including chronic irritation from harsh stimulants, undesirable microbes, pharmaceutical and recreational drugs, pesticides used on foods, and other environmental pollutants.

Once the nutrients have been transported into the bloodstream they are ushered into a large vein called the *portal vein* which flows into the liver and branches out into numerous capillaries. From this blood, cells in the liver begin to filter out the nutrients, processing them either to be sent out to cells in the rest of the body or to be stored in the liver for future use. Amino acids are reformed into new protein configurations and rereleased into the blood. Sugars that are not needed by the body at the moment are hooked together to create huge storage molecules called glycogen. When the liver is in a healthy condition, sugars are readily processed then released or stored while sugar content of the blood remains at a constant level. If the liver is not functioning properly, however, sugars may not be modified appropriately and can flood into the bloodstream unprocessed.

The liver not only processes nutrients but must detoxify all the harmful substances the villi were unable to prevent from being absorbed into the bloodstream. Other situations that can tax the liver considerably include overeating and eating foods that are refined. Refined foods are missing the nutrients they need to be properly metabolized. If the liver can no longer filter and cleanse the blood, or properly metabolize nutrients, or take care of its own health, it is because liver cells are damaged or begin to die. Liver damage is not easily detected by conventional testing and its condition may not be known until dysfunction becomes apparent through illness. Symptoms may range from headache, diarrhea, constipation, food sensitivities, flatulence, sleeplessness, and aching joints to cirrhosis and hepatitis.

On the lower right-hand side of the abdomen, the small intestine ends and the large intestine, or colon, begins via the ileocecal valve. The colon is mainly for elimination and contains a thriving population of bacteria. Most nutrients have been removed and what remains is fiber and water, which is soon absorbed. Bacteria, while simultaneously feeding on the food mass, begin to break down the tough fiber molecules, creating an appropriate texture for elimination.

The kinds of bacteria found in the colon determine what effects the last stage of the digestion process will have on health. A predominance of beneficial bacteria will protect the lining of the intestinal tract from damage and irritation or infection that can be caused by undesirable bacteria, and will detoxify or neutralize any harmful substances. A diet that includes plenty of whole grains, legumes, fruits, vegetables, and fermented products like miso, soy sauce, and yogurt or acidophilus encourage growth of these beneficial bacteria. They in turn exert their considerable influence in keeping the colon in a healthy and vibrant condition.

Macronutrients

Carbohydrates, fats, and protein are the three macronutrients the human body needs. Carbohydrates and fats supply energy while protein, in addition to energy, provides the structural components necessary for the growth and repair of tissues.

Carbohydrates

Carbohydrates are the chief source of energy for all body functions and muscular exertion. They are necessary for the digestion and assimilation of other foods. They help regulate protein and fat metabolism, and fats require carbohydrates to be broken down in the liver.

Carbohydrates are carbon, hydrogen, and oxygen molecules arranged structurally in the form of rings. Simple carbohydrates like glucose, fructose (fruit sugar), and galactose (milk sugar) are composed of one single ring and are called monosaccharides. Sucrose from sugar cane and sugar beets, maltose (which is a component of grains), and lactose (in milk) are composed of two rings linked together and are called disaccharides. The two rings in sucrose are made up of glucose plus fructose; maltose is glucose plus glucose; and lactose is glucose plus galactose. When individuals are said to be lactose-intolerant, it means that they lack the enzyme necessary to break the disaccharide links into a monosaccharide, an action necessary for further metabolism. Fiber is a carbohydrate but consists of very large molecules that are resistant to enzymatic action.

The human body, especially the brain, needs a constant supply of glucose. There are hormonal mechanisms that regulate glucose metabolism, a process that can go awry in cases of obesity and diabetes. Glucose levels that drop too low can result in weakness and fatigue. (A condition of low blood sugar is recognized as hypoglycemia. Minimizing sugar in the diet and eating small frequent meals focusing on whole grains, seeds, nuts, legumes, fresh fruits, and vegetables, low-fat dairy, yogurt, and fish can aid in stabilizing blood sugar levels. Blood sugar levels can be stabilized with 200 mcg of chromium GTF. Hypoglycemia is often an indication of an underlying health condition.)

The body converts some of these simple sugars into a starch in which the molecules are larger and structurally different. This starch is called *glycogen* and is stored in the liver and muscles as a short-term energy reserve. The starch we obtain from plants (which the plants have converted, just like the human body, from glucose) consists of two kinds, amylose and amylopectin. Both are similar in structure and are glucose rings linked together in long chains. Amylopectin starch chains also branch out on the sides, which provides more surface area for enzymes to work on. This makes it easier and faster for the human body to convert amylopectin starch back into glucose. Glycogen also has this branching structure.

The conversion rate, or how fast the body turns starches into sugars, is a measure of the glycemic index (GI). Amylopectyin starches have a higher GI. High GI carbohydrates raise blood sugar levels quite rapidly, providing bursts of energy that may be followed by an energy let-down. Low GI starches, because they take longer to be converted into glucose, maintain blood sugar at normal levels and provide energy at a more sustained pace. For the glycemic index of various foods see Section IV.

An important element in sugar processing is insulin. Insulin is a hormone released by the pancreas to manage blood glucose levels. The more the blood is flooded with glucose, the more insulin is required. Excess insulin can cause the body to store fat, damage the arteries, and accelerate the growth of tumors. In some individuals, if the release of insulin is too frequent, cells, which have receptor sites to receive the insulin, can eventually become desensitized to the hormone, a condition associated with cardiovascular disease, high blood pressure, adult-onset diabetes, blood fat abnormalities, and some cases of obesity. It is important to moderate high GI foods in the diet by eating foods that are low in GI value. The selection of higher GI foods should be nutrient-dense as opposed to the more refined ones like white bread and sugar. Whole-wheat bread and white bread are in the same GI range because when wheat is ground into the fine particles of flour, the surface area is much greater for digestive enzymes to work on and the yeast factor that puffs up the bread also increases surface area, so the result is faster glucose conversion. However, whole wheat is nutrient-dense and more wholesome in that it contains more vitamins, minerals, and fiber. A starch food that contains fiber and fat have a lower GI because these substances slow down the digestion process.

Although fiber is not digestible, it has important functions in the body. *Fiber* protects the health of the intestinal tract by increasing stool bulk and decreasing transit time, which minimizes the contact of carcinogenic and microbial elements with the intestinal walls. Colon and rectal cancers are not caused by a lack of fiber, but in susceptible individuals fiber may help prevent the diseases. A diet that supplies 40 g of fiber per day is suggested for most people; estimates are that most people ingest only 20 g.

There are two kinds of fiber, soluble and insoluble. Water-soluble fibers are gums, found in grains such as oats, seeds, and legumes, and pectins, which make up part of the edible portions of seeds, vegetables, and fruits, notably apples. Soluble fibers can lower cholesterol and they do this by binding up cholesterol-containing bile acids and cholesterol, preventing their absorption. Insoluble fibers are cellulose and lignins, found in the bran of wheat and other whole grains, and hemicellulose, found in whole grains, nuts, seeds, fruits, and vegetables. Insoluble fibers may help alleviate diverticulitis and irritable bowel syndrome.

Increasing fiber foods in the diet may cause flatulence in some individuals because as complex carbohydrates are digested by bacteria in the intestine, methane gas is released. Eating smaller amounts frequently helps eliminate the problem; so does selecting complex carbohydrates, through experimentation, that are better tolerated. Sometimes foods in combination cause gas while eating them singly does not. Ginger, garlic, peppermint, and fennel are carminatives or gas expellers and can be eaten or drunk as tea with or after meals. If a fiber supplement is necessary, a mucilaginous kind like psyllium husks or flaxseed is less irritating than crude bran fiber.

Fats

Fats are converted for storage in the body from glucose. We also derive fats directly from foods. Fats are a mixture of fatty acids composed of carbon molecules linked together with attached hydrogen and oxygen atoms. The carbon–carbon configuration is of high-energy and therefore twice the caloric value of carbohydrates. Fats are our energy reserve; they insulate the body and cushion vital organs. Almost all the cells in the body can convert fats into energy, a process called fatty-acid oxidation. Most fatty acids are in the form of triglycerides, a combination of fatty acids and a carrier molecule, glycerol. When we eat fats and oils, the body separates the fatty acids from their carrier; likewise when triglycerides in fat tissue are taken out of storage for conversion to energy. Every cell in the body needs fatty acids to produce and build new cells. They are critical in the transmission of nerve impulses and for normal brain development.

There are three kinds of fatty acids. Saturated fatty acids (SFAs) are comprised of carbon bonds that are saturated with hydrogen molecules. The body prefers these fats to burn as energy. Monounsaturated fats (MUFAs) have a link in their carbon chain where two carbon molecules share, not one, but two bonds with each other. Body fat contains MUFAs and can be converted into energy that the body burns as easily as

saturated fats. Polyunsaturated fats (PUFAs) have two or more double bonds in their carbon chain. Some PUFAs are used for energy but most have other vital functions in the body. All fats and oils are a mixture of fatty acids; for example, beef fat is 51% SFA, 44% MUFA, and 4% PUFA. Olive oil is 14% SFA, 77% MUFA, and 9% PUFA. Safflower oil is 9% SFA, 12% MUFA, and 78% PUFA. Whichever fatty acid predominates determines classification. For a list of foods containing the three kinds of fatty acids, see Section IV.

There are two fatty acids that are from the PUFA category and that the body cannot make, therefore called essential fatty acids (EFAs). They are linoleic acid (LA) and linolenic acid (LNA). LA has two double bonds in its carbon chain, the first being between the numbers 6 and 7 carbon. LNA contains three double bonds, the first being between the 3 and 4 carbon. Because the human body does not have the enzyme that is necessary for inserting these obligatory double bonds, it needs to obtain them from an outside source. The presence of a double bond in a carbon chain is noted by the Greek letter for omega, hence, LA is in the omega-6 series and LNA is in the omega-3 series. Once the body has omega-3 and omega-6 fatty acids, it can make other necessary fatty acids from them. The ability of the omega-3s to make other fatty acids can be interfered with, however, if the ratio of omega-6s are too high in the diet as they both compete for the same enzymes in performing their conversions. Omega-6s are more prevalent in the diet principally because of the extensive use of polyunsaturated oils in cooking and food processing. For a list of foods containing omega-3 and omega-6 fatty acids, see Section IV.

EFAs are invaluable for the production and movement of energy throughout the body. They regulate the transport of oxygen and are vital in maintaining the integrity of cell structure. They are crucial for blood clotting, for support of the immune system, and for synthesizing hormones such as prostaglandins which regulate numerous biological processes including the healing mechanism. Omega-3s are particularly important in protecting the nervous system and the integrity of cell membranes in the brain, especially important to fetal and early childhood development. A deficiency can impair mental functions like learning and intelligence; and there may be an association with depression, attention deficit disorder, and autism.

The chemical configuration of PUFAs, the double bonds in the carbon chain, tend to be unstable making them very susceptible to oxidation, a process that can create free radicals. Free radicals are highly reactive molecules that can cause extensive damage in the body involving enzymes, DNA, cellular structure, and the immune system. As a result, premature aging of cells and tissues, arterial disease, and even cancer are some of the conditions that can develop.

When fatty acids oxidize they begin to turn rancid. Most PUFAs oxidize quickly when exposed to heat or air. Oils that are not commercially cold-processed are exposed to heat as well as chemical solvents. Safflower and flaxseed oils oxidize most rapidly when heated; grapeseed oil can be heated to 485 degrees before damage occurs. Once nuts and seeds have been roasted or chopped, they begin to oxidize. Buying them raw and toasting them in a fry pan right before eating minimizes harmful effects. Never reuse fat in cooking; deep fried foods in restaurants are especially hazardous. A recent study showed significant damage to the lining of arteries in participants soon after they ate foods cooked with used fat in restaurants.[1]

MUFAs are more resistant to oxidation, supply fat needed by the body for energy, and are rich in omega-3s. They also lower blood cholesterol. Extra-virgin olive oil, which is the first pressing, or cold-pressed canola oil, are good oils to use in cooking. Pesticide use is heavy on crops of its source, rape.

Hydrogenated fats or partially hydrogenated fats contain trans fatty acids (TFAs). TFAs are unnatural forms of fatty acids that develop when unsaturated fatty acids are exposed to heat during commercial extraction to make oils, when exposed to heat and light after extraction, and when hydrogen is added to their molecular structure, as in the making of margarine. TFAs increase cholesterol levels in the body, which can result in atherosclerosis. TFAs can have damaging effects on cell membranes, the immune system, hormonal function, and can promote heart disease and cancer.

Cholesterol is a hard waxy substance critical to many body functions. Made by the liver, it is involved in the synthesis of hormones including estrogen, testosterone, and cortisone, which helps regulate metabolism. While EFAs keep cell membranes pliable, cholesterol gives them enough rigidity to prevent their collapse. If the cell structure becomes too stiff, the body removes any excess cholesterol from it; if too soft, more cholesterol is added. Vitamin D and bile are made from cholesterol and cholesterol is an important component in secretions of the oil glands.

Too much cholesterol in the body has definite adverse effects. It is the main component of the plaque that builds up on the walls of arteries. This buildup leads to heart attacks, strokes, and other problems from poor blood circulation. Except for those individuals whose genes prevent cholesterol from building up no matter what they eat, diet is the major influence on cholesterol's production. The body uses carbon or acetate fragments to make cholesterol. Acetate fragments are the end-product of fatty-acid oxidation and an intermediate product of carbohydrate metabolism. Saturated fats are the main source of acetate fragments because they are the preferred fuel of the body for energy. High GI carbohydrates produce acetate fragments rather quickly and so diets high in saturated fats and refined carbohydrates have great influence on cholesterol production. Comparatively, cholesterol in foods actually has a lesser effect on blood cholesterol levels.

Another important aspect of cholesterol is how it is transported throughout the body. When fat droplets are absorbed through the walls of the small intestine, they are picked up by protein-coated carriers called lipoproteins. These particular lipoproteins are called high-density lipoproteins, or HDL. They carry the fat globules composed of both cholesterol and triglycerides to the liver. The liver then metabolizes the fat. Some of the cholesterol is deposited in the bile. The fats that are sent out to various parts of the body are carried by low-density lipoproteins, or LDL.

All cells in the body have receptors for LDL, but when each cell has absorbed enough fat and cholesterol for its needs, the receptor closes. The remaining LDL keeps circulating in the blood and eventually is either stored as fat or transferred back to an HDL carrier for return to the liver. HDL is known as good cholesterol and LDL as bad cholesterol. The reason is that when it's in the form of LDL, cholesterol can damage arterial walls, which increases the risk for atherosclerosis and heart attack. Diets high in saturated fats and refined carbohydrates increases the amount of LDL circulating in the blood, elevates blood serum triglycerides and cholesterol, and places extra burden on HDL as it tries to carry the excess back to the liver. PUFAs lower LDL but lower HDL as well. MUFAs moderately lower LDL but do not affect HDL.

Protein

Proteins are more complex than carbohydrates or fats. They make up most of the body weight after water. When a protein food is ingested, the body breaks it down into amino acids. Ribosomes in each cell receive coded messages from DNA in the cell nucleus on how to put these amino acids together in chains. There are 20 amino acids and they can be combined in numerous ways, like the letters in the alphabet. When a protein chain is finished, its chemical, electrical, and sequential (the sequence of amino acids) characteristics result in a unique coiled three-dimensional shape which is important because the shape alone enables the protein to perform a specific function. For example, the distinctive shape of the proteins that make up muscle fibers allows them to easily slide back and forth over one another during muscle contraction.

Proteins are of primary importance in the growth and development of all body tissues. They are the major source of building material for muscles, blood, skin, hair, nails, and internal organs, including the heart and brain. Most of the transmitters relayed by the brain that affect muscular and emotional activity are composed of amino acids. Protein is needed for the formation of hormones which control a variety of body functions such as growth, sexual development, and rate of metabolism. Protein also helps prevent the blood and tissues from becoming either too acid or too alkaline and helps regulate the body's water balance.

Enzymes are proteins that act as catalysts for all chemical reactions in the body. If it were not for enzymes, life would not continue because these reactions would not happen fast enough. Enzymes are essential for digestion, cellular energy, tissue and organ repair, and brain activity. Each enzyme, with its specialized configuration, binds with another specific molecule known as a *substrate*. The enzyme attaches to a specific site on that substrate that is geometrically and electrically compatible. The enzyme, highly energetic, initiates a reaction in the substrate that often forces it to change its chemical configuration in order to effect a desired result. Enzymes divide, snip off pieces, put parts together, and do whatever it takes; all with maximum speed and precise orchestration. There is a unique enzyme for every substrate, so the body needs to produce a substantial number of different enzymes. Specific enzymes are also obtained directly from foods in the diet.

A deficient or defective enzyme can have significant consequences. For example, a deficiency of one or more pancreatic enzymes (amylase, protease, or lipase) results in incomplete digestion of food. An enzyme that is defective or slightly off in its configuration is not able to bind with its substrate, and, consequently, the intended chemical reaction will not be able to proceed.

Enzymes are also carriers of information within and between cells by playing the role of receptors. Receptors are found on almost every cell in the body. For example, once the hormone insulin gets a pass from its receptor, the cells allow glucose to enter and the production of energy begins. If there is a deficiency of insulin receptors, the cells will not respond to the insulin and energy production is hindered; meanwhile there will be an elevation of blood glucose.

Protein that is not needed for construction, maintenance, or repair of the body's structure can be used for energy production. Excess protein in the diet, once broken down into amino acids, is turned into glucose or glycogen, or put into storage as fat. When protein is burned for energy, it does not burn clean like carbohydrates and fat but leaves a toxic residue, ammonia. This the body must eliminate. First, the liver turns ammonia into urea, which is less toxic. Then the kidneys remove the urea from the bloodstream, using extra amounts of water in the flushing process. This in turn causes an increased loss of minerals, especially calcium. If there is insufficient carbohydrate in the diet, in order to meet energy demands especially of the brain, protein in muscle tissue is used, which results in a loss of lean body mass. High dietary intake of protein can also exacerbate allergies and autoimmune diseases by aggravating the immune system.

Amino acids are synthesized by the body except for eight of them which are called the essential amino acids. Meats, fish, poultry, eggs, and dairy products furnish the eight essential amino acids. From the vegetable kingdom, soybeans contain them as well. All essential amino acids can be obtained by combining vegetable proteins: serving beans with brown rice, corn, nuts, seeds, or wheat; or by combining brown rice with beans, nuts, seeds, or wheat, for example. It is also possible for the body to find the deficient or missing amino acid in a meal from amino acids in the small intestine or those that naturally slough off the walls of the digestive tract.

Micronutrients

Vitamins and minerals are needed in minute quantities by the body but are essential for normal growth, muscle response, health of the nervous system, digestion, production of hormones, and metabolism of nutrients. Vitamins often act as coenzymes and minerals are constituents of bones, teeth, soft tissue, muscles, blood, and nerve cells. There are two kinds of vitamins: water-soluble—B complex, C, the bioflavonoids, and beta carotene—that are easily eliminated from the body; and fat soluble—A, D, E, and K—that can accumulate if an excess is ingested. Vitamins and minerals can be supplied by a varied diet of fresh fruits and vegetables, whole grains, legumes, nuts and seeds, fish, and low-fat animal products.

Phytochemicals are a recently discovered compound that shows the importance of eating a nutrient-dense whole foods diet, for it is inevitable that more nutrients are yet to be discovered. These elements are powerful antioxidants that protect the body from the oxidative effects of, for example, environmental pollution, and contain protective properties against illnesses including cancer and coronary heart disease.

The pigments in fruits, vegetables, and some beans and grains contain a group of phytochemicals called polyphenols; polyphenols are also found in olive oil. The red and purple pigments called anthocyanins and proanthocyanidins found in such foods as grapes, cherries, berries, plums, and red cabbage act to prevent degenerative diseases of the heart, blood vessels, and lungs. The carotenoids in yellow and orange fruits and vegetables and, invisibly, in dark green leafy vegetables have strong anticancer properties. Lutein and zeaxanthin are protective of the eyes and help prevent macular degeneration and cataract formation; and lycopene lowers the risk of prostate cancer. Polysaccharides are another group of phytochemicals found in plants, especially the mushrooms, shiitake, oyster, enoki, and maitake, that improve the effectiveness of the immune system. Phytoestrogens found in plants like soybeans and flax interrelate with estrogen receptors on the cellular level and are beneficial for women during menopause and may help prevent breast cancer; and for men in reducing the risk of prostate cancer; and for both in preventing coronary heart disease.

Vitamins

VITAMIN A

Vitamin A is essential in the formation of visual purple, a pigment found in the retina of the eye that is needed for vision at night. Health and the resiliency against infection of the outer skin, and internally of the mucous membranes that line the respiratory, gastrointestinal, and urinary tracts as well as the mouth, nose, and ears depend on vitamin A. The vitamin is an antioxidant and may be important in preventing cancer of the lungs and cervix in women. It helps cells reproduce normally. Vitamin A is fat-soluble and can accumulate in the body becoming toxic if more than 50,000 IU are ingested daily. *Pregnant women should not take more than 10,000 IU each day.*

Approximately 90% of the body's vitamin A is stored in the liver with small amounts deposited in the fatty tissues, lungs, kidneys, and retinas. Under stressful conditions the body uses this reserve supply if it doesn't receiving enough of the vitamin from the diet. The liver needs a sufficient supply of zinc in order to mobilize and release stored vitamin A into the bloodstream.

The liver converts beta carotene obtained from foods into vitamin A. Carotene is nontoxic and along with other carotenoids is an antioxidant and offers more protection against cancer than vitamin A by itself. These other phytochemicals include alpha carotene, lutein, lycopene, zeaxanthin, and cryptoxanthin and are found in the red, yellow, and orange pigments of fruits and vegetables.

B COMPLEX

Foods that are especially rich in one of the B vitamins will also contain several other members of the complex as their functions in the body are closely interrelated. The B vitamins are also made by bacteria in the intestinal tract. The complex is most important for the health of the nervous system. B vitamins have a role in the metabolism of carbohydrates, fats, and protein, and are essential for maintaining the muscle tone of the gastrointestinal tract and heart.

The B vitamins are water-soluble. They are not stored in the body in any great quantity and need to be supplied daily by the diet. The need for the complex increases during chronic illnesses, stress, and when alcohol, tobacco, and recreational drugs are used. Taking a single B vitamin should be accompanied by the complex in order to avoid an imbalance or deficiency of the others.

THIAMINE (VITAMIN B₁)

Mental efficiency, health, and a feeling of well-being are dependent on thiamine. It is required for nerve cells to function normally. It is essential for the formation in every cell of adenosine triphosphate (ATP), the energy fuel that the body runs on. The vitamin easily dissolves in water, is vulnerable to heat during cooking, and to baking soda and powder in baked goods. It is a component of the germ and bran of wheat, the husk of rice, and that portion of all grains that is commercially milled out to give the grain a lighter color and finer texture.

RIBOFLAVIN (VITAMIN B₂)

Riboflavin is a constituent of enzymes involved in cell respiration. It is also necessary for the maintenance of good vision and healthy skin. The vitamin helps convert carbohydrates to ATP, the energy fuel. It has a yellow pigment and colors the urine.

NIACIN (VITAMIN B₃)

Niacin is a coenzyme involved in the metabolism of proteins, fats, and carbohydrates. Besides its presence in food, the vitamin is manufactured in the body from the essential amino acid tryptophan. It is important for blood circulation and reducing cholesterol levels in the blood.

Large doses cause a flushing of the skin as a result of the dilation of blood vessels but the effect is not harmful. A form of niacin, niacinamide, does not cause any skin sensations, however, large doses can damage the liver and cause depression in some people. The form inositol hexanicotinate lowers serum cholesterol without harming the liver. Doses of the vitamin should not exceed 1000 mg a day, unless under the supervision of a physician. High doses of niacin should not be taken during pregnancy, or in cases of ulcers, gout, diabetes, gallbladder or liver diseases, or recent heart attack.

PYRIDOXINE (VITAMIN B₆)

Pyridoxine is extremely important in the development of the nervous system. It helps process amino acids and is involved in the production of serotonin, melatonin, and dopamine. The vitamin has been used to reduce morning sickness during pregnancy. A hormonal shift leading to PMS (premenstrual syndrome) in women, and nerve compression injuries such as carpal tunnel syndrome, have been helped by the vitamin. Because of its role in fat metabolism, a deficiency is associated with atherosclerosis. A lack of the vitamin can cause depression.

Oral contraceptives can create a pyridoxine deficiency, and much of the vitamin is lost in the processing of foods and is not one of the vitamins that is replaced in so-called "enrichment." Nerve damage has been observed in individuals taking more than 300 mg a day.

VITAMIN B$_{12}$

Absorption of B$_{12}$ depends on the presence in the stomach of the intrinsic factor, a mucoprotein enzyme. Autoimmune reactions in the body may either bind the intrinsic factor to prevent B$_{12}$ absorption or prevent cellular ability to produce the enzyme. B$_{12}$ is closely related to the activity of four amino acids, pantothenic acid, and vitamin C. It also helps iron function better in the body and aids folic acid in the synthesis of choline. It has a role in the production of DNA and RNA, which are the body's genetic material, and in s-adenosyl-L-methionine (SAMe), a mood altering substance. The vitamin, along with folic acid, regulates homocysteine levels. Homocysteine is an amino acid which, in excess, is associated with heart disease, stroke, osteoporosis, and Alzheimer's disease.

The vitamin is found in meats, fish, eggs, and milk and is not provided in vegetarian diets. Sublingual and nasal forms are effective as supplements. The daily recommended dose is 2 to 3 mcg.

FOLIC ACID

Folic acid is involved in the duplication of chromosomes during cell reproduction, a process that is accelerated during pregnancy when new tissue is being formed. The vitamin is important in preventing birth abnormalities such as neural tube defect which involves poor brain and spinal cord development, and mental disorders that may be obvious or may be subtle in effect and not noticed at birth or in infancy but become evident later in life. It can help in preventing cleft palate. Folic acid regulates blood homocysteine levels, an amino acid associated with risk of heart disease, strokes, osteoporosis, and Alzheimer's disease. It is necessary for the production of the mood related substance SAMe.

Birth control pills and diets high in fat and refined carbohydrates can cause a folic acid deficiency. The vitamin is easily destroyed by high temperatures.

PANTOTHENIC ACID

There is a close correlation between pantothenic acid tissue levels and function of the adrenal glands. The adrenals are, for example, important in responding to stress. Pantothenic acid is a part of the energy cycle and the production of acetylcholine, a neurotransmitter. It is involved in cholesterol and hormone synthesis. The vitamin is widely available in almost all natural foods; however, food processing destroys substantial amounts. Fifty percent of pantothenic acid is lost in the milling of grains and 37% in meat during cooking.

BIOTIN, CHOLINE, INOSITOL, AND PABA

These vitamins have been isolated in foods and their chemical structures identified as part of the B group, although the activity of para amino benzoic acid (PABA) is quite different from other B vitamins. Biotin acts as a coenzyme in the metabolism of fats, carbohydrates, and protein. Prolonged use of antibiotics and antiseizure medicines interfere with its production. It is destroyed by raw egg white. The vitamin strengthens brittle nails and lowers blood glucose levels preventing diabetic neuropathy. Deficiency symptoms include fatigue, lack of appetite, dermatitis, hair loss, anemia, nausea, and depression.

Choline and inositol are constituents of lecithin and are primarily associated with the use of fats and cholesterol in the body and for cell membrane integrity. Choline is a component of acetylcholine, a neurotransmitter in the brain, and has been helpful in treating neurological and psychological disorders. Inositol is also involved in nerve transmissions. Diabetics excrete the vitamin at a rate greater than normal. PABA occurs in combination with folic acid and plays an important role in determining skin health, hair pigmentation, and health of the intestines.

VITAMIN C (ASCORBIC ACID)

Vitamin C is necessary for the formation of collagen, the connective tissue in skin, ligaments, and bones, and is important for the healing of wounds. The vitamin aids in forming red blood cells and preventing hemorrhaging and bleeding gums. It maintains the activity of white blood cells which act as bacteria fighters, but too high amounts of C reverses that effect and white blood cells actually become less active. Vitamin C acts as an inhibitor of histamine, a compound that is released during allergic reactions.

Vitamin C has shown protective effects against heavy metal exposure, pesticides, and food additives such as nitrates which have been associated with cancer. The vitamin is an antioxidant, protects LDL cholesterol from oxidative damage, supports the immune system, and helps prevent cancer. Recent studies have shown vitamin C affects nitric oxide activity, which is important in the dilation of blood vessels beneficial in preventing artery spasms leading to heart attacks and in lowering blood pressure.[2]

Birth control pills and aspirin deplete the tissues of vitamin C. Ingestion of above 100 mg at one time results in decreased efficiency of absorption and an increased rate of excretion of unmetabolized ascorbic acid. Tissues reach saturation at 200 to 250 mg. Large doses may inactivate vitamin B_{12}, have caused demineralization of bones in animals, may prevent the absorption of calcium, interfere with the absorption of copper, and result in the formation of kidney stones.

The bioflavonoids are part of the C complex and enhance the effectiveness of vitamin C. They are important in increasing the strength of the capillaries and regulating their permeability. Some act as antihistamines, have antiviral, anti-cancer, and anti-inflammatory properties, and protect LDL cholesterol from oxidative damage. Bioflavonoids are categorized as isoflavones, anthocyanins, flavans, flavonols, flavones, and flavanones. Subcategories include rutin, hesperetin, eriodictyol, quercetin (in onions), quercetrin, hesperidin, and genistein (in soy), and are found in the edible portions of fruits and vegetables and in the white segments of citrus fruits.

VITAMIN D

Vitamin D is necessary for the absorption of calcium from the intestinal tract reducing its urinary loss, and for the assimilation of phosphorus which is required in bone formation. The vitamin aids in the synthesis of enzymes in the mucous membranes that are involved in the transport of calcium. When the skin is exposed to ultraviolet radiation, vitamin D is formed from a cholesterol derivative and absorbed into the circulatory system. The more pigment there is in the skin, the less of the vitamin is produced. Vitamin D is involved in cell reproduction, blood cell formation, and enhances the immune system. It is needed for regulating glucose. Dietary sources of vitamin D are egg yolks, butter, fortified milk, and fish livers or oil. After absorption, vitamin D is transported to the liver for storage and deposits are found in the skin, brain, spleen, and bones.

Excessive amounts may cause a rise of calcium and phosphorus in the blood and excessive excretion of calcium in the urine. This may lead to calcification of soft tissues and of the walls of the blood vessels and kidney tubules, a condition called hypercalcemia. Too much vitamin D for prolonged periods can result in weight loss, headaches, and kidney stones.

VITAMIN E

Vitamin E plays an essential role in cellular respiration of all muscles. This makes it possible for muscles and their nerves to function with less oxygen, thereby increasing endurance and stamina. Studies have shown that vitamin E can reduce the stickiness of blood preventing its tendency to form blood clots. It also acts as a powerful antioxidant and protects LDL cholesterol from oxidation. Recent studies have shown vitamin E supplementation of 100 IU daily for 2 years reduced the risk of heart attack[3] and in another, 400 to 800 IU daily produced a 77% drop in nonfatal heart attacks.[4] The *d*-alpha form of supplemental E is natural and more effective than the synthetic *dl* form. The gamma tocopherol may better protect against oxidation and supplements should include the mixed tocopherols.

In animal studies, rats were exposed to ozone levels that are normally found in industrial areas. Ozone is a single reactive oxygen molecule that does much injury to cellular structures. Those that received little of the vitamin had the most damage, those given larger doses essentially had no damage. Tissue damage can also occur from the diet; the same reactive oxygen molecules are present when unsaturated vegetable oils are exposed to air and heat and become rancid. The antioxidant properties of vitamin E may retard the aging process. Topically the vitamin can reduce scar formation (applied after the wound has closed) from burns, surgery, or other injuries.

Vitamin E is a fat-soluble vitamin, absorbed in the presence of bile salts and fat. From the intestine, it is absorbed into the lymph and transported in the bloodstream as tocopherol to the liver where high concentrations are stored. It is also stored in the fatty tissues, heart, muscles, testes, uterus, blood, and adrenal and pituitary glands. The vitamin is one of a group of compounds called tocopherols which include beta, delta, epsilon, gamma, and zeta.

Vitamin E is mainly found in the oily portions of foods like whole grains and seeds. The milling process reduces vitamin E content by as much as 85%. The vitamin has a tendency to raise blood pressure if given in supplemental form, therefore, initial intake should be low and gradually increased. High doses can interfere with iron metabolism; at dosages of 300 to 400 IU a day, nausea, intestinal distress, fatigue, weakness, and urinary abnormalities may be experienced in some individuals.

VITAMIN K

Vitamin K is necessary for the formation of prothrombin, a chemical required in blood clotting. It is also involved in a body process, phosphorylation, in which phosphate, when combined with glucose, passes through the cell membranes and is converted into glycogen. It is involved in bone formation by transporting calcium. The vitamin is absorbed in the upper intestinal tract with the aid of bile salts, transported to the liver and stored in small quantities. Besides dietary sources, it is manufactured in the intestinal tract by certain bacteria. Synthetic vitamin K can be toxic. Supplemental vitamin K can interfere with the actions of some blood thinners.

Minerals

CALCIUM

Calcium is the most abundant mineral in the body. Ninety-eight percent is found in the bones, 1% in teeth, and 1% in other tissues. When the body is at rest, calcium is pulled out of the bones to be used elsewhere, establishing the importance of daily adequate intake of the mineral and of exercise. Calcium helps regulate nerve transmissions and along with magnesium, is important for cardiovascular health. If muscles do not have enough calcium, they cannot contract or if contracted, do not relax, which results in cramps. The mineral is good for relaxation and improves the quality of sleep. During the hormonal shifts of menopause, the dominance of the parathyroid hormone causes calcium to be removed from bone resulting in osteoporosis.

Requirements for calcium may vary depending on how much each individual absorbs and retains. Pregnant women need to ingest at least 1200 mg a day, especially in the last two months because over half of the calcium in an infants body is deposited at that time. Moderate amounts of protein, lactose, and butterfat enhance absorption of calcium, therefore, low-fat rather than nonfat milk products should be part of the diet, especially for children.

Excess protein in the diet causes a urinary loss of calcium. High intakes of calcium interfere with the absorption of other minerals including iron, zinc, and manganese, disrupt the functioning of the nervous and muscular systems, and may prevent blood coagulation.

CHROMIUM

A trace element, chromium is essential in producing a substance called glucose tolerance factor (GTF) which is important in the utilization of insulin, a hormone that stabilizes blood sugar levels. The mineral is also involved in the synthesis of fatty acids and cholesterol. Eating refined sugar can cause depletion of body chromium as sugar lacks sufficient amounts of the mineral for its own digestion. The chromium content of refined sugar is 0.02 parts per million (ppm) whereas the by-product, molasses, has 0.2 ppm; sugar cane juice has approximately 0.1 ppm.

COPPER

Copper assists in the formation of hemoglobin and red blood cells by facilitating the absorption of iron and may protect against atherosclerosis. Iron metabolism depends on copper. Zinc and copper have similar elemental properties and have a balancing effect on each other. Both are related to the functioning of the nervous system and compete in the intestinal tract for absorption. Excess zinc supplementation affects the absorption of copper. Too much vitamin C can impair its metabolism. Copper is a component of superoxide dismutase (SOD), an antioxidant enzyme; and it is necessary for the production of ATP, adenosine triphosphate, the body's energy source. Synthesis of collagen, certain hormones, and enzymes depend on copper.

High levels of copper may aggravate PMS and it can be increased by the use of birth control pills. Excess copper can cause mental and emotional problems and may be prominent in schizophrenia. Anemia not helped by iron may be an indication of elevated copper levels. Serum copper, elevated by estrogens, rises progressively during pregnancy and takes several months to return to normal after delivery, during which time the mineral could be a factor in the depression and psychosis women often experience right after giving birth. Excess copper may be getting into the diet from contaminated food and water and copper pipes through which drinking water flows.

IODINE

Iodine aids in the development and functioning of the thyroid gland and is an integral part of thyroxine, a principal hormone produced by the thyroid gland. Thyroid hormones are important for normal cellular metabolism. Sea plants and animals absorb iodine from seawater and are good sources of the mineral.

IRON

At the center of a hemoglobin molecule is iron and when combined with oxygen, it gives arterial blood its bright red color. Hemoglobin transports oxygen in the blood from the lungs to the tissues which need oxygen to maintain basic life functions. Iron is also necessary for the formation of myoglobin, found only in muscle tissue, which supplies oxygen to the muscle cells.

Significant amounts of iron can be lost during menstruation and needs are higher for pregnant women. Protein and vitamin C aid in the absorption of iron by chelating or attaching onto the iron ion and carrying it across the intestinal walls. Excess iron can accumulate in the body to toxic levels. Take iron supplements only on the advice of a physician.

MAGNESIUM

Along with calcium, magnesium is found in bones and is important in the conduction of electrical impulses of the muscles and nerves. Magnesium, like calcium, is a relaxant yet either one in excess causes a malfunction of the nervous system. Keeping both minerals in balance is important. Most magnesium is found in the cell where it activates the enzymes necessary for the metabolism of carbohydrates and amino acids. It is involved in insulin secretion and function. Magnesium has been shown to reduce hyperactivity in children who had low magnesium levels. It may improve vision in glaucoma patients, lower blood pressure, and may be a factor in chronic fatigue syndrome. The mineral is refined out of many foods and amounts are lost during cooking of foods.

MANGANESE

Manganese plays a role in activating numerous enzymes and in skeletal development involving connective tissue which provides the framework for bone and its growth. Along with zinc, the mineral lowers serum copper levels and balances histamine levels, a substance that is released during allergic reaction. Manganese stimulates activity of the antioxidant enzyme SOD, or superoxide dismutase, and helps maintain glucose levels.

POTASSIUM AND SODIUM

Potassium and sodium exist in important ratios, potassium concentrated inside the cell and sodium remaining outside. They regulate water balance in the body and their equilibrium enables them to stimulate nerve impulses for the heart and other muscle contractions. Depletion of either element would depress cell response. The typical American diet of processed and convenience foods do not contain sufficient amounts of potassium creating an imbalance between the two minerals. Diuretics can cause an excessive urinary loss of potassium. An excess of sodium is related to high blood pressure and fluid retention which taxes the heart and kidneys.

SELENIUM

Selenium is a natural antioxidant and appears to preserve the elasticity of tissues by delaying oxidation of polyunsaturated fatty acids. It supports the immune system, protects against cancer, is a factor in fertility, and is necessary for the production of prostaglandin, a substance that affects blood pressure.

Selenium content of foods depends on the extent of its presence in soil whether directly as plant food or indirectly as animal products when selenium levels are derived from feed. Sulfur content in commercial fertilizers inhibits plant absorption of the mineral. Refining, processing, and cooking of foods reduce selenium levels. High doses are toxic and no more than 300 mcg a day are recommended.

ZINC

Zinc is a constituent of at least 25 enzymes involved in digestion and metabolism. It is a component of insulin and essential in the synthesis of nucleic acids which control the formation of different proteins in the cell. Zinc is important for the proper development of the reproductive organs and normal functioning of the prostate gland. The mineral speeds the healing of wounds and bone fractures, keeps the skin healthy, and is involved in the formation of keratin, a substance in hair and nails. It supports the immune system and protects against free radicals.

Zinc content of foods depends on soil content. Chemical fertilizers impair its absorption into plants. The milling process removes substantial amounts of the mineral. Although moderate doses enhance immunity, excessive amounts depress it. It is recommended that no more than 100 mg be taken daily.

Water

Respiration, digestion, assimilation, metabolism, elimination, waste removal, and temperature regulation are bodily functions that can only be accomplished in the presence of water. Water is essential in dissolving and transporting nutrients such as oxygen and mineral salts via the blood, lymph, and other bodily fluids. Water also keeps the pressure, acidity, and composition of all chemical reactions in equilibrium.

Only oxygen is more essential than water in sustaining the life of all organisms. Human beings can live around 5 weeks without protein, carbohydrates, and fats but just 5 days without water in a moderate climate. Its circulation between the blood and bodily organs is perpetual and always maintained in proper balance; however, a certain amount is eliminated daily through evaporation or excretion and must be replaced.

Most of this water is removed by the kidneys, through which the entire blood supply passes and is filtered 15 times each hour. Whenever the body becomes overheated, two million sweat glands excrete perspiration which is 99% water. The heat of the blood evaporates the sweat, cooling the body and keeping the internal organs at a constant temperature. A minimal but consistent loss of water occurs during the processes of breathing and tearing. Moisture is breathed out from the water-lined nasal passages and the lungs. Dry air draws off more water than humid air. Tiny tear ducts carry a liquid solution to the upper eyelids, which lubricate the eyes 25 times every minute. The tears then pass down to the nose where they evaporate.

To replace lost water, approximately 3 qt is needed by the body each day under normal conditions. More strenuous activity, a high climate temperature or a diet too high in salt may increase this requirement. The sense of thirst is controlled by a part of the forebrain called the hypothalamus. Metabolic water is produced as a by-product of the food combustion process yielding as much as a pint per day. Foods can provide up to 1½ qt. For example, fruits and vegetables are more than 90% distilled water. Even dry foods like bread and crackers are 35 and 5% water, respectively. Drinking water is the other source of replenishment.

Municipal water treatment systems are mainly concerned with disinfection and do not remove most chemicals. Because of environmental pollution, there is probably not a water source that is not contaminated to some degree. The most efficient removal and reduction of the widest range of contaminants is in bottled water, purified by ozone, reverse osmosis, and distillation, or a combination. Needed minerals do not have to be obtained from drinking water as they are found in a wide range of foods in a varied and wholesome diet.

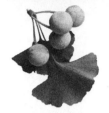

Alternative Medicine and Therapies

Alternative medicine asks the questions: What are the underlying reasons for an illness? And, why was the body not able to stimulate its own intrinsic mechanisms in defense? The human body has immense resources for healing and rejuvenation. Alternative medicine and therapies assist in this endeavor. The body is viewed as an integrated whole with all aspects of life having an influence on health—lifestyle, work, diet, genetics, and mental and emotional constitution. For this reason, although a particular health condition may appear the same, the cause may be different, and therefore each individual is treated accordingly. Conventional or allopathic medicine is superior for trauma, emergencies, and complex surgical procedures, but alternative medicine is often better at managing common illnesses, degenerative diseases, mental illnesses, stress, and cancer. Alternative disciplines place great emphasis on prevention and encourage changes in diet, exercise, reducing stress, and becoming an active participant in one's own health and well-being.

Aromatherapy

Genuine essential oils contain diverse complex substances comprising active ingredients, secondary components, and trace compounds. The oily volatile compounds are the result of plant metabolism and each plant has a particular organ for producing then storing an oil. The oil can be produced in the flowers, leaves, seeds, fruit, rinds, roots, or in wood like cedar. They are also found in grasses, herbs, needles, and branches of trees, in resin, balsam, and bark. The oils are extracted from the plant through a variation of distillation processes or by cold pressing. Different components can come from different parts of a single plant. Sometimes there are a number of varieties of the same plant; for example, there are hundreds of eucalyptus varieties throughout the world, each with a different oil, chemical composition, and therapeutic use.

The pharmaceutical effects of essential oils are due to their inherent chemical constituents and to the fact that these constituents work synergistically. Their specific effects are determined by their structures, whether they have lipophilic or hydrophilic properties, and if they attract or repel electrons. They are so complex on the molecular level that one oil can have many different uses. The physical nature of oils, a low molecular weight, and an affinity for lipids or fats allow them to penetrate body tissues with great ease. When an oil is inhaled, it is absorbed in the nasal cavity and picked up by smell receptors that pass information to the limbic system of the brain where emotions and memory are controlled and to the hypothalamus which controls digestion, heart rate, blood pressure, hormone balance, sexuality, and stress. Placed on the tongue or taken in gelatin capsules, the oil is absorbed along the digestive tract and travels to the liver where it is metabolized. Rubbing oils into the skin or inhaling them can be more effective delivery systems because they bypass liver processing. Massaging an oil into the feet is particularly efficacious.

High potency oils are expensive; however, they tend to be cost-effective because results can be obtained with smaller doses. The interaction of all the various compounds within an oil are qualitatively more effective than the isolation of a particular component or components. The oils can be inhaled, ingested, or applied topically. When delivered through a vaporizer, microparticles of the oil are dispersed into the air and inhaled. This system is effective for respiratory illnesses, to calm nerves, or to clear airborne infectious microbes. The oils can be used for massage, dispersed in the bath, mixed with water and sprayed into the air or on the skin, applied as a compress, or placed directly on the skin full strength or diluted with vegetable oil. When using a base or carrier oil for combining with the essential oil, use a cold-pressed unrefined vegetable, nut, or seed oil; essential oils can also be added to creams or lotions. *Internal ingestion should be done only under the supervision of an aromatherapist. Essential oils can be toxic when taken internally; as little as one teaspoon of some oils can be fatal.*

Aromatherapy is especially effective for infectious illnesses, for maintaining hormonal balance, and for psychological and nervous system conditions. Essential oils can harmonize moods and emotions and alter brain waves in such a manner as to have a tranquilizing effect that produces a sense of well-being and calm. Certain oils act as stimulants and have an energizing effect. Treatments may be less effectual for diseases that are genetic or have been chronic for a number of years; metabolic and degenerative illnesses may not respond at all. Extensive studies, many of which have been conducted in Germany, have shown the beneficial effects of essential oils. For example, as antibacterial agents, certain oils were found to prevent the spread, and eliminate the presence, of a number of pathogens including E. coli, Streptococcus, Staphylococcus, and Candida albicans in an enclosed room.[5] Their ability to prevent microorganism proliferation in the body may be through their ability to penetrate cellular membranes and influence cell metabolism. At the same time, they do not destroy valuable intestinal flora as conventional antibiotics tend to do.

Certain essential oils have antiviral properties, act as expectorants for respiratory ailments, have sedative and antispasmodic qualities, and give support to the immune system. Some oils have an effect on the autonomic nervous system, moderating an overactive sympathetic system. In a clinical study, 80% of the participants reported positive improvement for symptoms affecting the nervous system including depression, tension, headache, fatigue, insomnia, and loss of appetite.[6] Some oils have shown in studies to have an anti-inflammatory effect by stimulating the adrenal glands and releasing cortisone-like substances. Brain waves were shown to be altered on another group who experienced improved visual search tasks.

The manner in which the oils are taken is very important. Sometimes oral ingestion has no effect while inhalation presents clear results. If doses are too high, a secretion-stimulating effect reverts to a secretion-inhibiting one. The most effective dosages are usually the lowest (1 mg per kilogram of body weight), while raising the dosage reduces efficacy. An individual weighing approximately 150 lb would normally use between two and five drops. In a clinical study, blood samples were taken from participants after they had inhaled certain essential oils. Therapeutic levels of the compounds were found but within an hour levels decreased by half, showing that the oils did not accumulate in the blood.[7]

Some essential oils can cause a reaction in certain individuals who are susceptible to allergies. To test for potential sensitivity, place a small amount of oil on the inside of the elbow for 24 hours. If no reaction is evident, it is advisable to repeat the process in 20 to 48 hours. Certain oils are to be used either externally or internally exclusively; some can exacerbate or complicate existing health conditions; and yet others are poisonous, although those are not usually available commercially.

Ketones are the toxic elements in essential oils and these molecules can penetrate the blood-brain barrier causing damage to the nervous system and irreversible liver damage. The ketone most widely found in oils is thujone, a component in mugwort, sage, thuja, wormwood, and yarrow oils. Although sage oil has a high content of the ketone, it appears to have low toxicity and can be used by adults with caution. The toxic effects of ketones depend on how it is administered; inhalation being the safest, followed by skin contact, vaginal, rectal, and oral ingestion.

Anise, atlas cedar, eucalyptus dives, yarrow, clary sage, chamomile, pennyroyal, and rosemary oils are not to be used during pregnancy; spike lavender and niaouli, which have hormone-like properties, should be used with caution. Fennel oil stimulates the production of estrogen and is not to be used if an individual has breast cancer or if there is a family history of the disease. Basil and possibly tarragon oils can be carcinogenic in large quantities. Thuja, wormwood, mugwort, tansy, and hyssop are toxic when taken internally. Pine is not to be used internally. Hyssop and thuja should be administered only in small doses externally. Pennyroyal is poisonous in large doses. Savory and oregano dosages are not to exceed three drops taken internally and not to be used for more than a 21-day period. Oregano, thyme, and savory are not for external use; although thyme and oregano are well tolerated if rubbed into the soles of the feet. Internal use of thyme should not exceed three drops per day. Clove oil, clove leaf oil, cinnamon bark oil, and cinnamon leaf oil can cause skin irritation and may cause swelling of the entire body and severe shortness of breath in susceptible individuals. Bergamot, bitter orange rind, khella, lemon, and mandarin should not be applied to the skin. Juniper oil can be damaging to the kidneys whereas the berries of the juniper are not irritating. Crested lavender, anise, atlas cedar, basil, cinnamon, eucalyptus dives, eucalyptus globulus, rosemary, sage, and yarrow are not suitable for children. Niaouli and peppermint should be used with caution. Spike lavender should be mixed with benign oils. Camphor induces abortion and is toxic to the nerves.

If the following health conditions are present do not take the listed oils:

Abdominal pain—clove

Asthma—marjoram, oregano, rosemary, yarrow

Breast cancer—angelica, anise, caraway, cypress, fennel, sage

Epilepsy—anise, fennel, hyssop, nutmeg, parsley, sage

Glaucoma—cypress, hyssop, lemon balm, tarragon, thyme

Hemorrhaging—lavender if taking an anticoagulant

High blood pressure—hyssop, lemon

Hypothyroidism—fennel

Insomnia—peppermint, pine

Menstrual complaints—angelica, anise, caraway, cypress, sage

Prostate cancer—angelica, cypress, hyssop, *Thymus serpyllum*

Tumors—anise, caraway, fennel

Urinary tract infection—eucalyptus, juniper

For more information contact: National Association for Holistic Aromatherapy, P.O. Box 17622, Boulder, Colorado 80308–0622, 303-258-3791; Lotus Light, P.O. Box 1008, Wilmot, Wisconsin 53170, 414-889-8501; The Pacific Institute of Aromatherapy, P.O. Box 6842, San Rafael, California 94903, 415-479-9121.

Ayurvedic Medicine

Ayurvedic means the *science of life,* and is probably the oldest system of healing. It encompasses a philosophy that is both subtle and complex. In treating an individual, an assessment is first made of metabolic body type or *dosha.* There are three doshas: vata, pitta, and kapha, and the dominance of one over the others determines classification. *Doshas* are blueprints, or a health profile of an individual, encompassing physiology, innate tendencies, strengths, weaknesses, and susceptibilities to ill health. Once a diagnosis of the illness has been made, the methods of treatment may include cleansing the body of toxins, whether of an environmental, bacterial or viral nature, appropriate changes in diet, herbal and mineral preparations to rebuild and rejuvenate body tissues, and stress management through activities such as meditation, deep breathing, and sound therapy. The purpose is to balance the doshas within the individual.

Several factors are believed to be at the basis of physiological imbalance and disorder. There may be a genetic predisposition to an illness that is prompted by something in the surrounding environment or triggered while still in the womb by the activities of the mother. Individuals usually have natural tendencies toward a particular habit or behavior such as alcoholism, overeating, or overworking. A disease may be the result of a congenital defect acquired during development in the uterus. Environmental pollutants, poor diet, or eating the wrong foods according to dosha type can cause illness; and each dosha may be susceptible to seasonal influences. Other conditions affecting health are physical and emotional trauma, and electrical or magnetic imbalances along the spinal cord.

The foremost characteristic of the vata metabolic type is changeability. People of this type are active, energetic, moody, imaginative, and impulsive; prone to erratic sleep patterns, intestinal problems, nervous disorders, and premenstrual syndrome. There is a sensitivity to cold and dry and their vulnerable season is autumn. Pitta types are predictable, aggressive, intense, efficient, articulate, moderate in daily habits, short-tempered, and impatient. They tend to perspire more and may be open to poor digestion, ulcers, skin inflammations, hemorrhoids, and heartburn. In summer they are sensitive to the sun and heat. Kapha is relaxed, stable, conservative, with a tendency to laziness and procrastination. They sleep long and move, eat, and digest food slowly. There is an inclination toward overweight, allergies, sinus, and lung congestion and they are highly susceptible to the cold of winter.

An important aspect of Ayurvedic medicine is the categorization of food according to taste and other inherent properties, then using that information to establish the proper diet for each dosha. Ayurvedic medical schools often teach pharmacology and cooking in the same course. Whether a food is sweet, sour, salty, pungent, bitter or astringent, heavy or light, solid or liquid, dry or oily as well as its hot or cold-producing abilities, all have an effect on the health of an individual.

There is also a consideration of food transformation once digested, for example, from sweet to pungent, as is the case with honey. Honey is sweet when eaten but once processed in the body becomes pungent. From a health aspect it would not have the affect that sweet foods do. The pharmacological effect of a meal can be altered by adding or subtracting a spice or herb. The Ayurvedic method of nutrition is ultimately to observe the reactions that different foods have on each patient.

Ayurvedic medicine is very effective in treating metabolic, stress related, or chronic conditions and for relieving the deleterious effects of surgery and debilitating treatments such as chemotherapy. Many Ayurvedic herbal preparations have been clinically tested and documented as improving a wide range of health conditions. A number of studies have shown guggul (an extract from the mukul myrrh tree) to lower cholesterol. For example, in a study of 40 patients with high cholesterol, the herb was shown to reduce in a 16-week period, serum cholesterol levels by 21%, triglycerides by 27%, a 35% rise of HDL cholesterol, and a decrease in LDL levels.[8] Guggul properties have an anticoagulating effect on blood platelets and prevent LDL cholesterol from oxidizing.[9] Other illnesses that have responded to therapy in studies are metabolic and endocrine gland dysfunctions, neurological disorders, gastrointestinal diseases, mental disorders, inflammation of the musculoskeletal system, and the prevention of cancer.

For more information contact: American Association of Ayurvedic Medicine, P.O. Box 598, South Lancaster, Massachusetts, 01561, 1-800-843-8332; American School of Ayurvedic Sciences, 10025 NE 4th Street, Bellevue, Washington 98004, 206-453-8022; Sharp Institute for Human Potential and Mind-Body Medicine,

8010 Frost Street, Suite 300, San Diego, California 92123, 1-800-82SHARP; The College of Maharishi Ayur-Veda Health Center, P.O. Box 282, Fairfield, Iowa 52556, 515-472-5866; Canadian Association of Ayurvedic Medicine, P.O. Box 749 Station 'B', Ottawa, Ontario Canada K1P 5P8, 613-837-5737; Ayurvedic Institute, 11311 Menaul NE, Suite A, Albuquerque, New Mexico 87112, 505-291-9698.

Bodywork

Therapeutic massage, deep tissue manipulation, movement therapies, and energy balancing are forms of bodywork that are used to correct the structure and improve the functioning of the human body. The various techniques increase the energy flow throughout the system, thereby stimulating natural physiological healing mechanisms.

Therapeutic Massage

Manipulation of the soft tissues of the body affects the skin, blood vessels, nerves, lymph systems, and muscles as well as some internal organs. When nerve endings in the dermis, the inner layer of the skin, are stimulated, they send nerve impulses to the spinal cord and brain. Touch nerve impulses can prevent pain nerve impulses from reaching the brain. Endorphins are also released. These are the body's own pain killers that can minimize or alleviate pain.

There are four basic movements in soft-tissue massage. Effleurage relaxes superficial muscles. Pettrisage releases tension from superficial and deep-muscle tissue and increases blood flow to the area. The third stroke, friction, breaks down adhesions between tissues and releases the tension of muscle spasm. The fourth, tapotement, has a stimulating effect on the skin and soft tissues and increases blood circulation. A familiar method of this technique appears like a karate chop—a movement that is swift and rhythmical.

Massage is beneficial for numerous health conditions including pain, respiratory ailments, circulatory and digestive problems, and psycho-logical and stress-related illnesses. The therapy aids in the elimination of toxins from the body, for example, by stimulating the lymphatic glands. It acts as a sedative on the nervous system, and is the most frequently used therapy for musculoskeletal (muscle and skeleton) disorders. Muscle nerve fibers can become compressed by tension and stress, which causes muscle fatigue and pain. If prolonged, this contraction can interfere with the elimination of metabolic waste in muscle and surrounding tissue. Tension can also cause headaches and neck, shoulder, and lower back pain. At the University of Miami School of Medicine, a study found that premature babies who received a daily massage gained weight faster than those who did not. Another study found that individuals with eating disorders felt better about themselves and their bodies after massage treatments.

For more information contact: American Massage Therapy Association, 820 Davis Street, Suite 100, Evanston, Illinois 60201, 312-761-2682; National Association of Massage Therapy, P.O. Box 1400, Westminster, Colorado 80030, 800-776-6268.

Deep Tissue Manipulation

Manipulation and stretching of the fascia, which is the thin, elastic membrane that envelops every muscle, connects muscles and muscle fibers, and creates bands to form tendons and ligaments, is the primary focus of deep-tissue massage. *Rolfing, Hellerwork,* and *Aston-Patterning* are the better known methods of this therapy.

Dr. Ida Rolf compared the body to a stack of bricks, each one squarely and firmly on top of one another. If just one of the bricks was out of alignment, the entire structure would be unstable and under duress. When the body is properly aligned, the muscles use little tension in maintaining any given position; however, improper posture puts such stress on the muscles, especially of the back, neck, and legs, that the muscles become over-contracted. After months or years in this condition, the movement of fascial tissues, because they have to hold everything in an out-of-balance state, become shortened and inflexible, and eventually lose their pliability. The muscles underneath become stiff and rigid. Because the neuromuscular system adapts, the body does not know it is in misalignment. Meanwhile, the stress factor depletes energy and interferes with the intrinsic healing abilities of the body.

The belief is that physical or mental trauma can also affect the mobility of the fascia and prevent the muscles from full-range movement. Deep-tissue massage loosens the fascial tissues so that muscles underneath can move more freely. The muscles lengthen, become relaxed, and posture is realigned. A University of Maryland study found that rolfing reduced stress and improved the body's neuromuscular function in the participants.

For more information contact: Rolf Institute, 205 Canyon Boulevard, P.O. 1868, Boulder, Colorado 80302, 303-449-5903. The Body of Knowledge/Hellerwork, 406 Berry Street, Mt. Shasta, California 96067, 916-926-2500. The Aston Training Center, P.O. Box 3568, Incline Village, Nevada 89450, 702-831-8228.

Movement Therapies

The *Alexander technique, Feldenkrais method,* and *Trager approach* reeducate muscle movements to improve body flexibility, balance, coordination, and release of muscle tension. There is an increase in energy level and breathing becomes easier and deeper. Children move with great ease and grace but as adults, poor posture and incorrect movements eventually become natural habits. Meanwhile, the body is misaligned and muscles are tense and over-stretched. These unconscious habits can be reprogrammed and new messages relayed to the brain by practicing new patterns of movement that eventually become involuntary and automatic.

Movement therapies are especially effective for the prevention of illness, and their techniques have improved conditions such as stress, chronic pain, neuromuscular (nerve and muscle) and musculoskeletal disorders, and respiratory and digestive problems.

For more information contact: North American Society of Teachers of the Alexander Technique, P.O. Box 517, Urbana, Illinois 61801, 1-217-367-6956 or 800-473-0620. Feldenkrais Guild, P.O. Box 489, Albany, Oregon 97321, 503-926-0981.

Trager Institute, 21 Locust Avenue, Mill Valley, California 94941, 415-388-2688.

Energy Balancing

Meridians are invisible pathways through which energy or life force flows in the human body. These channels are connected to specific organs that can become diseased if the energy to them is blocked. *Acupressure, shiatsu, qigong, t'ai chi,* and *polarity therapy* use various techniques in restoring energy flow.

Acupressure manipulates the same points as acupuncture but uses the hands and fingers instead of needles. Shiatsu is a Japanese therapy and a form of acupressure. Qigong is practiced by millions in China. It is a system of gentle exercise and breathing techniques that restore the circulation of energy. The theory behind qigong is that the energy or life force that is inherent in all matter has two aspects, yin and yang. Illness, whether physical or emotional, develops when the energy flow between these two opposites moves out of balance or is depleted. Because of its ease and slowness, qigong can be practiced by all ages including the elderly, helping them maintain their strength and agility. Among the conditions that are benefited by the discipline are gastrointestinal ailments, ulcers, arthritis, high blood pressure, and heart disease.

T'ai chi also incorporates the life force and yin-yang principles in its exercise program and can be practiced by all age groups as well as the disabled. Research compiled in Atlanta, Georgia, showed that a group of elderly individuals who practiced t'ai chi had improvements in the functioning of the nervous, cardiovascular, and musculoskeletal systems and delays in osteoporosis development. Polarity therapy uses both Eastern and Western philosophies of energy. The right side and head of the body represent the positive electric pole, and the left side and feet the negative; the spine is neutral. The practitioner uses a light touch on specific points in the body in order to encourage the free flow of energy and facilitate the process of healing.

For more information contact: Acupressure Institute, 1533 Shattuck Avenue, Berkeley, California 94709, 510-845-1059; American Oriental

Bodywork Association, 6801 Jericho Turnpike, Syosset, New York 11791, 516-364-5533. American Shiatsu Association, P.O. Box 718, Jamaica Plain, Massachusetts 02130. National Qigong Association of the USA, P.O. Box 20218, Boulder, Colorado 80308, 1-888-218-7788; Qigong Academy, 8103 Marlborough Avenue, Cleveland, Ohio 44129. American Polarity Therapy Association, 2888 Bluff Street, Suite 149, Boulder, Colorado 80301, 1-303-545-2080; Polarity Wellness Center, 10 Leonard Street, Suite A, New York, New York 10013, 212-334-8392.

Reflexology

Areas in the feet have reflex points that correspond to every part of the body, which can be affected when these points are stimulated. When pressure is applied to nerve endings in the feet, the spinal cord and the sensory cortex of the brain respond by sending information via the nervous system to other parts of the body. Lactic acid and calcium crystals can accumulate at reflex points in the feet, and massage can break them up allowing nerve energy to flow more freely. The treatment is relaxing and beneficial as an adjunct to a number of health conditions including PMS, anxiety, hypertension, stress, headache, and skin inflammations. The belief is that reflexology encourages the body's own healing mechanisms.

For more information contact: International Institute of Reflexology, P.O. Box 12462, St. Petersburg, Florida 33733, 813-343-4811; Reflexology Association of America, 4012 S. Rainbow Boulevard, Box K585, Las Vegas, Nevada 89103-2509.

Chinese Medicine

Chinese medicine, or traditional Chinese medicine, is thousands of years old and one of the most traditional healing systems on earth. Central to Chinese medicine is the principle of *qi*, or energy, which travels along invisible meridians, on the surface of the body, and through internal organs. A balance of this energy is crucial for maintaining good health. To a physician of Chinese medicine,

visible illness is preceded by invisible illness, and detection of nascent diseases is a main focus and a potentially powerful approach to health care.

The polarities of yin and yang are an important aspect of Chinese medicine, describing the interdependence and relationship of opposites. Yin refers to the tissue of an organ and yang to its activity. A yin deficiency means the organ does not have enough raw materials to function; in a yang deficiency, the organ does not react adequately when needed. The organs of the body work synergistically, each one either nourishes or inhibits the proper functioning of another.

The methods of diagnosis are observing the patient's outward appearance, demeanor, body language, complexion, and tongue; the smell of the breath, skin, and secretions; and the tone and strength of the voice. Questions are asked regarding symptoms, medical history, diet, and lifestyle. A palpation test, which is the taking of the pulse, is conducted at six different locations at three depths on each wrist, with an analysis involving 28 different qualities. Once a diagnosis is made, the treatments involve one or more of the following: acupuncture which reestablishes the flow of energy to affected organs through needle stimulation, herbs and herbal combinations, diet adjustments, massage and manipulation, and therapeutic exercise specifically qigong.

In China, methods for conducting clinical studies differ from the West in that they consider giving a placebo to a sick person unethical. If they do use a placebo, they first offer the patient a choice. When double-blind studies are conducted, there is an application of two substances in which both are presumed to be effective. They believe the West relies too much on laboratory tests and not enough on how patients feel and their quality of life. Chinese medicine therapy is individualized and so there is not a standard treatment for any one condition. Studies in both the East and West have proven Chinese medicine to be effective in the treatment or prevention of nearly all common health conditions including infertility, digestive problems, respiratory ailments, cancer, brain dysfunctions, cardiovascular irregularities, and AIDS.

For more information contact: American Association of Acupuncture and Oriental Medicine,

4101 Lake Boone Trail, Suite 201, Raleigh, North Carolina 27607, 919-787-5181; National Acupuncture and Oriental Medicine Alliance, P.O. Box 77511, Seattle Washington 98177.

Chiropractic

Chiropractic means doing by hand which is the method chiropractic practitioners use in adjusting misaligned vertebrae and other joints. Vertebrae are the 26 bones that make up the spinal column or backbone. The vertebrae surround and protect the spinal cord. Between each vertebrae are disks made of cartilage with a gelatinous center that enables them to act as shock absorbers. Spinal nerves branch out from the spinal cord from which they send messages throughout the body, to the muscles, glands, organs, and bones.

The spinal column is the central station for the nervous system. The nervous system consists of three parts: the central nervous system which is the brain and spinal cord; the autonomic nervous system which controls involuntary functions such as digestion, heart rate, and breathing; and the peripheral nervous system which connects the central nervous system to voluntary muscles and other body tissues.

When the vertebrae are in proper alignment, nerve impulses flow freely along the spinal cord and out to other parts of the body. However, if a vertebrae falls out of alignment, called a subluxation, it impinges on the spinal nerves as they try to leave the spinal cord. Consequently, the nerves are unable to continue their functions properly and the recipient organs are adversely affected. A subluxation can occur from a physical trauma or injury, poor posture, muscle spasm or weakness, or birth defect. Stress, chemical toxicity, temperature extremes, and a genetic predisposition are also possible conditions that can have an affect on the vertebrae and nerve transmission.

Methods used in treatment involve several types of adjustments including the manipulation of a joint by stretching it beyond its normal range in which an audible click can be heard due to the release of gases from the joint fluid. There are also nonforce techniques applied along the spine, skull, or pelvis. Some chiropractors give additional advice on nutrition and exercise.

Chiropractic treatment has been used for the neuromusculoskeletal (nerve, muscle, and skeleton) system, lower back, upper back, neck and head pain, and for extremity, joint, and muscle problems. It has also been beneficial for respiratory illnesses, the common cold, sinusitis, bronchial asthma, gastrointestinal disorders, high blood pressure, heart trouble, menstrual difficulties, and emotional problems such as depression and schizophrenia.

For more information contact: American Chiropractic Association, 1701 Clarendon Boulevard, Arlington, Virginia 22209, 703-276-8800; International Chiropractors Association, 1110 North Glebe Road, Suite 1000, Arlington, Virginia 22201, 703-528-5000; World Chiropractic Alliance, 2950 N. Dobson Road, Suite 1, Chandler, Arizona 85224, 800-347-1011; Association for Network Chiropractic Spinal Analysis, P.O. Box 7682, Longmont, Colorado 80501, 303-678-8086; The American College of Addictionology and Compulsive Disorders, 5990 Bird Road, Miami, Florida 33155, 305-661-3474.

Herbal Therapy

Approximately 25% of all prescription drugs are an extract of an herb or a synthetic replica. Although they work rapidly, enter the bloodstream quickly, and have dramatic responses, these derivatives are of short duration and often have toxic side effects. The whole plant, on the other hand, has chemical properties that work synergistically, containing secondary compounds that not only have their own pharmacological effects but that modify or mitigate the reactions of the more dominant active ingredients. They enter the bloodstream more slowly because they are bound up in inert compounds that take longer to break down. Herbs may take several days, weeks, or even months for their effects to be fully experienced but the result will be more qualitative and lasting than many comparable conventional drugs.

Extensive documentation shows the usefulness of herbs in a wide variety of health conditions including respiratory tract infections, gastrointestinal disturbances, PMS, insomnia, heart disease, cancer, and for immune system support. The definitive text on herbal medicine is the German government's Commission E, an extensive compendium on herbs and their efficacy and safety. Efficacy was determined in most cases by two or three different constituents of the plant. For example, in St. John's wort, the three compounds in the flowers and leaves used are hyericins, hyperforins, and flavonoids. The Commission stressed the greater therapeutic range of activity and effects of standardized extracts that contain not only the primary active components but secondary and accompanying compounds as well, as opposed to individual isolated compounds, for example, found in conventional drugs.

They also emphasize that variations in dosage of phytomedicines have differing effects. For example, extracts of goldenrod in low doses have no diuretic effect but adequate doses do, while too high doses have a diuretic-inhibiting effect. The Commission also cautions that the quality of the plant material affects intended results. Certain herbs contain compounds that can be toxic, so herbal therapy should be conducted under the supervision of an herbal practitioner.

The most popular way to ingest herbs is by infusion—pour one cup of boiling water over one or two teaspoons of dried herb or one or two tablespoons of fresh herb. Infusions are appropriate for leaves, flowers, or stems. Steep 10 to 20 minutes to allow the phytochemicals to seep into the water. Decoctions are used for roots, twigs, bark, nuts, or certain seeds; prepare by simmering the plant material for 10 to 20 minutes. Herbal capsules, tablets, and ointments are commercially available. Extracts and tinctures are advantageous since the body assimilates them rather quickly. A poultice is made by moistening dried or cut up fresh herbs and applying them directly to the wound or infection and then covering the wound with a bandage. Compresses are cloths that have been dipped in infusions, decoctions, or tinctures and placed directly on the skin.

Do not take the following herbs under the listed conditions:

Aloe vera—may cause allergic reaction in some people; test on skin and if stinging or rash appears do not use.

Barberry—do not use during pregnancy or lactation.

Bitter melon—do not take in the presence of hypoglycemia.

Black Cohosh—do not take during pregnancy or lactation.

Bloodroot—do not use during pregnancy or lactation; take only small amounts internally; long-term use has been linked to glaucoma.

Blue Cohosh—do not use during pregnancy; should only be used in limited amounts.

Boneset—do not use during pregnancy or lactation; do not use in the presence of liver disease; do not use for more than 6 months consecutively.

Buchu—do not use during pregnancy or lactation.

Cat's claw—do not use during pregnancy or lactation; do not use in combination with hormonal drugs, insulin, or vaccines.

Celery—do not use in large amounts during pregnancy.

Chamomile—may cause ragweed allergy if used for long periods of time; do not use in presence of ragweed allergy.

Chaparral—large amounts taken internally or for long periods of time can be toxic to the liver.

Cinnamon—do not use during pregnancy.

Clove—clove oil can cause irritation, dilute with vegetable oil.

Comfrey—do not use during pregnancy or lactation; taken internally can be toxic to the liver, use only under the supervision of a professional.

Dandelion—do not use in the presence of gallstones; use cautiously in the presence of stomach ulcer or gastritis.

Devil's claw—do not use in the presence of ulcers, heartburn, or gastritis; in the presence of gallstones consult a physician.

Dong quai—do not take during pregnancy or lactation; may cause sensitivity to sunlight in some individuals if taken for long periods of time.

Echinacea—do not take in the presence of lupus, tuberculosis, multiple sclerosis, or HIV infection; do not take if allergic to plants in the daisy family.

Ephedra or ma huang—do not use during pregnancy or lactation; do not use in the presence of an anxiety disorder, glaucoma, high blood pressure, diabetes, or heart disease; do not use if monoamine oxidase (MAO) inhibitor drugs commonly prescribed for depression are being taken.

Eucalyptus—for external use only; do not put on broken skin or open cuts and wounds.

Feverfew—do not use during pregnancy or lactation.

Garlic—if taking anticoagulants or preparing for surgery, consult with a physician.

Ginger—in the presence of gallstones consult a physician; may cause stomach distress if taken in large amounts.

Ginseng—Siberian, American, and Korean/Chinese have similar properties; do not use during pregnancy or lactation or in the presence high blood pressure.

Goldenseal—do not use during pregnancy or lactation.

Horse chestnut—do not use in the presence of liver or kidney disease unless under the supervision of a physician.

Hydrangea—do not ingest the leaves as they contain cyanide and are toxic.

Juniper—do not use during pregnancy or in the presence of kidney disease.

Kava kava—do not use during pregnancy or lactation; can cause drowsiness, if so, adjust dosage; do not take with alcohol, barbiturates, antidepressants, or antipsychotic drugs.

Licorice—do not use during pregnancy; do not use in large doses or for long periods of time as it can cause high blood pressure in sensitive individuals.

Lobelia—do not use during pregnancy or lactation or internally for more than one month consecutively.

Meadowsweet—do not use if sensitive to aspirin; not to be used by children to lower fever.

Mustard—can irritate skin if applied topically.

Oak—do not bath in water with oak bark in the presence of open sores or high fever or infection.

Oregon grape—do not use more than 2 or 3 weeks consecutively; use with caution during pregnancy or lactation.

Passion flower—do not use during pregnancy or lactation or with MAO inhibiting antidepressant drugs.

Pau d'arco—do not use during pregnancy or lactation.

Peppermint—in the presence of gallstones, consult a physician.

Primrose—do not take in the presence of breast cancer if estrogen related as the herb promotes the production of estrogen.

Red clover—do not use fermented red clover.

Rhubarb—do not take during pregnancy.

Sage—decreases milk supply in lactating women; do not use alcohol extract internally during pregnancy; do not take in the presence of fever.

Sandalwood—do not use internally in the presence of kidney disease.

Sarsaparilla—do not use with digitalis or bismuth.

Scullcap—do not use during pregnancy or lactation.

St. John's wort—may interact with selective serotonin reuptake inhibitor drugs such as Prozac causing side effects, use only under the supervision of a practioner; do not use during pregnancy or lactation; taken internally in large amounts can cause a heightened sensitivity to the sun especially in fair skinned people.

Tea tree—may cause skin irritation in sensitive individuals if used topically, if so, dilute with vegetable oil.

Turmeric—do not take in the presence of gallstones.

Uva ursi—do not use during pregnancy or lactation; do not use for more than 2 or 3 weeks consecutively.

Vitex—do not use during pregnancy.

White willow—because of the aspirinlike properties, caution should be used in the presence of gastritis and ulcers or those allergic to aspirin; do not use to treat fever in children.

Wild indigo—do not use for more than 2 or 3 weeks consecutively.

Wormwood—do not take during pregnancy or lactation; do not use for long periods of time.

Yarrow—may increase sensitivity to sunlight.

Yohimbe—do not use during pregnancy or lactation or in the presence of kidney disease, peptic ulcer or psychological disorders; do not combine with antidepressant drugs unless under the supervision of a physician; may cause elevated blood pressure, heart rate, headache, dizziness, skin flushing; may precipitate anxiety attacks and hallucinations in some people.

Yucca—do not use for more than 3 months consecutively.

For more information contact: American Botanical Council, P.O. Box 201660, Austin, Texas 78720, 512-331-8868; Herb Research Foundation, 1007 Pearl Street, Suite 200, Boulder, Colorado 80302, 303-449-2265; American Association of Acupuncture and Oriental Medicine, 4101 Lake Boone Trail, Suite 201, Raleigh, North Carolina 27607, 919-787-5181; American Association of Naturopathic Physicians, 2366 Eastlake Avenue, Suite 322, Seattle, Washington 98102, 206-323-7610.

Homeopathy

Homeopathy is a complete health care system that can therapeutically effect a wide range of illnesses and dysfunctions. The principle behind homeopathy is the Law of Similars—the same substance that in large doses produces a symptom of an illness will cure the same symptom by using a small dose (the theory behind vaccines and allergy desensitizing); and the Law of Infinitesimal Dose—the higher the dilution, the more potent the remedy. Remedies can be diluted to such an extent that no molecule of the original substance remains, which is where homeopathy enters the realm of quantum physics. In a study of 23 different homeopathic remedies, through the use of nuclear magnetic resonance imaging, subatomic activity was observed in all samples tested.

Homeopathic remedies are prepared by diluting a substance with pure water or alcohol, then shaken vigorously by a process called succussion. The procedure is repeated a number of times which not only dilutes the substance but removes any risk of toxicity. A remedy diluted more than 24 times will no longer have an original molecule present but the electromagnetic frequencies of the substance will have been stored in the water molecules.

Homeopathic treatment is individual and specific. For example, chronic headaches are conventionally treated with analgesics or anti-inflammatory drugs, but in homeopathy, there are over 200 symptom patterns of headache with corresponding remedies for each one. A patient is profiled according to physical, emotional, and mental qualities before a remedy is prescribed. If an incorrect remedy is taken, it will work either superficially or not at all, so it is recommended that therapy be conducted under the supervision of a homeopathic practitioner.

Homeopathy can reverse and benefit many acute or chronic diseases including allergies, vascular diseases, autoimmune disorders, viral and bacterial infections, arthritis, flu, respiratory illnesses, female health problems like PMS, epilepsy, mental and emotional disorders, skin eruptions, and digestive disorders. The therapy is especially effective for children in cases such as ear and bladder infections, teething, colic, diarrhea, hyperactivity, emotional problems, and learning disabilities. Pregnant and lactating women benefit as well in not passing on toxic elements from conventional drugs to the fetus or infant.

For more information contact: National Center for Homeopathy, 801 North Fairfax, Suite

306, Alexandria, Virginia 22314, 703-548-7790; International Foundation for Homeopathy, 2366 Eastlake Avenue, East, Suite 301, Seattle, Washington 98102, 206-324-8230; Homeopathic Educational Services, 2124 Kittredge Street, Berkeley, California 94704, 800-359-9051; British Institute of Homeopathy and College of Homeopathy, 520 Washington Boulevard, Suite 423, Marina Del Rey, California 90292, 310-306-5408.

Mindbody Therapy

Mindbody therapy recognizes the connection between the mind and the body. How individuals think and feel, their attitudes and habits are a determining factor in either wellness or ill health. Researchers in the new science field of psychoneuroimmunology have found that peptides and neuropeptides, amino acids that act as biochemical messengers in the body and influence pain, pleasure, and mood, are found not only in the brain but in other parts of the body as well including the immune system and the endocrine system which produces secretions that are distributed throughout the body via the bloodstream. Therefore, emotional states and fluctuations affect the ability of the immune system to defend against diseases and of the endocrine glands to produce hormones.

It has also been discovered that the immune system has memory and can learn, which means that there is intelligence in every cell and that individuals can influence that intelligence by conscious effort. Studies have shown that attitude, emotions, thoughts, stress, depression, lifestyle, as well as food, exercise, and environment, can have a direct affect on health conditions from chronic pain and coronary heart disease to cancer and AIDS.

Disciplines in mindbody therapy include meditation and yoga, biofeedback, imagery, and hypnotherapy. They are often used as an adjunct to other healing systems and are practiced in many clinics and hospitals across the country and around the world.

Meditation

Meditation is a state of relaxed yet alert awareness in which control of the autonomic nervous system that regulates involuntary actions such as heartbeat, secretion, and peristalsis, can be turned over to its parasympathetic system which induces secretion, increases muscle tone and slows heart rate as opposed to its sympathetic system, which depresses endocrine secretions, decreases tone, and increases heart rate. Meditation can lower heart and respiration rates, reduce plasma cortisol which is a stress hormone, slow the pulse rate, and promote the relaxed brain wave state of alpha.

Meditation techniques have been used in clinical setting to enhance the immune system, reduce stress, manage pain, lower blood pressure, reduce anxiety and depression, and improve blood circulation. Those adept at yoga have learned to control the digestive, respiratory, and circulatory systems.

Biofeedback

In biofeedback, patients are taught to consciously regulate unconscious body functions. By learning to depress the activity of the sympathetic nervous system, improvements can be realized in blood circulation and pressure, heart rate, digestion, and spastic conditions of the stomach and colon. The sympathetic system is for emergencies, a fight-or-flight situation, and it is thought that this system is also activated when anger and anxiety remain unexpressed which can keep the body in a constant state of tension. As a result, organs become chronically stressed and eventually give way to illness and disease.

Biofeedback uses computers to give instant feedback on brain wave activity, respiration, skin temperature, electric resistance of skin and muscle tension, and can also monitor conditions of the bladder, esophagus motility, stomach acidity, and of the rectal sphincter in cases of incontinence. Patients are taught through various techniques to effect a desired response while computers reflect the progress that is being made. Once the patient has learned to stabilize and control body functions, the machine is no longer necessary and the exercises can be performed whenever needed. Hyperactivity and behavioral problems in children, poor muscle control, back pain, temporomandibular joint syndrome, brain and nerve damage, cerebral palsy, and insomnia are some of the health conditions that have responded to biofeedback training.

Imagery

Positron emission tomography, an advanced imaging technology, has recorded the effects of imagery. When individuals imagine, the same parts of the cerebral cortex are activated as when the situation is actually experienced; imaginary seeing, hearing, or feeling stimulates the same optic, auditory, and sensory cortexes. Consequently, messages are sent from the cerebral cortex to the limbic system of the brain that influence the endocrine and autonomic nervous system.

Imagery has helped reduce stress, lower heart rate, stimulate the production of immune cells, and in a study of elderly patients increase killer T-cells. The practice can reduce pain and anxiety, has helped cancer patients tolerate chemotherapy, managed chronic arthritic pain, and aided patients in preparing for surgery and post surgery.

Hypnotherapy

The hypnotic state is one of relaxation and increased alpha and theta brain wave activity which allows for the opportunity to control the autonomic nervous system and to make changes in thinking and behavior. Properly applied, hypnosis can be used for a variety of conditions including the reduction of stress, pain, and anxiety, in lowering blood pressure, slowing the heart rate, producing analgesia during surgery, supporting the immune system, and treating sleep disorders and depression.

For more information contact: The Center for Mindbody Studies, 5225 Connecticut Avenue NW, Suite 414, Washington, D.C. 20015, 202-966-7338; Mind-Body Clinic, New Deaconess Hospital, Harvard Medical School, 185 Pilgrim Road, Cambridge, Massachusetts 02215, 617-632-9530; Stress Reduction and Relaxation Program, University of Massachusetts Medical Center, 55 Lake Avenue, North, Worcester, Massachusetts 01655, 508-856-2656; The Center for Applied Psychophysiology, Menninger Clinic, P.O. Box 829, Topeka, Kansas 66601, 913-273-7500 ext. 5375; The Center for the Improvement of Human Functioning, 3100 North Hillside Avenue, Wichita, Kansas, 67219, 316-682-3100.

Institute of Transpersonal Psychology, P.O. Box 4437, Stanford, California 94305, 415-327-2066; Maharishi International University, 1000 North 4th Street, Fairfield, Iowa 52556, 515-472-5031; Himalayan Institute of Yoga, Science and Philosophy, RRI, Box 400, Honesdale, Pennsylvania 18431, 800-822-4547; International Association of Yoga Therapists, 109 Hillside Avenue, Mill Valley, California 94941, 415-383-4587.

Association for Applied Psychophysiology and Biofeedback, 10200 West 44th Avenue, Suite 304, Wheat Ridge, Colorado 80033, 303-422-8436; Center for Applied Psychophysiology, Menninger Clinic, P.O. Box 829, Topeka, Kansas 66601, 913-273-7500 ext. 5375; Tools for Exploration, 4460 Redwood Highway, Suite 2, San Rafael, California 94903, 415-499-9050.

The Academy for Guided Imagery, P.O. Box 2070, Mill Valley, California 94942, 800-726-2070; Exceptional Cancer Patients, 1302 Chapel Street, New Haven, Connecticut 06511, 203-865-8392; Simonton Cancer Center, P.O. Box 890, Pacific Palisades, California 90272, 310-459-4434. The American Society of Clinical Hypnosis, 2200 East Devon Avenue, Suite 291, Des Plaines, Illinois 60018, 708-297-3317; International Medical and Dental Hypnotherapy Association, 4110 Edgeland, Suite 800, Royal Oak, Michigan 48073, 313-549-5594; National Society of Hypnotherapists, 2175 North West 86th, Suite 6A, Des Moines, Iowa 50325, 515-270-2280.

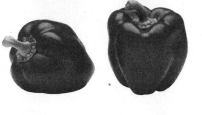

Health Conditions

Common health conditions are listed alphabetically with explanations regarding the nature of the condition and treatments that have been used by physicians in a clinical setting as well as research findings that have been shown to be efficacious. This section is designed to be a guide for individuals in finding the appropriate treatment or adjunct treatment for a particular health condition. The information here is not meant to be a substitute for the advice and care of a professional practitioner.

The foods listed contain nutrients that can be beneficial for the health condition under discussion. For a list of foods containing specific nutrients, see Section IV. For a complete nutrient breakdown of single foods, see the food composition chart in Section V. Health food stores and pharmacies that carry homeopathic remedies have literature that explains in detail the various symptoms for a particular remedy. William Boericke's *Materia Medica Repertory* is extensive and available in paperback. Combination formulas for common diseases are also available. For more complex situations, it is advisable to consult a homeopath to assure that the appropriate remedy is selected and the desired response results.

The amounts given of a treatment represent those that researchers have found to be effective in some people, but are not necessarily reflective of everyone's needs. *The amounts are not prescrip-* *tive.* If you are using a pharmaceutical drug or are pregnant, consult your physician before taking a nutrient supplement or herbal remedy as there may be contraindications. For more information on a specific type of therapy, see Section II.

Abscess

An abscess is a localized infection with a collection of pus in any part of the body, including the gums, externally or internally. A *boil* is an abscess. Pus is composed of dead tissue, living and dead bacteria, and white blood cells. The body responds to the bacteria by increasing blood flow to the area that results in redness and swelling as white blood cells from the bloodstream travel to the infection and engulf the bacteria. An abscess may be caused by lowered resistance to infection, bacterial contamination, or injury.

As a result of the large numbers of bacteria entering the bloodstream, symptoms of abscess may include fever, chills, vomiting, muscle aches, and headache. Recurrent abscess formation can indicate chronic conditions such as diabetes or kidney malfunction.

Antibiotics may be used to treat the infection and if conditions are severe, surgery is required to drain the pus. Antibiotics destroy intestinal flora so supplemental B complex and acidophilus may be necessary. Alternating hot and cold compresses can have a soothing affect and hasten natural discharge of the pus. Increase fluid intake.

Nutrients

Vitamin A—25,000 to 50,000 IU, also apply topically.

Carotenoid complex.

Vitamin B complex—if antibiotics are taken.

Vitamin C—250 mg four times a day.

Bioflavonoids—work synergistically with vitamin C.

Vitamin E—400 IU with mixed tocopherols.

Zinc—oxide, apply topically.

Foods

Fresh fruits

Fresh vegetables

Berries

Whole grains

Garlic

Raw honey—also apply topically, has antibacterial properties and heals wounds.

Juices

Fruits

Vegetables

Beet

Carrot

Celery

Cucumber

Spinach

Wheat grass

Herbal therapy

Tea tree oil—apply topically, contains the powerful antiseptic compound terpinen-4-ol.

Clove oil—an antiseptic and pain killer, dilute with vegetable oil.

Calendula—compress or cream, reduces inflammation and heals wounds.

Comfrey—cream, compress, or poultice, contains allantoin which heals wounds.

Goldenseal—tea and poultice, has antibacterial properties.

Echinacea—tea or tincture, for support of immune system.

Homeopathy

Take remedy according to symptoms:

Arsenicum album

Belladonna

Bryonia

Calendula

Echinacea angustifolia

Hepar sulphuris calcareum

Mercurius solubilis

Silicea

Tarentula cubensis

Aromatherapy

Lavender

Bergamot, chamomile, or lavender—hot compress.

Ayurvedic medicine

Kalanchoe

Chinese medicine

Consult a qualified practitioner.

Bodywork

Reflexology

Acne

Acne is a common disorder of the oil glands in the skin and can appear on the face, back, shoulders, chest, and arms. In adolescents during puberty, sex hormones stimulate the sebaceous glands resulting in excess secretion of sebum, a fatty oil that lubricates the skin. The glands become blocked and inflamed, which causes blackheads and pimples. If the glands become infected, sebum and pus build up under the skin and larger pimples and cysts appear which can eventually lead to scarring and pitting.

In adults, stress, hormonal fluctuations, and possibly food allergies may be the cause of acne. Oral contraceptives can cause breakouts. Excess dietary iodine irritates the pores and can induce flareups. Iodine is found in iodized salt, shellfish, seaweed, and fast foods in which an average meal can contain 30 times the RDA, and in milk, which can be contaminated from milking equipment and cow medication.[10] Acne may be caused by a deficiency in zinc.

It is important to keep the skin clean and free from oil. Facial steaming opens blocked skin pores and clears out sebum. Do not squeeze acne spots as they may become infected and leave scars. Reduce stress and avoid refined sugar and foods. For mild cases of acne, topical exfoliants and face washes are usually sufficient; for medium cases, beneficial preparations should contain benzoyl peroxide or salicylic acid; for severe acne, topical or oral antibiotics may be necessary or vitamin A derived drugs which include topical Retin A and Accutane taken internally. Long-term antibiotic use should be avoided and vitamin B complex and acidophilus supplemented as antibiotics destroy intestinal flora. Sunlight and ultraviolet light are beneficial if not undertaken excessively.

Rosacea is a chronic acnelike skin disorder. The nose and cheek areas are abnormally reddish in color and may be covered with pimples. Large doses of the B vitamins has shown to be very effective in treating rosacea patients, who often have a deficiency. Hydrochloric acid tablets have been effective for those that show a deficiency. Patients who have a low secretion of the pancreatic enzyme lipase can benefit from supplementation.

Nutrients

Vitamin B$_6$—50 mg, for premenstrual flareups.

Niacinamide—gel containing 4%, apply topically twice a day.

Zinc—30 mg two or three times daily for several months, reduce to once daily, has been found to be as effective as oral antibiotics; use a more absorbable form such as gluconate for maximum effectiveness.

Foods

Fresh fruits

Fresh vegetables

Dandelion greens

Whole grains

Brown rice

Legumes

Peanuts

Soybeans

Pecans

Sunflower seeds

Pumpkin seeds

Eggs

Poultry

Shellfish

Juices

Beet

Carrot

Celery

Cucumber

Dark green lettuce

Red lettuce

Spinach.

Herbal therapy

Calendula—cream and infusion as a face wash.

Calendula or tea tree soap.

Tea tree oil—5 to 15% dilution apply topically, contains terpinen-4-ol an antimicrobial agent, more effective overall than benzoyl peroxide.

Burdock—2 to 4 ml tincture or 1 to 2 g capsules three times daily, has a cleansing action on the skin.

Vitex—40 drops daily for premenstrual acne.

Chickweed, elderflower, and marigold—use as facial steam, add to boiling water, place towel over head and allow steam to penetrate face.

Homeopathy

Take remedy according to symptoms:

Antimonium tartaricum

Arsenicum album

Belladonna

Berberis vulgaris

Calcarea carbonica

Carbo vegetabilis

Hepar sulphuris calcareum

Ledum palustre

Pulsatilla

Silicea

Sulfur

Aromatherapy

Tea tree oil or lavender (Lavandula hybrida)—apply topically, both contain terpinen-4-ol and this particular lavender contains borneol, another strong antiseptic component.

Thyme (linalol type)—strong antiseptic properties, mild on skin.

Bergamot—has relaxing properties.

Rosemary (verbenone type)—has cell regenerating properties.

Ayurvedic medicine

Sunder Bati—for acne vulgaris not the severe cystic form.

Shanka bhasma—for vatta and pitta types.

Aloe vera—½ cup juice twice daily.

Chinese medicine

Effective topical treatments and capsules are prescribed.

Cai Feng Zhen Zhu an Chuang Wan/Margarite—acne pills, contain pearl, an effective remedy.

Cucumber, watermelon—apply juice topically.

Dandelion, honeysuckle—drink as tea.

Bodywork

Massage—assists in drainage of the lymphatic system.

Acupressure

Shiatsu

Reflexology

Mindbody therapy

Meditation—relieves tension and stress.

Yoga

Biofeedback

Imagery

AIDS

AIDS is thought to be caused by the human immunodeficiency virus, HIV. The virus destroys the body's infection fighting T-cells. After exposure to the virus, 3 to 6 months will elapse before tests show evidence that antibodies to the virus have or have not developed in the blood; until then tests read HIV negative. Early symptoms appear as flulike and may take 7 to 11 years to develop. Later stage symptoms are fatigue, appetite and weight loss, chronic diarrhea, fever, swollen lymph nodes, skin tumors, and night sweats.

Pneumonia, herpes, gastroenteritis, cancer, tuberculosis, and meningitis are associated with AIDS. HIV is transmitted through body fluids such as semen, breast milk, and blood; through sexual intercourse, sharing syringe needles, and from blood transfusions of unscreened blood. Mothers can pass the virus during pregnancy and at delivery. Some people do not develop AIDS from the virus and it is thought that the reason is a strong immune system.

A Chinese medical journal has reported success with administration of intravenous garlic against a fungal infection of the brain, cryptococcal meningitis,[11] found in some AIDS patients. A nutrient-dense diet, rest, and stress reduction are beneficial for the illness. Deep breathing aids relaxation, improves circulation, and increases oxygen intake. Drink pure water frequently. Resolve unexpressed emotional issues that may be suppressing the immune system.

Nutrients

Multivitamins and minerals

Vitamin A—a deficiency is common in HIV infected individuals.

Beta carotene—30 mg twice daily, low levels are often found in HIV infected individuals, can be taken with the carotonoid complex.

Vitamin B complex—low levels are often found in AIDS patients.

Vitamin C—500 to 1000 mg three times daily (larger doses may interfere with lymphocyte function) improves resistance against infection, inhibits HIV replication in test tubes.

Bioflavonoids—work synergistically with vitamin C.

Vitamin E—400 to 800 IU, with mixed tocopherols, reduces toxicity of AZT and improves its effectiveness in test tubes, an antioxidant, aids immune system.

Iron—for children if deficient.

Selenium—reduces infection, improves heart and intestinal function, stimulates appetite.

Zinc—reduces infections, commonly deficient in AIDS patients.

Coenzyme Q_{10}—200 mg, prevents infections, improves white blood cell counts.

N-acetyl cysteine—enhances function of immune system, taken with glutamine it stimulates production of glutathione, a powerful antioxidant many AIDS patients are deficient in.

Carnitine—6 g, often deficient in AIDS patients, increases white blood cell proliferation and levels of circulating tumor necrosis factor, supports immune system.

Acidophilus—encourages healthy bacteria in intestine.

Bromelain—enhances absorption of supplements and herbs, has protease inhibitor activity with less side effects than the drugs commonly prescribed.

Foods

Organic fresh fruits and vegetables—contain concentrated amounts of glutathione, carotenoids, and vitamin C

Whole foods—contain large amounts of valuable nutrients

Bitter melon

Dandelion greens

Shiitake mushrooms

Reishi mushrooms

Maitake mushrooms

Spinach

Whole grains

Legumes

Peanuts

Seafood

Tuna

Oysters

Crab

Sardines

Turkey

Low-fat yogurt

Nuts

Brazil nuts

Sunflower seeds

Pumpkin seeds

Flaxseed oil

Extra virgin olive oil

Turmeric

Garlic—a natural antibiotic against infections

Herbal therapy

Licorice root—2 g daily or 2 to 4 ml extract two to three times daily or 150 to 225 mg glycyrrhizin, inhibits the reproduction of HIV in test tubes and is shown in human studies to be beneficial taken orally due to the constituent glycyrrhizin; improves immune system, monitor blood pressure if taken for long periods of time.

Curcumin—1 to 2 g, from turmeric, inhibits replication of HIV virus, may increase CD_4 cell counts, an antioxidant with up to 300 times the activity of vitamin E.

Asian and Siberian ginseng—immune system boosters.

St. John's Wort—10 to 30 drops tincture, has antiviral properties; slows progression of mild HIV infection and reduces some symptoms.

Aloe vera—250 mg four times daily of acemannan, the constituent active against HIV in test tubes, or 2½ cups juice, minimizes side effects of AZT.

Bitter melon—increases CD_4 and T_4 cell counts and blocks HIV infected macrophage and lymphocytes.[12]

Boxwood extract—990 mg daily, delays progress of infection due to CD_4 cell count decline.[13]

Garlic—extract, reduces infections and relieves diarrhea.

Echinacea—stimulates production of white blood cells and antibodies, enhances immune system.

Homeopathy

Hypericum

Remedies available to support immune system according to individual symptoms.

Aromatherapy

Tea tree oil, eucalyptus or thyme—massage that benefits the lymphatic system, and stimulates the immune system.

Bergamot, lavender, and ylang ylang—help depression and relieves stress.

Ayurvedic medicine

Ashwagandha—enhances immune system.

Chinese medicine

Herbal combinations prescribed to reduce side effects and increase efficacy of conventional medicine.

Chinese Angelica—stimulates white blood cell and antibody formation, increases energy.

Acupuncture—increases white blood cells and T-cell production,[14] alleviates symptoms such as skin reactions, diarrhea, fatigue, and sweating, and the side effects from chemotherapy and radiation treatments.

Bodywork

Massage—reduces stress, improves circulation, and promotes toxin removal from lymph glands.

Acupressure—for diarrhea and gastroenteritis through the stomach and spleen meridians.

Shiatsu—restores energy to internal organs.

Qigong and T'ai chi—unblocks the flow of qi.

Reflexology

Mindbody therapy

Meditation

Biofeedback

Imagery

Allergy

An allergy is the body's reaction to a substance that may be harmless in itself but the immune system misidentifies and treats it as a pathogen. Antibodies, called immunoglobulin E or IgE, react by attacking the substance and in the process histamine is released by the surrounding cells which causes an allergic reaction. The allergic reaction may include itchy nose and throat, nausea, vomiting, diarrhea, skin irritations, hay fever, hives, asthma, high blood pressure, abnormal fatigue, constipation, or hyperactivity. A severe reaction called *anaphylactic shock* will swell the larynx, obstruct the airway, and may be fatal. This is an emergency situation and remedied by an injection of adrenalin.

Allergens can enter the body in numerous ways. They can be taken in by the mucous membranes of the nose from pollen or dust, absorbed through the intestinal tract from foods, bacteria, molds or drugs; they may be injected from drugs or vaccines; or they can enter through the skin from cosmetics, insect bites, or poison oak or ivy. (For spider bites, apply a comfrey poultice or compress; for stings and bites in general, apply a cold compress.)

Susceptibility to allergy can be genetic or precipitated by emotional stress. A wide range of chemicals in the environment can act as irritants. Common food allergens are peanuts, cow's milk, soy, egg whites, wheat, and shellfish. Excessive protein in the diet can exacerbate symptoms by causing the immune system to overreact. Rotating foods and eating a wide variety minimizes exposure to food allergens.

Skin and blood tests may be required to find the source of an allergy. For chronic hives, check with a physician that the thyroid is functioning properly and that there are no antithyroid antibodies present. Thyroid hormone replacement therapy may be necessary. Although they may be necessary in acute situations, commercial antihistamines merely suppress allergy symptoms and can cause drowsiness and depression. Vitamin C is a natural antihistamine. For *hives* and itching, a colloidal oatmeal product or cornstarch added to the bath can relieve symptoms.

Nutrients

Vitamin C—250 to 1000 mg several times a day, prevents secretion of histamine by white blood cells and helps break down the compound.

Bioflavonoids—work synergistically with vitamin C.

Quercetin—400 mg twice daily between meals, start taking 2 weeks before and throughout allergy season; also helpful for hives.

Bee pollen—from local bees, start slowly before season begins; *do not take if allergic to pollen.*

Foods

Organic foods

Fresh fruits

Citrus fruits

Fresh vegetables

Seeds

Nuts

Low-fat protein

Low-fat yogurt

Whole grains

Brown rice

Corn

Buckwheat

Amaranth

Legumes

Ginger, garlic, onions, black pepper, and cayenne pepper—stimulate the production of IgA, an antibody in the gastrointestinal tract that coats a potential allergen and prevents its absorption.

Juices

Beet

Carrot

Celery

Cucumber

Herbal therapy

Ephedra—20 mg capsules, relieves symptoms of hayfever.

Astragalus, echinacea—normalize immune function.

Stinging nettle—1 to 2 freeze dried capsules every 2 to 4 hours, relieves symptoms of hayfever, hives, and itching.

Garlic—has a high concentration of quercetin which retards inflammatory reactions.

Chamomile—topical preparations for hives and itching.

Yarrow, myrhh—contract tissues, reduce secretions, and discharges.

Calendula—lotion and compress, relieves itching eyes.

Tiger balm—relieves itching.

Witch hazel—apply topically, relieves itching.

Homeopathy

Remedies are often minute doses of the allergic substance that stimulates the body's natural healing mechanism and neutralizes the allergic reaction.

Take remedy according to symptoms:

Aconite, veratrum, arnica—helpful for anaphylactic shock until help arrives.

Allium cepa

Apis—for bee stings

Arsenicum album

Eurphrasia officinalis

Ferrum phosphoricum

Gelsemium

Natrum muriaticum

Nux vomica

Sabadilla

Similisan—relieves redness and itching.

Wyethia

Aromatherapy

Lavender—dilute with vegetable oil and massage on chest or sinus area around eyes.

German chamomile (Matricaria recutita)—has strong anti-inflammatory properties and soothes allergic rashes, is nontoxic and can be used topically in undiluted form.

Khella—relieves spasms in smooth muscle of the bronchi in hayfever, do not use on skin.

Moroccan chamomile—apply externally or through inhalation, relieves allergic reactions.

Melissa—relieves stress and soothes reactions.

Myrtle hydrosol (myrtle water)—spray on eyelid or into eye, relieves allergic reactions and inflammation of eyes, do not use after expiration date on label.

Niaouli—a strong antiallergenic.

Ayurvedic medicine

Triphala—aids digestion and eliminates toxins from the body as allergies are believed to be a result of faulty digestion; also use daily as a preventive.

Harithaki—for eczema.

Bitter orange—for respiratory allergies.

Stramonium—supports immune system.

Pancha karma—a cleansing and detoxifying program.

Chinese medicine

Herbal prescriptions prescribed for specific symptoms.

Acupuncture—strengthens immune system response on a systemic level.

Bodywork

Acupressure—alleviates allergic responses.

Shiatsu

Reflexology

Polarity therapy

Imagery

Mindbody therapy

Hypnotherapy—very effective in desensitizing allergic reactions and reducing stress.

Biofeedback—training to recognize the body's response to an allergy.

Alzheimer's Disease

Alzheimer's is a progressive brain disease characterized by impaired memory, mood swings, confusion, and mental deterioration in how the brain receives and processes information. Symptoms include fatigue, depression, fear, aggressive behavior, restlessness, and repetitive actions. An accurate medical diagnosis is important because other diseases can have the same symptoms. The cause of Alzheimer's is unknown. Oxidative damage is part of the disease progression. Patients often have an acetylcholine deficiency. Acetylcholine is a neurotransmitter that plays a role in cognition and reasoning.

The only treatment now available for Alzheimer's is to maintain quality of life. Relaxation and deep breathing improve circulation and help memory. Ginkgo biloba has been found to increase the blood flow to the brain affecting cognitive function. High blood levels of vitamin E correlate with improved brain function in older individuals.[15] Music therapy has been found to be of great benefit; as other abilities decline, sensory stimulation promotes emotional well-being and facilitates a way of communication.

For individuals with symptoms of *memory* or *attention problems* not diagnosed as Alzheimer's, the nutrients vitamin A, the carotenoid complex, vitamin E (400 to 800 IU) with mixed tocopherols, vitamin C (1 g), selenium (100 to 300 mcg) and ginkgo biloba (2 cups twice daily) are beneficial.

Nutrients

Phosphatidylserine—100 mg three times daily, a naturally occurring compound in the brain, improves mental function.[16]

Acetyl-L-carnitine—500 mg to 1 g three times daily, delays progression of the disease,[17] improves memory and performance, involved in the production of acetylcholine.

Vitamin E—400 to 800 IU with mixed tocopherols, an antioxidant, may slow progression of the disease.

Zinc—27 mg, if deficient, improves memory and communication skills.

Foods

The following are foods that contain lecithin or choline from which the body makes acetylcholine:

Brazil nuts

Legumes

Soybeans

Mung beans

Fava beans

Whole wheat

Eggs

Fish

Herbal therapy

Ginkgo biloba—80 mg extract three times daily, improves memory, and especially helpful during early stages of the disease.

Huperzine A—200 mcg twice daily, slows the progression of the disease improving memory and cognitive and behavioral function, inhibits the destruction of acetylcholine, a compound found in the Chinese medicinal herb Huperzia serrata.

Rosemary—an antioxidant and memory enhancer, contains compounds that prevent the breakdown of acetylcholine.

Dandelion flowers—contain lecithin.

Fenugreek leaves and shepherd's purse—contain choline.

Ginseng—improves mental concentration, memory and attention.

Aromatherapy

Rosemary

Balm

Fennel

Sage

Ayurvedic medicine

Dietary and herbal remedies prescribed depend on metabolic type and blood chemistry.

Ashwagandha—improves memory.

Chinese medicine

Acupuncture—treatments on the scalp that clear pathways in the brain.

Ginseng, dong quai, hoshou-wu—herbs that enhance energy and mobility.

Bodywork

T'ai chi—helps mental agility.

Qigong—improves circulation of the blood to the brain; stimulates mental activity due to the concentration and visualization involved in the exercise.

Mindbody therapy

Yoga—beneficial affects are relaxation and deep breathing which increases blood circulation and oxygen flow.

Anemia

Abnormally low numbers of red blood cells and a reduction in the amount of hemoglobin in those cells results in anemia. Because red blood cells are needed as carriers of oxygen to the tissues, oxygen supply to the body is subsequently interrupted. The exact cause of anemia must be diagnosed by a physician before any treatment can begin.

Anemia can be caused by an iron deficiency due to blood loss from excessive menstrual flow, gastrointestinal bleeding and ulcers, during pregnancy, breast-feeding, from frequent blood donations, colon cancer, or a lack of iron in the diet. It can result from autoimmunity, a condition in which the immune system mistakenly attacks itself, in this case the red blood cells; or from a malfunction of the bone marrow system when it is adversely affected by infection, cancer, or toxic chemical exposure or radiation. Anemia can also occur because of a deficiency of vitamins B_6, B_{12}, folic acid, or copper; and from certain anti-inflammatory drugs or antibiotics or an excessive consumption of alcohol. Genetics may also be a factor.

Symptoms of anemia include lethargy, fatigue, pale skin, weakness, dizziness or faintness, poor concentration, breathlessness, irritability, recurrent infections, or loss of appetite. In severe cases, there is irregular and increased heart rate because the body is pumping more blood to compensate for the lack of oxygen.

Pernicious anemia is a form of anemia resulting from a deficiency of vitamin B_{12} characterized by a gradual reduction in the number of mature red blood cells as the bone marrow fails to produce them. This form of anemia could be a genetic inability to secrete the intrinsic factor which is necessary for the absorption of vitamin B_{12}. Vegetarians are susceptible to pernicious anemia because vitamin B_{12} is found mainly in animal proteins. In addition, high levels of folic acid contained in vegetarian diets can mask a B_{12} deficiency. Symptoms of pernicious anemia include weakness and gastrointestinal disturbances causing a sore tongue, slight yellowing of the skin and tingling of extremities. Disturbances of the nervous system such as partial loss of coordination of the fingers, feet, and legs; some nerve deterioration; and disturbances of the digestive tract such as diarrhea and loss of appetite may occur.

Sickle cell anemia is characterized by red blood cells that become bent (sickled) and hard, and clog the circulation system, depriving the body tissues of oxygen. It has been observed that these patients seem to have a high requirement for folic acid.

Treatment for anemia depends on the cause of the disease. Black tea contains tannins that can interfere with the absorption of iron as can excessive amounts of dietary fiber.

Nutrients

Depending on cause:

Iron—follow physician advice.

Vitamin A—10,000 IU, helps effectiveness of iron.

Vitamin C—100 to 500 mg, aids absorption of iron.

Vitamin B_6—50 to 100 mg, if deficient.

Vitamin B_{12}—20 to 100 mcg, injections or sublingual.

Folic acid—0.5 to 1.5 mg, if deficient.

Copper—2 mg, if deficient.

Foods

Fresh fruits

Dried apricots

Raisins

Dried fruit

Dark berries

Fresh vegetables

Green leafy vegetables

Watercress

Asparagus

Beets

Legumes

Soymilk

Whole grains

Oats

Pumpkin seeds

Low-fat dairy

Fish

Eggs

Poultry

Meats

Liver

Juices

Dark berry, cherry—contain iron

Beet

Carrot

Aromatherapy

Roman chamomile—as massage oil.

Herbal therapy

Alfalfa, dandelion, nettle—contain iron.

Homeopathy

Take remedy according to symptoms:

Calcarea phosphorica

Ferrum phosphoricum—helps assimilation of iron in food.

Natrum muriaticum

Picric acid

Ayurvedic medicine

Anemia is due to an imbalance of pitta.

Kalyaraka ghritha

Kishor

Avipathi choorna

Pancha karma

Chinese medicine

Chinese Angelica

Gui Pi Wan

Acupuncture—acupoints on back, arm, lower trunk, and legs are stimulated.

Bodywork

Shiatsu—energies are rebalanced along the spleen and stomach meridians.

Mindbody therapy

Yoga—helps to restore hormonal imbalance that leads to heavy menstruation; inverted asanas should not be practiced during menstruation, pregnancy, or in the presence of high blood pressure.

Arthritis

Arthritis means fire in the joints and is a condition characterized by joint inflammation, pain, swelling, and redness and causes a limitation in joint movement. The two most common forms are osteoarthritis and rheumatoid arthritis.

Osteoarthritis is a deterioration of the cartilage that cushions the ends of bones; consequently, bone begins to move against bone causing pain. A buildup of synovial fluid in the joint causes swelling and inflammation. Symptoms are intermittent pain at affected joints that becomes more frequent, an audible creaking sound, swelling, inflammation, and restricted movement. Osteoarthritis is age-related, a normal wearing and tearing process, but may also be genetic or caused by injury. Psychological stress and allergies can exacerbate the disease.

Rheumatoid arthritis is considered an autoimmune disease and can be caused by a viral infection. Dysfunctional antibodies attack the lining of the joints which secrete the lubricant necessary to keep bones moving smoothly against each other. Joints become swollen, stiff, and painful. Stress and food allergies are possible triggers of the disease. Symptoms include vague joint pain, morning stiffness, fatigue, low-grade fever, night sweats, and poor circulation. Inflammation of the tendons, eyes, lining of the heart, and fibrosis of the lungs can also occur.

Overweight is a risk factor in arthritis because of the pressure put on weight-bearing joints increasing the pain. Early diagnosis is essential in limiting the long-term effects of the disease. The kind of fat in the diet influences the symptoms. Omega-3-fatty acids help regulate hormone-like substances called eicosanoids that control inflammation and pain. The fats in meat have the opposite effect by stimulating the production of inflammatory agents. Food allergies may play a prominent role in precipitating arthritis. Common allergens are milk products, refined sugar, citrus fruits, and nightshade vegetables such as tomatoes, potatoes, eggplant, peppers, and chili. It is recommended that these foods or any food suspected of causing an allergic reaction be eliminated from the diet for a period of 2 months and then be reintroduced to observe the reaction. Moderate exercise is very beneficial for arthritic individuals in relieving stress, improving circulation, and increasing mobility. An electrical nerve stimulating unit (TENS) can effectively reduce chronic pain.

Nutrients

Glucosamine sulfate—500 mg three times a day, repairs joint cartilage, reduces symptoms of osteoarthritis.[18]

Chondroitin sulfate—400 mg two or three times a day, reduces pain, increases mobility and healing of joints,[19] a major component of the lining of the joints.

SAMe—400 mg three times a day, reduces pain, stiffness, and swelling.

Niacinamide—250 mg four times a day, improves joint mobility, muscle strength and reduces fatigue.

Vitamin B$_6$—100 mg twice a day, for osteoarthritis.

Pantothenic acid—1 mg, relieves symptoms of rheumatoid arthritis.

Vitamin E—400 to 600 IU with mixed tocopherols, reduces symptoms.

Selenium—if deficient, take with vitamin E, for rheumatoid arthritis.

Boron—3 to 6 mg, helps relieve symptoms of osteoarthritis, aids the retention of calcium in the bones.

Evening primrose or black currant oil—for rheumatoid arthritis, if taking anti-inflammatory drugs, contains gamma linolenic acid which is a precursor to anti-inflammatory prostaglandins.

Flaxseed oil—1 T, for rheumatoid arthritis.

Bromelain—250 to 750 mg three times daily between meals, helps reduce symptoms of rheumatoid arthritis.

DMSO—apply topically, alleviates pain.

Copper—1 mg, has anti-inflammatory activity.

Foods

Fatty fish

Salmon

Herring

Sardines

Albacore tuna

Extra virgin olive oil

Cold pressed organic canola oil

Fresh fruits

Pineapple

Cherries

Dark berries

Raisins

Grapes

Fresh vegetables

Asparagus

Broccoli

Brussel sprouts

Cabbage

Celery

Mustard greens

Yams

Onions

Nuts

Brazil nuts

Sunflower seeds

Whole grains

Legumes

Eggs

Garlic

Turmeric

Ginger

Cinnamon

Cayenne

Oregano

Juices

Beet

Cabbage

Carrot

Celery

Cherry

Cucumber

Parsley

Pineapple

Watermelon

Herbal therapy

White willow—containing 100 mg salicin daily, has anti-inflammatory and pain relieving properties; slower acting but lasts longer than aspirin.

Turmeric—400 mg curcumin three times daily for rheumatoid arthritis; has an anti-inflammatory effect due to the compound curcumin.

Garlic—has anti-inflammatory properties.

Ginger—⅙ oz fresh or ⅓ tsp powdered three times a day, an anti-inflammatory agent, relieves pain and increases mobility, superior to the NSAIDs with no side effects.[20]

Feverfew—1 to 2 capsules twice a day, prohibits the synthesis of inflammatory agents.

Devil's claw—1 to 2 g root powder or 4 to 5 ml tincture three times daily, an anti-inflammatory and analgesic.

Cayenne—cream, capsaicin compound relieves pain.

Yucca—2 to 4 g three times daily, saponin content reduces symptoms.

Burdock root—relieves pain in the joints.

Horsetail—silicon content strengthens connective tissue.

Homeopathy

Take remedy according to the symptoms:

Aconitum napellus

Apis mellifica

Arnica montana

Aurum metallicum

Belladonna

Benzoicum acidum

Bryonia

Calcarea carbonica

Calcarea fluorica

Calcarea phosphorica

Causticum

Cimicifuga

Colchicum

Dulcamara

Kali bichromicum

Kali carbonicum

Kalmia latifolia

Ledum palustre

Medorrhinum

Pulsatilla

Rhus toxicodendrum

Rhododendron

Ruta graveolens

Aromatherapy

Juniper berry, black pepper, Roman chamomile, lavender—mix together as massage oil with carrier oil, omit juniper berry if pregnant.

Rosemary, lavender, marigold—mix together as massage oil.

Rosemary, chamomile—place 10 drops in bath water.

Lavender, rose, eucalyptus, juniper berry—mix together as warm compress.

Moroccan thyme—borneal content beneficial for autoimmune disease.

Everlasting—high content of sesquiterpene hydrocarbons which are effective anti-inflammatory compounds, relieves joint pain.

Ayurvedic medicine

Vata types are prone to arthritis.

Guggul—reduces swelling and pain.

Boswellia—400 mg boswellic acids three times daily, prevents further damage of joints and increases mobility.

Sesame or mustard oil—whole body massage as well as specific joint areas; relieves pain.

Calmus oil—massage, improves circulation and drainage.

Chinese medicine

Herbal formulations prescribed for arthritis.

Chinese throroughwax—2 to 4 g dried root or 5 to 10 ml tincture or 2 to 4 ml extract three times daily, contains the anti-inflammatory compounds saikosaponins, increases release of cortisone and other adrenal hormones, prevents adrenal gland atrophy caused by corticosteroids.

Licorice and ginseng—2 to 4 g dried root or 10 to 20 ml tincture or 4 to 6 ml extract three times daily and 4 to 6 g or 500 mg extract, respectively, enchances effectiveness of thoroughwax, have anti-inflammatory properties.

Acupuncture—relieves pain; improves immune system functioning.

Chiropractic

Consult a qualified practitioner.

Bodywork

Massage—soothing to sore areas; see practitioner who is knowledgeable about arthritis.

Movement therapies

Acupressure

Shiatsu—adjusts flow of qi.

Qigong—reduces stress.

T'ai chi—deep breathing is beneficial; helps stiffness and keeps joints supple; reduces stress.

Polarity therapy

Reflexology—relieves pain and inflammation.

Mindbody therapy

Meditation—reduces stress.

Yoga—relaxes muscles and keeps joints supple, specific poses for various joints.

Imagery

Hypnotherapy

Asthma

Asthma is caused by spasms of the bronchial passages restricting the flow of air in and out of the lungs. The bronchi are chronically inflamed and hypersensitive. Asthmatic attacks can be triggered by allergens such as food, tobacco smoke, pet hair, or chemicals; or by stress, viral infection, physical exertion, or inhaling cold air. The body also releases histamines in reaction to an allergen which results in coughing and further constricting of the bronchial muscles.

Treatment involves managing acute attacks and long-term prevention and control. In acute attacks, the herbs ephedra and lobelia have been used. Caffeine can help prevent asthmatic attacks; up to three cups of coffee a day have a bronchodilating effect relaxing the bronchial muscles. Finding and eliminating allergens is important. Some allergic reactions may not occur for a day or more after exposure to an allergen. Milk, besides being a possible allergen, contains a protein that causes an increase in mucus secretion. In asthmatics, airways in the lungs become clogged with mucus and other secretions. Other possible allergens are food additives, eggs, colas, nuts, chocolate, and MSG. Meat and dairy products contain fats that are inflammatory. Regular exercise expands lung capacity and strengthens the heart. Ionized air can help counteract allergenic reactions. Drinking plenty of water keeps the respiratory tract secretions in a fluid condition.

Nutrients

Vitamin B_6—50 to 200 mg, decreases frequency of attacks.

Vitamin B_{12}—1 g, especially effective for sulfite sensitive asthmatics.

Vitamin C—10 to 30 mg per 2-lb body weight, taken in divided doses, an antihistamine.

Quercetin—400 to 1000 mg three times daily, an antihistamine.

Magnesium—200 to 400 mg, prevents spasms of the bronchial passages.

Selenium—45 to 200 mcg, if deficient.

Bromelain—an anti-inflammatory.

Foods

Fresh fruits, vegetables—especially those high in vitamin C

Pineapple

Apricots

Jerusalem artichokes

Yams

Nuts

Seeds

Whole grains

Legumes

Fatty fish

Sardines

Salmon

Albacore tuna

Mackerel

Chili peppers, garlic, onions, horseradish, and mustard—open air passages by thinning mucus

Ginger

Turmeric

Juices

Carrot

Celery

Grapefruit

Lemon

Orange

Radish

Spinach

Tomato

Pineapple

Herbal therapy

Ephedra—12 to 25 mg capsules every 4 hours or 1 to 2 cups tea or tincture every 2 to 4 hours for an asthma attack;[21] *do not overdo amounts as ephedra has side effects including insomnia, anxiety, restlessness and possible high blood pressure.*

Lobelia—mix three parts tincture to one part tincture of capsicum and take 20 drops in water at start of attack and repeat every 30 minutes three or four times.[22]

Stinging nettle—an antihistamine.

Anise, fennel—have compounds that loosen bronchial secretions.

Marshmallow, mullein, licorice—have soothing actions on the respiratory tract.

Ginkgo biloba—120 to 140 mg extract or 3 to 4 ml tincture three times daily, contains compounds that block the action of a platelet activating factor that can cause asthmatic symptoms.

Homeopathy

Take remedy according to symptoms:

Arsenicum album

Carbo vegetabilis

Chamomilla

Ipecacuanha

Lachesis

Lobelia

Natrum sulphuricum

Nux vomica

Pulsatilla

Spongia tosta

Aromatherapy

Eucalyptus, juniper, wintergreen—dilute mixture with carrier oil and apply to chest nightly.

Moroccan chamomile—an anti-inflammatory and antiasthmatic; relieves allergic symptoms.

Chamomile, lavender or eucalyptus—can be used as steam inhalation during and after attack, opens airways and relieves panic.

Khella—relieves spasms of the bronchial muscles; can be combined with creeping hyssop to prevent attacks; do not apply to skin.

Frankincense—an antiasthmatic; strengthens immune system.

Ayurvedic medicine

Tylophora asthmatica—200 mg dried or 40 mg extract twice daily, has antihistamine and antispasmodic activity.

Sida cordifolia

Triphala

Ashwagandha

Licorice—1 to 2 g powdered root or 2 to 4 ml extract three times daily, has anti-inflammatory and antiallergenic properties, an expectorant, glycyrrhetinic acid component has cortisol-like activity, can be taken with ephedra or tylophora.

Ginger

Chinese medicine

Ephedra

Almond

Acupuncture—relieves symptoms; controls bronchial spasms.

Chiropractic

Upper thoracic vertebrae may be out of alignment putting pressure on the lungs.

Bodywork

Massage

Deep tissue manipulation

Rolfing—breaks up restriction patterns of the nerves and muscles.

Movement therapies

Alexander technique—improves posture and allows chest to expand fully thereby relieving strain; breathing is easier and airways are cleared.

Acupressure

Shiatsu

T'ai chi

Qigong

Mindbody therapy

Meditation—lowers body tension.

Yoga—improves respiratory endurance; encourages relaxed breathing.

Biofeedback—lessens number of attacks and use of medicines.

Imagery

Hypnotherapy

Atherosclerosis

At birth, human arteries are smooth and elastic and the blood flows freely. In as little as a year, streaks of fat can begin to appear under the layer of cells that line the arteries. Turning into plaque, fatty deposits build up and bulge into the arterial cavity and restrict the circulation of blood. The plaque attracts cholesterol and calcium, which have a solidifying effect. Arteries become thick and lose their elasticity preventing the blood from passing through easily and allowing clots to develop.

Symptoms of atherosclerosis are not apparent until the arteries are nearly 90% blocked in diameter. If the coronary artery is narrow, chest pains result from exertion, an effect called *angina;* if coronary arteries become blocked, there is a sudden, severe, and persistent chest pain that can lead to heart attack. If the cerebral arteries are narrow, there is a temporary disturbance in balance, speech, vision, and the use of arms and legs, or the symptom may be a transient ischemic attack (TIA). In a blocked cerebral artery, loss in the use of limbs, speech impairment or stroke, and sometimes unconsciousness develop.

Reduction in blood flow can also cause abnormal heart rhythms that may result in sudden death. Atherosclerosis of the legs can cause *intermittent claudication* or leg pain in the calf while walking or a sudden pain of the femoral artery. An inherited defect that creates high levels of the amino acid homocysteine may cause atherosclerosis by increasing the rate of low-density lipoprotein (LDL) cholesterol damage. Treatment involves the administration of vitamins B_6, B_{12}, and folic acid. If levels are not reduced, adding 6 g of betaine (not HCl) may be efficacious.

Factors that increase the risk of atherosclerosis include high blood LDL cholesterol, which becomes dangerous when oxidized by free radicals, high blood pressure, smoking, diabetes, and a family history of the disease. Overeating, which results in food being deposited as fat, stress, physical inactivity, and type A personalities, people who tend to be impatient and aggressive, are contributing factors. Stress results in the formation of free radicals and stimulates the release of adrenalin that can increase platelet aggregation and blood viscosity.

Autopsy studies have shown that individuals who had the clearest arteries had the highest levels of omega-3 fatty acids in their tissues; and the most clogged arteries had the least amount of omega-3 in body tissues. The higher the proportion of omega-3 to omega-6 in the diet, the lower the risk of the disease. Omega-3s are found most abundantly in fatty fish; and omega-6s are found in margarine, vegetable oils including safflower, sunflower, and corn, and processed foods made with vegetable oils. Saturated fats, most abundant in meats and full fat dairy products, and trans-fatty acids, from margarine and processed foods using vegetable oils, promote atherosclerosis. Foods containing cholesterol do not increase serum cholesterol as much as saturated fats, nor do they increase serum cholesterol if the diet is low in fat.

Atherosclerosis can be reversed by eating a low-fat, basically vegetarian diet, exercise, and yoga, meditation, or other forms of stress reduction.

Nutrients

Vitamin C—100 to 200 mg, an antioxidant, protects LDL cholesterol from oxidation, reduces high homocysteine levels.

Bioflavonoids—work synergistically with vitamin C.

Vitamin E—100 to 200 IU with mixed tocopherols, protects LDL cholesterol from oxidative damage, prevents abnormal blood clot formation; increases walking distance and blood flow in cases of intermittent claudication.

Selenium—100 to 200 mcg, an antioxidant, reduces platelet aggregation.

Quercetin—35 mg, protects LDL cholesterol from oxidation.

Inositol hexaniacinate—1500 mg to 3 g, lowers serum cholesterol and triglycerides;[23] 2 g twice daily, improves walking distance in intermittent claudication.

L-carnitine—1 to 3 g, reduces serum cholesterol and triglycerides; 4 g, increases walking distance in cases of intermittent claudication.[24]

Evening primrose oil—3 to 4 g, lowers cholesterol levels; increases exercise tolerance in intermittent claudication.

Chromium—200 mcg or 2 T brewers yeast, reduces LDL cholesterol and increases HDL cholesterol.

If homocysteine levels are high:

Vitamin B_6—50 mg

Vitamin B_{12}—100 to 300 mcg

Folic acid—500 to 800 mcg

Foods

Fatty fish

Salmon

Sardines

Mackerel

Herring

Albacore tuna

Anchovies

Atlantic sturgeon

Fresh fruits

Prunes

Fresh vegetables

Reishi mushrooms

Shiitake mushrooms

Cucumber

Artichokes

Onion

Whole grains

Oats

Legumes

Soybeans

Soymilk

Lentils

Almonds

Low-fat yogurt

Extra virgin olive oil

Cold pressed organic canola oil

Garlic

Fenugreek

Ground flaxseeds—1 to 2 T

Juices

Beet

Carrot

Celery

Cucumber

Dark berries

Herbal therapy

Gingko biloba—interferes with the chemical PAF that the body can make in excess and that causes platelets to stick together,[25] increases blood circulation to the brain and legs; 120 mg extract, increases walking distance in cases of intermittent claudication and reduces pain; protects LDL cholesterol from oxidation.

Garlic—protects LDL cholesterol and reduces triglycerides; prevents excessive platelet adhesion due to its components, allicin and ajoene;[26] 400 mg extract twice daily, improves walking distance in cases of intermittent claudication.

Turmeric—the component curcumin has high antiplatelet activity.

Bilberry—prevents platelet aggregation.

Hawthorne—increases blood circulation to the heart.

Motherwort—tincture helps palpitations.

Wild yam—2 to 3 ml tincture or 1 to 2 capsules three times daily; raises HDL cholesterol and reduces triglycerides.[27]

Fenugreek, green tea—reduce triglycerides.

Homeopathy

Take remedy according to symptoms:

Baryta carbonica

Glonoinum

Vanadium

Aromatherapy

Juniper and lemon—massage can help break up fatty deposits.

Peppermint, rose, lavender, marjoram, rosemary—massage may help strengthen heart muscle; if pregnant avoid marjoram.

Lavender, melissa, neroli, ylang-ylang—for palpitations.

Ayurvedic medicine

Guggul—lowers cholesterol and triglyceride levels, prevents oxidation of LDL cholesterol.[28]

Pancha karma and specific prescribed herbs—reduces free radicals and oxidized fats.

Chinese medicine

Herbs prescribed and acupuncture—dissolve plaque, lower cholesterol, increase circulation.

Fo-ti—3 to 5 g, lowers blood cholesterol.

Bodywork

Massage—reduces stress and stimulates circulation.

Movement therapies

Acupressure

Shiatsu

Qigong—improves memory, insomnia, dizziness, numbness, and tinnitus.

T'ai chi—encourages flow of qi, does not strain the heart.

Reflexology

Mindbody therapy

Meditation—focuses mind in calmness and reduces stress.

Yoga—relaxes, reduces stress, and improves circulation.

Biofeedback—training in anticipating stress and modes of relaxation.

Imagery

Hypnotherapy

Athlete's Foot

Athlete's foot is a fungal infection related to *ringworm* and *jock itch,* and grows in warm dark moist places. Keep affected areas clean and dry and exposed to air and sunlight as much as possible. Tea tree oil is as effective as pharmaceutical antifungal products. Herbal drying powders such as arrowroot can be placed in shoes or socks.

Herbal therapy

Tea tree oil—apply directly to skin or dilute with water or vegetable oil three or four times a day, keep applying for 2 weeks after fungus has cleared; also effective for fungal infection under the nails.

Grapefruit seed extract—apply as above.

Garlic—contains ajoene, a potent antifungal component, eat one or two cloves a day with meals; steep several cloves fresh crushed garlic in olive oil for 3 days, strain, and apply to affected area with a cotton ball once or twice a day.

Chamomile oil—apply topically, has antifungal properties.

Myrrh—tincture, apply topically.

Ginger, licorice—contain numerous antifungal compounds.

Back Pain

Acute back pain can result from lifting a heavy object, from a misstep, falling, or a sudden motion. Chronic back pain can develop from a viral infection, stress, muscle tension, emotional problems, poor posture and movement, weak muscle strength, as a result of pregnancy, or a congenital defect. Smokers often have back pain that may possibly be due to a deficiency of vitamin C that is destroyed by tobacco. The brain can sometimes mistake signals from another part of the body such as the kidney, prostate gland, or uterus as originating from the back;[29] back pain may also be an indication of cancer somewhere in the body. If back pain is accompanied by numbness or tingling in the legs, pain shooting down a leg to the knee or foot, inability to move legs and feet, urinary incontinence or stomach cramps, chest pain or fever, see a physician immediately. Otherwise, most back pain will subside in a matter of days, weeks, or possibly several months with proper rest and care.

In most cases, acute back pain results from a muscle spasm and not from a pinched nerve, slipped disk, torn muscle or ligament, or spinal subluxation. Because there is a complex relationship between the mind, brain, nerves, and muscles, chronic back pain is often psychosomatic in origin.

For acute pain, immediately apply an ice pack for 15 to 20 minutes and repeat every hour or two. Alternating cold and heat may be helpful. Remain immobilized for at least a day or two. Avoid any positions that add pain or stress to the injury. A nonsteroidal anti-inflammatory such as aspirin may be necessary. Because of the emotion-brain-nerve interplay, participate in activities that encourage a pleasant state of mind. After pain diminishes, apply heat compresses, or bathe in warm water.

Chronic pain may require changes in mental and emotional attitude and lifestyle. An osteopathic method called counterstrain may be helpful in correcting nerve patterns.[30] Drinking lots of water for back pain is beneficial because dehydration, which occurs even though not thirsty, allows acidic wastes to build up in muscles, causing pain. Avoid animal fat in the diet as it contains substances that are inflammatory.

Prevention is the best way to guard against back pain by lifting properly—always bend knees, improve posture, lose excess weight, and strengthen the abdominal muscles and the extensor muscles of the back. Stretching promotes flexibility and nonjarring exercises are beneficial.

Nutrients

Vitamin C—1 to 3 g, strengthens connective tissues.

Bioflavonoids—work synergistically with vitamin C.

Calcium, magnesium—500 mg, relaxes muscles.

Foods

Fatty fish, salmon, mackerel, herring, sardines, albacore tuna—contain omega-3 fats which are anti-inflammatory

Fresh fruits

Vegetables

Dark green leafy vegetables

Whole grains

Nuts

Walnuts

Seeds

Pumpkin seeds

Black sesame seeds

Legumes

Low-fat dairy

Extra virgin olive oil

Cold pressed organic canola oi

Ground flaxseeds—1 to 2 T

Ginger

Cayenne

Black pepper

Herbal therapy

Willow bark—contains salicylate, the pain-relieving compound from which aspirin is derived.

German chamomile—has anti-inflammatory properties.

Wintergreen oil—apply topically, contains salicylate, relieves pain.

Capsaicin—cream or balm apply topically, compound from hot peppers that relieves pain; crush hot pepper and apply directly to affected area or can be mixed in cream.

Peppermint—contains menthol, eases muscle tightness.

Homeopathy

Arnica montana—for acute muscle spasm; 30× potency—take four tablets every hour on the first day while awake, four tablets every two hours the second day, and four tablets four times a day for four to five days.

Take remedy according to symptoms:

Aconite napellus

Aesculus hippocastanum

Arsenicum album

Bryonia

Calcarea carbonica

Calcarea phosphorica

Cimicifuga

Dulcamara

Ignatia amara

Kali carbonicum

Natrum muriaticum

Nux vomica

Rhus toxicodendron

Ruta graveolens

Sulfur

Aromatherapy

Sage, rosemary—add several drops to carrier oil and massage, contain compounds that relax muscles.

Birch, lavender, clary sage—massage, help relieve pain; add lavender to warm bath.

Ayurvedic medicine

Kaishore guggula—200 mg twice daily after meals.

Dashamoola basti

Mahanarayan oil—use as massage on affected area.

Mustard oil—use as massage, reduces pain and aching.

Chinese medicine

Teasel root, ginseng, acanthopanax—can relieve pain.

Jing Jie, pseudoginseng root—helps relieve swelling and pain.

Acupuncture—stimulates certain acupoints to relieve pain.

Chiropractic

Corrects misalignment of the vertebrae that can press on a nerve causing pain; restores normal movement to joints of the back.

Bodywork

Massage—relieves pain of muscle spasms.

Deep tissue massage—reduces spinal curvature and eases back pain; massage may not be possible until severe pain diminishes.

Movement therapies—correct postural defects; teach how to use body correctly; prevent or alleviate pain; develop body awareness, flexibility, and coordination.

Acupressure—stimulates points to ease pain.

Shiatsu

Qigong—relaxes muscles and reduces stress.

Reflexology

Mindbody therapy

Meditation—reduces stress.

Yoga—strengthens back, promotes flexibility, and reduces stress; deep breathing acts beneficially on the nervous system.

Biofeedback—training to recognize and anticipate habitual muscle contraction and learn relaxation techniques.

Imagery

Hypnotherapy

Bronchitis

Bronchitis is an inflammation of the mucous membrane that lines the breathing, or bronchial, tubes. Acute bronchitis follows a cold or flu when the viral infection moves to the chest. Chronic bronchitis is a result of smoking or exposure to polluted air or allergens. Bacteria is present if phlegm is yellow-green in color. Eating spicy foods liquifies the mucus and helps to open air passages. Identify allergens if they are the cause. Avoid dairy products as they contain components that suppress fluid secretions that thin mucus in the respiratory tract.

Nutrients

N-acetyl-cysteine—200 mg twice daily, breaks up mucus and protects lung tissue, an antioxidant.

Vitamin A—25,000 IU, protects lung tissue.

Beta carotene—an antioxidant.

Vitamin C—300 to 500 mg, has mucus thinning properties, neutralizes free radicals.

Bioflavonoids—work synergistically with vitamin C.

Vitamin E—with mixed tocopherols, protects lung tissue and increases oxygen supply.

Carnitine—2 g twice daily, eases breathing during exercise.

Magnesium—if deficient, deficiency may not be reflected in blood tests; needed for normal lung function.

Bromelain—decreases bronchial secretions.

Foods

Fresh fruits

Citrus fruits

Pineapple

Raspberries

Apricots

Fresh vegetables

Onions

Shiitake mushrooms

Legumes

Soybeans

Whole grains

Amaranth

Flaxseeds

Nuts

Seeds

Fatty fish

Salmon

Herring

Mackerel

Sardines

Albacore tuna

Garlic

Horseradish

Hot mustard

Chili peppers

Ginger

Juices

Beet

Carrot

Celery

Cucumber

Hot lemon and honey

Radish

Spinach

Wheatgrass

Herbal therapy

Eucalyptus—steam inhalation or tea, an expectorant (loosens phlegm).

Garlic—has antiviral and antibacterial properties.

Mullein—tincture in steam or tea, an expectorant; soothes throat, helps prevent coughing and has antibacterial activity; also for bacteria infected bronchitis.

Stinging nettle—infusion with raw honey, relieves symptoms.

Couchgrass—relieves symptoms of respiratory inflammation.

Ginger—use as tea.

Elecampane—an expectorant and antiseptic.

Horehound, wild cherry, yerba santa, lobelia—expectorants.

Marshmallow—a demulcent and anti-inflammatory, soothes respiratory tract.

Homeopathy

Take remedy according to symptoms:

Aconitum napellus

Antimonium tartaricum

Arsenicum album

Bryonia

Calcarea carbonica

Calcarea phosphorica

Causticum

Ferrum phosphoricum

Hepar sulphuris calcareum

Kali bichromicum

Phosphorus

Pulsatilla

Silicea

Sulfur

Aromatherapy

Cypress—an antibiotic, use at first sign of sore throat; can prevent development of bronchitis; take one drop on tongue, repeat when soreness returns.

Eucalyptus dives—thins mucus; mix with eucalyptus radiata to enhance affects.

Thyme—contains antiviral properties.

Marjoram—for acute bronchitis with accompanying cough.

Oregano—1 to 2 drops, has high concentrations of carvacol, an antibacterial; for acute bacterial infection of the bronchi.

Pine—use in diffusor, has strong antiseptic effect.

Rosemary (verbenone type)—has mucolytic effect.

Marjoram—has spasmolytic esters and the antiseptic terpinen-4-ol.

Ayurvedic medicine

Kapha type most susceptible to bronchitis.

Herbal mixture of the following, take one quarter tsp with raw honey twice a day after meals:

Sitopaladi—500 mg

Punarnava—300 mg

Trikatu—100 mg

Mahasudarshan—300 mg

Ginger—grate root and add honey and lemon or lime juice.

Chinese medicine

Effective treatments prescribed.

Honeysuckle, forsythia, and scullcap—reduce symptoms of cough, fever, and wheezing.

Ephedra

Fritillary bulb, plantain seed, balloon flower root—for acute conditions.

Gardenia fruit, honeysuckle flowers, mulberry leaves—for chronic conditions.

Acupuncture—dilates throat muscle walls.

Bodywork

Massage—helps dislodge phlegm; improves breathing.

Acupressure

Reflexology

Mindbody therapy

Yoga—for relaxation and deep breathing.

Bruises

Sufficient trauma to the skin causes a bruise in anyone as blood leaks out of the capillary walls underneath the skin. As soon as possible after injury, apply a cold compress and reapply for most of the next 12 hours. Cold constricts the blood vessels allowing less blood flow to the area. Bruising easily can mean a deficiency of vitamin C and the bioflavonoids which are necessary for strong capillary walls. Sudden bruising may indicate a defective clotting system and should be checked by a physician.

For *sprains,* apply ice immediately. The homeopathic remedy, arnica, is helpful. Topically apply DMSO and/or tincture of arnica, bandage, and alternate heat and cold for the next 24 hours. Comfrey helps mend *broken bones.* Consult a physician to make sure the bone is properly set. Homeopathic remedies listed below can help pain, swelling, and the healing process. If there is a *cut* in the skin, disinfect with hydrogen peroxide. Goldenseal powder can be mixed to a paste with water and placed on cut. Cover with bandage. Vitamin E applied topically after wound has closed will help prevent scarring.

Nutrients

Vitamin C—1 to 3 g, helps capillary walls to heal more rapidly.

Bioflavonoids—200 mg, works synergistically with vitamin C.

Rutin—a bioflavonoid, helps strengthen capillary walls.

Bromelain—200 to 400 mg three times a day on empty stomach, stimulates production of prostaglandin E_1, an anti-inflammatory agent.

Foods

Fresh fruits

Pineapple

Blueberries

Fresh vegetables

Green leafy vegetables

Green peppers

Whole grains

Buckwheat

Legumes

Juices

Beet

Carrot

Citrus fruits

Dark berries

Green leafy vegetables

Herbal therapy

Horsechestnut—gel, apply topically twice daily; contains active ingredient, aescin.

Comfrey—apply topically as salve or compress; contains allantoin for its healing property; do not take internally.

Sweet clover—ointment or compress, apply topically.

Witch hazel—apply topically several times daily, disperses blood and facilitates healing.

Homeopathy

Arnica—salve, apply topically, tincture, or compress; massage tincture directly on injury; if there is irritation, dilute with rubbing alcohol; do not use on broken skin.

Take remedy according to symptoms:

Arnica montana

Bellis perennis

Calcarea phosphorica

Hamamelis

Hypericum perforatum

Ledum palustre

Millefolium

Phosphorus

Ruta graveolens

Symphytum officinale

Sulphuricum acidum

For broken bones:

Arnica montana

Bryonia

Calcarea phosphorica

Eupatorium perfoliatum

Hypericum perforatum

Ruta graveolens

Symphytum officinale

Aromatherapy

Everlasting—apply topically immediately to injury to prevent swelling and bruising; mix with comfrey ointment to increase effectiveness; apply directly or dilute in vegetable oil; also reduces pain.

Lavender—apply topically, place several drops on compress.

Chinese medicine

Effective treatments are prescribed.

Acupuncture—bruising responds well; relief for acute and chronic pain.

Mindbody therapy

Imagery

Burns

Immerse burned area immediately in cold water for 5 to 10 minutes then intermittently for another 10 or 15 minutes. This helps prevent blisters. Wash with soap and dry. Apply herbal salve or raw honey. Honey is a soothing antiseptic and has healing properties. First degree burns are superficial like a sunburn; second degree burns develop blisters; third degree burns penetrate deeper and can destroy nerve tissue. If burns are third degree, cover a large area, have a charred appearance or become infected, see a physician. To remove melted substances such as tar or plastic, use ice water.

Nutrients

Vitamin C—stimulates collagen synthesis and tissue repair.

Bioflavonoids—work synergistically with vitamin C.

Vitamin E—ointment, apply topically, an antioxidant (damage to skin is oxidative), helps prevent scarring.

Foods

Fresh fruits

Raisins

Fresh vegetables

Seafood

Oysters

Crab

Low-fat dairy

Eggs

Whole grains

Legumes

Almonds

Pumpkin seeds

Turkey

Lean meat

Garlic

Juices

Berry

Cantaloupe

Carrot

Herbal therapy

Aloe vera—gel, apply topically, soothes minor burns.

Calendula—cream or tincture, apply topically three times daily, an anti-inflammatory, aids tissue repair and soothes pain.

Garlic—poultice, apply topically, mash several cloves.

St. John's wort—tincture, apply topically, an anti-inflammatory, accelerates healing and reduces scarring.

Slippery elm powder—poultice, apply topically, mix with water.

Gotu Kola—tea, 3 cups daily or 10 to 20 ml tincture three times daily or 60 mg extract, saponin content inhibits buildup of scar tissue.

Homeopathy

Calendula or Hypericum—tincture, apply topically several times daily, 10 drops in 1 oz water, soothes burns and promotes healing of tissues.

Take remedy according to symptoms:

Arnica montana

Belladonna

Cantharis

Causticum

Hepar sulphuris calcareum

Hypericum perforatum

Phosphorus

Urtic urens

Natrum muriaticum—helps prevent sunburn.

Aromatherapy

Lavender—apply topically and cool with ice, very effective in preventing blisters and loss of skin; reduces pain.

German chamomile—apply topically and cool with ice, an anti-inflammatory, very effective.

Moroccan chamomile—an anti-inflammatory; for burns and sunburn.

Ayurvedic medicine

Aloe vera gel, coconut oil, tikta ghee—mix into paste and apply topically.

Chinese medicine

Ginger juice—apply topically.

Zicao and black sesame oil—apply topically.

Mindbody therapy

Imagery

Bursitis

Bursitis is the inflammation of the bursae, which are fluid-filled sacs that act as cushions in reducing the friction where muscle and tendon meet bone. Excess fluid collects in the sacs resulting in pain, swelling, heat, and restricted movement. Bursitis is most often caused by overuse; other causes include infection, injury, arthritis, or gout. Areas most affected are the shoulder, elbow, knees, hips, and heels. *Tendonitis* is a similar condition affecting the tendons, which are the fibrous tissues that connect muscle and bone, also caused by overuse and responds to the same treatments as bursitis.

Immobilize and rest the affected area, although once the swelling has diminished, exercise is advisable to prevent a permanent situation from developing. Applying a cold compress (such as a bag of frozen peas or ice pack after rubbing skin with oil to prevent frostbite) is helpful and then alternate or use just hot compresses when pain and swelling subside. TENS, an electrical nerve-stimulation unit, is beneficial in alleviating the pain.

Nutrients

Vitamin B_{12}—by intramuscular injection, relieves symptoms, prevents calcification in chronic bursitis.

Niacin—by intramuscular injection, with vitamin B_{12}, nicotinic acid form.

Bromelain—250 mg three times a day between meals, from pineapple, has anti-inflammatory properties, reduces bruising, pain, and swelling, and promotes healing.

Curcumin—250 to 500 mg, from turmeric, an anti-inflammatory, as effective as cortisone treatments.

DMSO—apply topically, 70% solution two or three times a day for 10 days, promotes healing of affected tissues.

Bioflavonoids—500 to 100 mg two or three times daily, stabilizes collagen structures, have anti-inflammatory properties, an antioxidant preventing free radical damage.

Foods

Fresh fruits

Pineapple

Papaya

Fresh vegetables

Dark green leafy vegetables

Extra virgin olive oil

Soybeans

Pumpkin seeds

Walnuts

Fatty fish

Salmon

Mackerel

Albacore tuna

Herring

Sardines

Ginger

Red pepper

Turmeric

Juices

Beet

Carrot

Celery

Cucumber

Leafy greens

Pineapple

Spinach

Herbal therapy

Ginger—tea or tincture, has anti-inflammatory properties, grate ½ tsp fresh, steep in one cup boiling water 15 minutes.

Willow bark, meadow sweet, wintergreen—tea or tincture, have anti-inflammatory properties, contain salicylate, the precursor of aspirin.

Turmeric—tea or tincture, has anti-inflammatory properties.

Capsaicin—ointment, apply topically, compound from hot pepper, soothes and reduces pain.

Homeopathy

Take remedy according to symptoms:

Apis

Arnica montana

Belladonna

Bryonia

Ferrum phosphoricum

Kalmia latifolia

Pulsatilla

Rhus toxicodendron

Ruta graveolens

Sanguinaria canadensis

Silicea

Sticta

Sulfur

Aromatherapy

Lavender—dilute with carrier oil, massage every day, soothes inflamed tissue and relieves pain.

German chamomile—has anti-inflammatory properties.

Ayurvedic medicine

Boswellia—has anti-inflammatory properties.

Barberry—as tea or compress, alleviates pain and inflammation.

Calamus oil—improves circulation and facilitates drainage.

Ginger

Coriander

Aloe vera

Chinese medicine

Pupleuri root, licorice, Chinese skullcap—have anti-inflammatory properties.

Acupuncture—relieves pain, increases mobility, promotes healing.

Bodywork

Deep tissue massage

Movement therapy

Acupressure

Reflexology

Cancer

Cancer develops when changes to DNA, nucleic acids that are the basis of heredity and contain the genetic blueprint, result in the production of malignant cells that replicate but are not controlled or killed by natural defense mechanisms in the body. Cells are most vulnerable to intrusion and damage from cancer-causing agents when cells normally divide and their DNA uncoils so that the gene information can be copied.

Often cancers are hereditary, meaning there is a predisposition to the disease but that it needs to be triggered by an environmental factor. Cancers can develop from free radicals that harm DNA or the immune system. Free radicals are created as the result of an oxidative process triggered by sources such as chemical toxins and certain fats in the diet; from viruses, exposure to industrial pollutants and chemicals including pesticides, herbicides, toxins in household products, food dyes and cigarette smoke; and as a result of radiation exposure from, for example, X-rays, nuclear waste, electronic instruments and dental enamel caps. No exposure is too small to initiate cellular damage. The cumulative effect from various sources of cancer-causing substances stresses the immune system. It may take 5 to 30 years from the time of exposure to a carcinogen before a cancer actually appears.

Ultraviolet rays can cause *skin cancer;* especially hazardous are midday sun and high altitudes because the rays have a shorter path to travel and less time to be filtered. The thinness of the ozone layer allows for stronger sun exposure. The kind of light used in tanning beds is also not safe. Topical applications for skin cancer that are beneficial are tea tree oil, a hot comfrey compress, or dry mustard poultice.

For women, *breast* and *reproductive cancers* can be caused by high levels of estrogen in the blood. Estrogen stimulates cell reproduction. Contributing to estrogen in the body are birth control pills and hormone replacement at menopause. Meat, poultry, and dairy foods may contain traces from animals that have been given the hormone for growth; and pesticides and industrial pollutants contain what are called xenoestrogens or foreign estrogens.

Cervical dysplasia is usually a precancerous lesion that if not treated can become cancerous. It is a condition of abnormal cells on the cervix surface. Pap smears, a sampling of cells, are taken to detect cancer of the cervix. Women susceptible to cervical cancer often have low nutrient levels such as vitamin C, the carotenoids, vitamin B_6, and selenium. A folic acid deficiency can cause an abnormal papsmear; 10 mg daily for three months then 2.5 mg daily until Pap smears are normal is recommended.

Diet is a big factor in cancer. Foods can either promote or prevent the disease. Meats, high-fat foods, polyunsaturated fatty acids, trans-fatty acids, and excess alcohol are major cancer causers. Frying, grilling, broiling, and barbecuing foods produce cancer-causing chemicals. Studies have shown the more fruits and vegetables in the diet, the less the risk of cancer. Foods rich in antioxidants prevent free radicals from forming and can repair cellular damage. Practicing safe sex prevents the viral transmission that damages DNA or weakens the immune system. Exercise stimulates immune system function and for women, lowers the level of estrogen in the blood.

Nutrients

Vitamin A—for lung and cervical cancer.

Carotenoid complex—enchances effectiveness of vitamin A.

Vitamin C—an antioxidant, protects immune system.

Bioflavonoids—work synergistically with vitamin C.

Vitamin E—400 IU with mixed tocopherols, an antioxidant, take with meals as fat is needed for absorption.

Selenium—100 to 300 mcg, an antioxidant, interferes with the absorption of vitamin C so take separately.

Coenzyme Q_{10}—300 mg, for breast cancer.

Foods

Organic whole foods, fresh fruits—especially citrus

Apples, mandarins, fresh vegetables, shiitake mushrooms, carrots, tomatoes, green, and yellow vegetables, broccoli, cauliflower, cabbage, cruciferous vegetables, asparagus, dandelion greens, enoki mushrooms, spinach, kale, whole grains, legumes, peanuts, soybeans—contain numerous anticancer agents

Fatty fish

Salmon

Albacore tuna

Herring

Mackerel

Sardines

Nuts

Brazil nuts

Walnuts

Almonds

Low-fat dairy

Low-fat yogurt

Eggs

Extra virgin olive oil

Cold pressed organic canola oil

Cold pressed flaxseed oil

Fennel

Garlic

Onions

Ginger

Juices

Apple

Beet

Carrot

Cabbage

Celery

Cherry

Grape

Berries

Spinach

Wheatgrass

Fruits

Vegetables

Herbal therapy

The following have anticancer or immune supporting properties:

Garlic

Green, black, and oolong tea

Licorice

Rosemary

Turmeric

Ginger

Thyme

Sage

Echinacea

Ginseng

Homeopathy

Take remedy according to symptoms:

Arsenicum album

Cadmium sulfuratum

Carbo animalis

Carcinosin

Conium maculatum

Cundurango

Hydrastis canadensis

Phytolacca

Thuja

For chemotherapy support:

Cadmium sulphuratum

Gelsemium

Ipecacuanha

Kali phosphoricum

Nux vomica

Sepia

Aromatherapy

Do not massage prior to or right after chemotherapy as it may cause the spread of cancer cells. Use a vaporizer or drops in the bath at the early stages of cancer.

Geranium, rose—helps depression.

Rosemary, sandalwood, bergamot—for fatigue.

Fennel—for nausea.

Ayurvedic medicine

Treatments prescribed for various forms of cancer.

Chinese medicine

Herbal treatments prescribed for symptoms of cancer.

Fu Zheng therapy—includes ginseng and astragalus.

Huang Qi—stimulates immune system, acts as a tonic on the nervous system.

Acupuncture—adjunct therapy to cancer, reduces side effects of chemotherapy and radiation treatments.

Bodywork

Massage—releases anxiety, promotes well-being and helps relieve pain.

Qigong

Mindbody therapy

Meditation—reduces stress supporting immune system; deep breathing increases blood circulation and oxygen supply.

Biofeedback

Imagery

Hypnotherapy

Canker Sores

Canker sores are small often painful ulcers inside the lip and mouth. The cause is unknown but may be exacerbated by allergies and food sensitivities. Stress may also be a factor. A component in some toothpastes, sodium lauryl sulfate, may be a cause of recurrent canker sores. Adding acidophilus to the diet has been beneficial for some individuals who experience recurrent episodes. Rinsing the mouth with salt water is helpful and placing ice on sore relieves pain. Bee propolis has healing and antiseptic properties; put tincture directly on sore.

Nutrients

Vitamin B complex—50 to 100 mg, if deficient.

Iron—if deficient.

Foods

Fresh fruits

Fresh vegetables

Whole grains

Nuts

Seeds

Legumes

Low-fat yogurt

Juices

Cantaloupe

Carrot

Celery

Herbal therapy

Myrrh—tincture, extract, or powder as mouthwash; tannin component is an antiseptic with antibacterial and antiviral properties; place powder directly on sore.

Goldenseal—as mouthwash, an antiseptic, heals wounds and infections; steep 2 tsp in one cup boiling water, cool and rinse mouth several times a day; 2 tsp powdered with ¼ tsp salt in one cup warm water as mouthwash.

Licorice—200 mg powdered DGL (glycyrrhizic acid) as mouthwash; contains the wound healing component, glycyrrhizic acid.

Aloe vera—1 to 3 T as mouthwash.

Echinacea—4 ml, swish in mouth 2 to 3 minutes then swallow three times daily, has antiviral and wound healing properties, supports immune system.

Chamomile—tincture, swish in mouth, soothes mucous membranes.

Homeopathy

Take remedy according to symptoms:

Arsenicum album

Borax

Calcarea carbonica

Hepar sulphuris calcareum

Mercurius solubilis

Natrum muriaticum

Nux vomica

Sulfur

Chinese medicine

Watermelon frost powder

Mindbody therapy

Imagery

Carpal Tunnel Syndrome

Carpal tunnel syndrome is the compression of a nerve as a result of repetitive motions of the fingers and wrist. Numbness, tingling, and pain may be felt along the entire arm and neck. Osteopathic therapy may be beneficial. The condition can be helped by reducing stress and massaging the affected areas.

Nutrients

Vitamin B_6—80 to 100 mg two or three times daily, relieves symptoms,[31] and may eliminate the need for surgery; in some individuals 300 mg taken for long periods of time may cause numbness and difficulty walking; discontinue use.

Vitamin B complex—enhances effectiveness of B_6.

Bromelain—250 to 1500 mg between meals, an anti-inflammatory, from pineapple.

Foods

Whole grains

Legumes

Soybeans

Fresh fruits

Bananas

Pineapple

Fresh vegetables

Green leafy vegetables

Cauliflower

Okra

Seeds

Nuts

Fatty fish

Salmon

Sardines

Mackerel

Albacore tuna

Cumin

Cayenne

Turmeric

Ginger

Herbal therapy

Willow bark—relieves pain and inflammation, contains salicylate, precursor of aspirin.

Meadowsweet, wintergreen—pain relievers, contain salicylate.

Chamomile—an anti-inflammatory.

Capsaicin—ointment, relieves pain and inflammation, from red pepper.

Comfrey—add 2 tsp powder to hand cream, relieves pain, inflammation, and swelling.

Turmeric—an anti-inflammatory from the component, curcumin.

Ginger, cumin, sage—have anti-inflammatory properties.

Homeopathy

Take remedy according to symptoms:

Aconitum napellus

Arnica montana

Calcarea phosphorica

Causticum

Guaiacum

Hypericum perforatum

Rhus toxicodendron

Ruta graveolens

Viola odorata

Aromatherapy

Use as massage oil, mix several drops with carrier oil:

   Lavender—relieves pain, a relaxant.

   Chamomile, yarrow, lemon verbena—have anti-inflammatory properties.

Chinese medicine

Acupuncture—relieves pain and discomfort.

Chiropractic

Consult a qualified practitioner

Bodywork

Deep tissue massage

Movement therapies

Acupressure

Qigong

Mindbody therapy

Biofeedback

Chronic Fatigue Syndrome

Chronic fatigue syndrome is characterized by profound fatigue that is not alleviated by sleep, and a myriad of other symptoms including impairment of memory and concentration, muscle pain, and swollen lymph nodes. There is no single cause of the illness and a physician should be consulted to explore all possibilities. Causes may be a viral infection, adrenal gland dysfunction, chemical sensitivity, autonomic nervous system disorder, or food allergy.

Common allergens are found to be wheat, corn, and milk. It is important to exercise daily and reduce stress. Home oxygen therapy may be helpful.

Nutrients

Vitamin B complex

Vitamin B_{12}—injections, increases energy.

Magnesium—200 to 300 mg, if deficient, take with potassium; in aspartate form.

Carnitine—1 g three times a day, necessary for energy production in the mitochondria of cells.

Foods

Whole organic foods

Fresh fruits

Fresh vegetables

Green leafy vegetables

Shiitake mushrooms

Maitake mushrooms

Oyster mushrooms

Whole grains

Legumes

Low-fat yogurt

Fatty fish

Albacore tuna

Herring

Sardines

Salmon

Mackerel

Garlic

Ginger

Basil

Juices

Wheatgrass

Herbal therapy

Astragalus—has antiviral properties, enhances the immune system.

Echinacea—supports the immune system.

Garlic—has antiviral properties, supports the immune system.

Ginseng—2 to 4 g dried root, 10 to 20 ml tincture, or 2 to 4 ml extract three times daily, improves stamina and energy; alternate after 6 to 8 weeks of licorice.

Licorice root—2 to 3 g powdered root or 2 to 4 ml extract, strengthens adrenal gland function which may be weak in individuals with the illness, has antiviral properties.

Homeopathy

Take remedy according to symptoms:

Baptisia

China

Gelsemium

Mercurius corrosivus

Aromatherapy

Bergamot, rose, neroli—use for massage or drops in bath, enhances mood.

Tea tree, niaouli—use for massage or in bath, strengthens immune system.

Ayurvedic medicine

Effective treatments are prescribed.

Ashwaganda

Amla

Bala

Triphala

Lomatium

Cluster fig

Ginger

Chinese medicine

Chinese angelica—restores energy.

Acupuncture

Chiropractic

Consult a qualified practitioner.

Bodywork

Massage—stimulates drainage of lymph systems.

Deep tissue massage

Movement therapy

Qigong

T'ai chi

Mindbody therapy

Meditation

Colds and Flu

A cold is a viral infection of the upper respiratory tract; flu is an infection of the upper and lower respiratory tracts. Both are caused by the same viruses of which there are 200 known. The walls of the upper respiratory tract swell and produce excess mucus resulting in a stuffy nose. Symptoms of cold are a runny nose, sore throat, and general malaise. The flu is more debilitating with symptoms that include diarrhea, vomiting, fever, chills, and fatigue.

The mucus that forms is full of viruses infecting the surrounding air when coughing and sneezing. Viruses can survive for several hours to several days outside the body and on inanimate objects. Individuals who do not develop colds after contact with a virus may have stronger immune systems; and susceptibility to the illness is closely related to stress levels.

Drink lots of fluids to hydrate the mucus membranes as viruses prefer dry environments; hot liquids are best at killing viruses. Avoid milk because it contains components that suppress secretions that thin mucus; hot spicy foods have the opposite effect. Take a hot bath and rest.

Nutrients

Vitamin C—1 to 3 g, lessens severity of symptoms and has antibacterial and antiviral properties, stimulates the immune system.

Zinc—15 to 25 mg lozenges for several days, gluconate form.

Foods

Fresh fruits

Citrus fruits

Acerola

Pineapple

Fresh vegetables

Leafy greens

Bell peppers

Asparagus

Mustard greens

Shiitake mushrooms

Onions

Low-fat yogurt

Garlic

Basil

Ginger

Horseradish

Chili peppers

Juices

Beet

Berry

Carrot

Citrus fruits

Cucumber

Hot lemon and honey—for sore throat

Spinach

Tomato

Fruits

Vegetables

Herbal therapy

Echinacea—3 ml tincture three times daily or 300 to 600 mg capsules three times daily, use at first sign of symptoms daily for 10 to 14 days, has antiviral properties, reduces symptoms; may be combined with wild indigo, boneset, and homeopathic arnica that effectively reduce cold symptoms.[32]

Ginger—tea, grate fresh, steep and strain, add cayenne and honey.

Goldenseal—tincture or 4 to 6 g powder three times daily, soothes mucous membranes of the throat, tea helps sore throat, has antiviral properties.

Garlic—has antiviral properties, strengthens immune system.

Licorice—has antiviral properties, enhances immune system.

Elderberry—has antiviral properties.

Willow bark, meadowsweet—relieve symptoms of cold and flu, have aspirinlike components.

Slippery elm, marshmallow—mucilagents, soothe mucous membranes.

Red raspberry, sage, yarrow—for sore throat.

Homeopathy

Oscillococcinum—take at first sign of illness, reduces the symptoms.

Take remedy according to symptoms:

Aconitum napellus

Allium cepa

Arsenicum album

Baptisia

Baryta carbonica

Belladonna

Bryonia

Dulcamara

Eupatorium perfoliatum

Euphrasia officinalis

Ferrum phosphoricum

Gelsemium

Kali bichromicum

Mercurius solubilis

Natrum muriaticum

Nux vomica

Phosphorus

Pulsatilla

Rhus toxicodendron

Aromatherapy

Tea tree, peppermint, rosemary—massage face and throat.

Eucalyptus, lavender, tea tree, peppermint—as steam inhalation; add several drops to bath water.

Cypress—one drop at sign of sore throat, repeat when soreness returns, an antibiotic.

Lemon—use diffusor, an antiseptic, has calming effect.

Thyme—has antiviral properties.

Ayurvedic medicine

Various treatments are used including ginger tea and breathing exercises.

Chinese medicine

Yinqiao—effective for the first stage.

Loquat syrup—relieves cough with phlegm and congestion.

Bo ying powder—relieves symptoms for infants and children.

Forsythia, honeysuckle—herbs have antiviral properties.

Plantain seed

Peppermint

Mulberry

Skullcap

Acupuncture—improves functioning of the immune system.

Bodywork

Acupressure—certain points relieve symptoms.

Shiatsu

Reflexology

Mindbody therapy

Yoga—boosts the immune system reducing frequency of colds; breathing exercises strengthen respiratory tract.

Constipation

Too little fiber and fluids are the most likely cause of constipation; others are drugs such as painkillers, antidepressants, antihistamines, and heart medications; lack of exercise, stress, anxiety, laxative overuse dull intestinal nerve reflexes; pregnancy, and aging due to the loss of muscle tone. If constipation develops suddenly, see a physician as it may be an indication of colon cancer or impaction. Chronic constipation may be triggered by food allergies.

Fiber acts like a sponge, absorbing water, producing softer stools, and allows quicker passage by stimulating nerve reflexes along the colon wall. However, fiber must be accompanied by plenty of fluids or further constipation could develop. Increase fiber foods gradually over a 4 to 6 week period. Coffee also stimulates bowel reflexes. Exercise increases muscular contraction along the intestinal tract.

Nutrients

Vitamin C—1 g, can encourage regular bowel movement.

Magnesium—400 to 800 mg, helps muscle contraction.

Folic acid—2 to 5 mg, if deficient.

Pectin—500 mg, source of fiber.

Foods

Whole grains

Legumes

Fresh vegetables

Cabbage

Carrots

Beets

Root vegetables

Asparagus

Celery

Chard

Jerusalem artichoke

Okra

Spinach

Fresh fruits

Banana

Pear

Persimmons

Prunes

Rhubarb

Dried fruits

Almonds

Pistachios

Pine nuts

Black sesame seeds

Sunflower seeds

Low-fat yogurt

Basil

Apples, peaches, pears, and berries—high in pectin

Ground flaxseeds—1 to 3 T daily with lots of water

Juices

Apple

Carrot

Celery

Pear

Prune

Black radish

Tomato

Spinach

Watercress

Herbal therapy

Psyllium, flaxseed, fenugreek—high fiber and mucilage content; mild, best for long-term use.

Senna, cascara bark, aloe, rhubarb root—high in anthraquinone glycosides that stimulate contractions; use occasionally.

Homeopathy

Take remedy according to symptoms:

Alumina

Bryonia

Calcarea carbonica

Causticum

Graphites

Lycopodium

Nux vomica

Opium

Sepia

Silicea

Sulfur

Aromatherapy

Marjoram, rosemary, or fennel—several drops in grapeseed or other carrier oil as massage.

Ayurvedic medicine

Treatments may include herbs, medicated enemas, massage, and steambaths.

Triphala

Chinese medicine

Fo-ti—roots are a mild laxative.

Ma Ren Wan

Run Chang Wan

Acupuncture—stimulates points along the large intestine and liver meridians.

Bodywork

Massage—stimulates bowel function.

Movement therapies

Acupressure

Shiatsu

Qigong

Reflexology—massage of areas relating to the intestine and liver.

Mindbody therapy

Yoga—certain asanas and deep breathing are beneficial.

Biofeedback

Hypnotherapy

Crohn's Disease

Crohn's disease is an inflammation of the wall of the colon and may affect the entire intestinal tract. *Colitis* is closely related but involves only the colon. Inflammations evolve in cycles and go into remission. Symptoms include abdominal cramps, fatigue, weight loss, fever, and often bloody diarrhea. The cause for both is unknown but could be stress-related or an autoimmune disorder. Food allergies are another possibility. The illness has been successfully treated when allergens have been removed from the diet. The most common offenders are wheat, dairy, yeast, sugar, eggs, corn, and vegetables of the cruciferous family—broccoli, brussel sprouts, cabbage, and cauliflower. Histamine that is released during an allergic response may not be broken down properly in affected individuals. Malabsorption can be a complication and a diagnosis should be made for any nutritional deficiencies. Smoking aggravates Crohn's disease. Avoid animal fats and omega-6 vegetable oils as they have an inflammatory effect on the system.

Nutrients

Multivitamins and minerals

Quercetin—400 mg, take 20 minutes before meals, for allergies, a bioflavonoid with anti-inflammatory and antihistamine properties.

EPA/DHA—2 to 3 g, enteric coated free fatty acid form, has anti-inflammatory properties, reduces recurrence rate.[33]

Folic acid—800 mcg, if deficient.

Vitamin B$_{12}$—800 mcg, if deficient.

Zinc—25 to 50 mg, if deficient; may need to be balanced with copper.

Vitamin D—if deficient.

Pancreatic enzymes—under the supervision of a physician.

Foods

Whole foods

Fresh fruits

Pineapple

Papaya

Underripe bananas

Fresh vegetables

Yams

Fatty fish

Salmon

Mackerel

Albacore tuna

Herring

Sardines

Low-fat yogurt

Garlic

Onions

Ginger

Cumin

Juices

Fruits

Vegetables

Green leafy vegetables

Apple

Beet

Carrot

Celery

Cucumber

Parsley

Papaya

Pineapple

Spinach

Wheatgrass

Herbal therapy

Slippery elm, marshmallow—has mucilaginous properties, soothes inflamed tissues.

Aloe vera—1 tsp juice after meals, contains healing properties.

Wild indigo—an astringent, inhibits growth of harmful bacteria in intestinal tract.

Goldenseal—antimicrobial, soothing to the intestines.

Green tea, raspberry—contains tannins that help clear up diarrhea; tannins have astringent qualities that contract tissues.

Licorice root—has anti-inflammatory properties.

Chamomile, peppermint—relieves muscle spasms and gas.

Echinacea—supports the immune system.

Hops—have antispasmodic activity; aid digestion.

Homeopathy

Take remedy according to symptoms:

Arsenicum album

Colocynthis

Nux vomica

Pulsatilla

Aromatherapy

Basil—an antispasmodic.

Roman chamomile—massage abdomen, helps relieve pain.

Ayurvedic medicine

Boswellia—350 mg three times a day.

Henbane—has sedative and antispasmodic properties.

Coriander—has anti-inflammatory properties.

Hollyhock—for bowel irritation.

Chinese medicine

Consult a qualified practitioner.

Bodywork

Qigong

Reflexology

Mindbody therapy

Meditation

Yoga

Biofeedback

Imagery

Hypnotherapy

Cystitis

Cystitis is a bacterial infection of the lining of the bladder affecting mainly women. It is usually caused by E. coli which travels from the anus through the urethra and into the bladder. Food allergies, vaginal yeast infections, chemical sensitivities, tissue abrasion from friction during intercourse, and a too large diaphragm may increase exposure to bacteria. Stress and oral contraceptives can lower resistance to infection.

Symptoms of cystitis include burning pain upon urination, pain in the lower abdomen, pressure, frequent urge to urinate but unable to do so, strong urinary odor, fever, and low back pain. If infection is recurrent, see a physician as the disease could spread to the kidneys. Drink plenty of fluids. Urinate frequently, completely, and always after intercourse. Wipe the genital area from front to back, wear cotton underwear, and avoid scented products.

Nutrients

Vitamin A—for infection.

Vitamin C—1 g, for infection, inhibits growth of E. coli.

Bioflavonoids—work synergistically with vitamin C.

Bromelain—for infection, has anti-inflammatory properties, from pineapple.

Cranberry extract—400 mg twice daily, decreases bacteria.

Foods

Fresh fruits

Blueberries

Watermelon

Fresh vegetables

Cilantro

Celery

Parsley

Barley

Low-fat yogurt

Horseradish

Garlic

Juices

Cranberry or blueberry—16 oz daily, contains substances that prevent bacteria from sticking to bladder walls[34] including arbutin which is an antibiotic and diuretic compound.

Sweeten cranberry juice with apple or grape juice.

Carrot

Celery

Cucumber

Parsley

Herbal therapy

Goldenseal—0.5 to 2 ml extract or 4 to 6 ml tincture or 1 to 2 g dried root three times daily, contains berberine which prevents bacteria from adhering to the walls of the bladder.

Uva ursi—3 to 5 ml tincture three times daily or 100 to 250 mg arbutin capsules three times daily, heals inflammation, arbutin content kills bacteria.

Corn silk—soothes inflammation.

Dandelion—a diuretic, helps flush urine out of the bladder.

Hibiscus—for painful urination.

Echinacea—supports immune system in fighting infection.

Homeopathy

Take remedy according to symptoms:

Aconitum napellus

Apis mellifica

Belladonna

Berberis vulgaris

Borax

Cantharis

Chimaphila umbellata

Clematis

Equisetum

Mercurius

Nux vomica

Pulsatilla

Sarsaparilla

Sepia

Staphysagria

Aromatherapy

Rosemary—massage legs.

Juniper

Lavender, bergamot, sandalwood—have antiseptic properties, add to bath.

Chamomile

Ayurvedic medicine

Shatavari 500 mg, punarnava 300 mg, guduchi 300 mg, kamadudha 100 mg—mix and take ¼ tsp twice daily after meals.

Hollyhock

Coriander

Chinese medicine

Plantain seeds

Bodywork

Acupressure—stimulates points along the stomach meridian.

Qigong

Mindbody therapy

Yoga

Depression

There are two general types of depression. Situational depression in which there are normal reactions to external events and endogenous depression, indicating an internal cause such as a biochemical or hormonal imbalance or nutritional deficiency. If depression is recurrent, constant, or severe, a physician should be consulted to find out the cause. Treating symptoms with antidepressants does not solve the underlying reason for the illness. Situational depressions can often be handled through psychotherapy or counseling.

Depression may be associated with low thyroid, hypoglycemia, PMS, or sensitivity or allergy to foods, chemicals, and pesticides; certain pharmaceutical drugs and recreational drugs can be a factor, as can addiction to caffeine, although moderate amounts for many individuals can lift depression and improve mood. Oral contraceptives can cause a depletion of vitamin B_6, which is necessary for mental health, and of tyrosine, an amino acid that converts to norepinephrine, a mood-affecting neurotransmitter. Depressed individuals not taking oral contraceptives may also be low in these nutrients. Symptoms of depression include weight loss or gain, insomnia or sleeping excessively, fatigue, hyperactivity or inactivity, loss of interest, poor concentration, feelings of guilt or worthlessness, and recurring thoughts of death and suicide.

Serotonin, melatonin, dopamine, epinephrine, and norepinephrine are neurotransmitters in the brain that affect mood. In some individuals, these chemicals may need to be replenished. Vitamins, minerals, and amino acids supply the building blocks for this process and because these compounds are found in foods, diet is important. Foods affect mental health. Exercise is beneficial as it increases the production of endorphins, the body's natural pain killers that increase a sense of well-being.

Nutrients

Assays on vitamin and mineral levels are helpful; supplement any that are deficient.

Take the following three nutrients with fruit juice or fruit before breakfast;[35] precursors to the synthesis of neurotransmitters that influence energy and alertness.

DL-phenylalanine—200 to 1500 mg

Vitamin B complex—100 mg

Vitamin C—500 mg

SAMe—raises dopamine and serotonin levels, improves binding of neurotransmitters to reception sites.

Vitamin B_6—20 mg twice daily, if deficient.

Folic acid—if deficient, often low in depressed individuals, improves efficacy of lithium.

Iron—if deficient.

Vitamin B_1—if deficient.

Vitamin B_{12}—if deficient.

Biotin—if deficient.

5-HTP—100 to 200 mg three times daily, an extract from the plant Griffonia simplicifolia, increases serotonin, endorphin, and other neurotransmitter levels.

Foods

Whole organic foods

Whole grains

Whole grain pasta

Whole grain cereal

Whole grain breads

Seafood

Fatty fish

Salmon

Albacore tuna

Herring

Mackerel

Sardines

Turkey

Nuts

Brazil nuts

Seeds

Sunflower seeds

Legumes

Dried beans

Vegetables

Green leafy vegetables

Mustard greens

Fresh fruits

Melons

Watermelon

Garlic

Cayenne

Ginger

Fennel

Dill

Coriander

Basil

Herbal therapy

St. John's wort—300 mg three times a day or two cups of tea daily, as effective as Prozac, for mild to moderate depression;[36] take 4 to 8 weeks to feel full effect. Take before or with meals to prevent stomach problems; can be combined with 5-HTP.

Licorice—has antidepressant compounds, add to other teas.

Siberian ginseng—promotes a sense of well-being.

Gingko biloba—80 mg extract three times daily, relieves depression especially in the elderly; can be combined with St. John's wort and/or 5-HTP.

Damiana—may relieve depression.

Yohimbe—has an MAO inhibitor compound; *can have side effects including increased heart rate and blood pressure, hallucinations, anxiety, and headache, use only under the supervision of a physician.*

Ginger—an antidepressant.

Cayenne—stimulates production of endorphins.

Kava kava—45 to 70 mg kavalactones three times daily, relieves depression and has a calming effect; reduce dose if drowsiness is experienced.

Valerian—relieves insomnia.

Walnut tea—high in serotonin.

Homeopathy

Take remedy according to symptoms:

Arsenicum album

Aurum metallicum

Calcarea carbonica

Causticum

Cimicifuga

Ignatia amara

Kali phosphoricum

Lycopodium

Natrum carbonicum

Natrum muriaticum

Phosphoric acid

Pulsatilla

Sepia

Staphysagria

Aromatherapy

Melissa—relieves depression.

Creeping hyssop—for nervous depression.

Lemon verbena—works on the psychohormonal level.

Frankincense—relieves depression.

Bergamot, chamomile, rosemary, clary sage, jasmine, geranium, lavender, orange, ylang ylang—antidepressants and sedatives; use several in combination as massage.

Ayurvedic medicine

Treatments prescribed have proven effective.

Chinese medicine

Angelica

Peony root

Licorice

Thorowax

Acupuncture—treatments are as effective as conventional antidepressant medications.

Chiropractic

Consult a qualified practitioner.

Bodywork

Massage—helps relieve symptoms.

Deep tissue manipulation

Movement therapies

Acupressure

Shiatsu

T'ai chi

Qigong

Reflexology

Mindbody therapy

Meditation

Yoga

Biofeedback

Imaging

Hypnotherapy

Diabetes

Diabetes is a condition in which there is too much sugar in the blood and the insulin that is required for processing it is either absent, insufficient, or ineffective. Diabetes is an inherited disease. There are two forms of diabetes, Type I, or juvenile-onset, and Type II, or adult-onset. *Type I* begins in childhood and is an autoimmune disorder in which the cells of the pancreas are eventually destroyed by the body's own immune system. Consequently, the pancreas cannot produce any insulin and the individual is dependent on insulin injections to prevent coma or death. Diet and lifestyle can at the most reduce the amount of insulin required.

Type II is less severe and affects adults usually over the age of 40. Insulin is available but there is either not enough to meet the demand, or the cells are resistant to accepting it, thereby not allowing the glucose to pass through the cell membrane. Type II can be controlled by diet, exercise, and maintaining proper weight. Oral medication may or may not be necessary, 90% of all diabetes is Type II, and half may not know they have it.

Symptoms of diabetes are excessive thirst and urination due to the excess of sugar in the blood, fatigue, weakness, and slow wound healing. Diabetics are more prone to cardiovascular disease because of faulty fat metabolism. They may have poor circulation, due to the narrowing of blood vessels, which leads to complications involving the feet, eyes, and kidneys, and susceptibility to infections. Inadequate diet, food allergies, viral infections, and stress can aggravate diabetes Type II. During stress, adrenaline levels increase, which causes a rise in blood sugar.

What is eaten can either cause blood sugar to rise or keep it at a moderate level. The more fiber in the diet, the lower the glycemic index of foods, the slower the rise in blood sugar. See Section IV for more information on glycemic index. Type II diabetes takes years to develop. Although genetically predisposed, diet will determine if the disease becomes manifest.

Studies have shown that a protein in milk can act as an antigen causing the immune system to dysfunction and begin to attack the beta cells of the pancreas. This process can trigger Type I diabetes when infants are fed cow's milk, especially in the first year. For infants from families who have a history of diabetes, breast-feeding is an alternative.

Maintaining proper weight is extremely important, because if too much food is eaten, all systems get overloaded. The pancreas overworks in trying to meet the insulin demand and the cells get weary of having to handle so much of the glucose that insulin brings to them. Eventually, diabetes is the result. Exercise is equally vital to the extent that it can actually prevent or stabilize diabetic conditions.

Nutrients

GTF chromium—200 mcg to 1 g, improves glucose tolerance and stabilizes blood sugar.

Coenzyme Q_{10}—100 mg, may stabilize blood sugar in some diabetics.

Vitamin C—1 to 3 g, improves glucose tolerance reducing insulin needs, fights infections, strengthens blood vessels. *In presence of renal insufficiency, see physician before taking megadoses.*

Bioflavonoids—1 to 2 g, work synergistically with vitamin C.

Vitamin E—800 IU with mixed tocopherols, prevents vascular complications, improves glucose tolerance;[37] supplement may keep Type II from needing insulin.

Vitamin B_6—improves glucose tolerance; levels are low in diabetic neuropathy.

Vitamin B_{12}—500 mcg three times daily, reduces nerve damage in diabetics.

Biotin—9 to 16 mg, can reduce blood sugar levels, helps diabetic neuropathy.

Vitamin B_1—if deficient.

Vitamin D—can increase insulin secretion and lower blood sugar levels.

Magnesium—300 to 400 mg, diabetics tend to be low in the mineral, can improve insulin production; for diabetics with normal kidney function.

Zinc—15 to 25 mg, diabetics are prone to deficiency, can lower blood sugar levels.

Inositol—500 mg twice daily; may reverse diabetic neuropathy.

Alpha-lipoic acid—600 mg, improves diabetic neuropathy and reduces pain.

Carnitine—1 g, reduces diabetic neuropathy pain, lowers blood fats.

Evening primrose oil—4 to 6 g, helps reduce nerve damage.

Foods

Whole foods

Whole grains

Buckwheat

Barley

Brown rice

Oats

Legumes

Soymilk

Lentils

Peanuts

Fish

Lean meats

Eggs

Fresh fruit

Avocado

Rhubarb

Blueberries

Plums

Mandarins

Pear

Fresh vegetables

Broccoli

Cabbage

Alfalfa

Onions

Mushrooms

Bitter melon

Water chestnuts

Jerusalem artichokes

Kohlrabi

Spinach

Dandelion greens

Winter squash

Nuts

Garlic

Fenugreek seeds

Cinnamon, cloves, turmeric, bay leaves—spices that stimulate production of insulin.

Herbal therapy

Blueberry leaf—two cups daily, morning and evening, lowers blood sugar levels.

Tea (Camellia sinensis)—reduces blood sugar levels.

Bilberry—40 to 80 mg extract three times daily, can improve diabetic retinopathy.

Aloe vera—1 T juice twice daily, lowers blood sugar.

Capsaicin—apply topically, reduces pain in diabetic neuropathy, from red peppers.

Fenugreek—50 g defatted powder, reduces fasting blood sugar levels and improves glucose tolerance.

Salt bush—3 g, improves glucose regulation and tolerance for Type II according to studies conducted in Israel.

Homeopathy

Take remedy according to symptoms:

Bovista lycoperdon

Lycopodium

Phosphoric acid

Phosphorus

Plumbum

Uranium nitricum

Aromatherapy

Camphor, eucalyptus, geranium, juniper, lemon, rosemary—mix and massage back, balance pancreatic secretions.

Juniper—mix with olive oil and massage spleen area.

Ayurvedic medicine

Pancha karma

Gymnema—400 mg extract, stimulates insulin production, reduces blood sugar levels.

Bitter melon—extract or 1 to 2 oz juice three times daily, stimulates pancreas, lowers blood sugar.

Karella—eat with seeds twice daily.

Chinese medicine

Herbal combinations prescribed that are effective.

Ginseng—200 mg extract, stimulates production of insulin and increases the number of cellular insulin receptors,[38] stabilizes blood sugar and increases energy.[39]

Astragalus

Wild yam

Lotus seed

Lilyturf root

Grassy privet

Rehmannia

Acupuncture—reduces autoimmune aspect and can reverse diabetic neuropathy, can lower insulin requirement.

Bodywork

Massage—relaxing and reduces stress.

Qigong

Reflexology

Mindbody therapy

Meditation—reduces stress.

Yoga—improves function of the pancreas, stabilizes blood sugar levels.

Biofeedback—reduces stress.

Imagery

Hypnotherapy—reduce stress and lower insulin requirements through suggestion.

Diarrhea

Diarrhea is the accumulation of too much water in the large intestine that the intestinal walls fail to absorb. The immediate concern is replacing lost fluids in order to prevent dehydration. The best way to do this is by eating thick starchy soups and cereals. Eating frequently leads to a faster recovery.

Diarrhea can be caused by bacteria, viruses, or parasites; antibiotics, allergies or food sensitivities, milk, caffeine, fructose and sorbitol from fruit juices especially apple, pear, and grape; dietetic foods that contain sorbitol; stress, large amounts of supplemental vitamin C or magnesium; or health conditions such as irritable bowel syndrome and Crohn's disease. If the illness lasts for more than several weeks or is accompanied by fever, severe cramps, or blood or mucus in the stool, call a physician. Because of diarrhea, beneficial bacteria are flushed out of the intestine and need to be replaced with acidophilus.

Nutrients

Multivitamins and minerals

S. boulardii—prevents antibiotic-induced and infectious diarrhea.[40]

Foods

Thick soups

Brown rice soup

Corn soup

Lentil soup

Carrot soup

Wheat soup

Barley soup

Potato soup

Chicken noodle soup

Tapioca pudding

Amaranth

Low-fat yogurt

Underripe bananas

Applesauce

Apples

Citrus fruits

Persimmons

Blackberries

Raspberries

Olives

Root vegetables

Tomatoes

Chestnuts

Nutmeg

Cumin

Fenugreek seeds—½ tsp with water three times a day, for adults.

Juices

Apple

Carrot

Celery

Coconut

Orange

Parsley

Spinach

Vegetable

Herbal therapy

Psyllium seed—9 to 30 g, solidifies stool.

Blackberry, raspberry, bilberry—tea or tincture, one cup every 2 to 4 hours, contains tannins that have an astringent or binding effect on the mucous membranes of the intestinal walls reducing inflammation.

Aloe vera—soothes inflamed intestines.

Goldenseal—has antimicrobial properties.

Carob—powder, mix 1 T with applesauce and take on empty stomach, contains tannins that have a binding effect on mucous membranes; for children and adults.

Chamomile—2 to 3 g powder or 3 to 5 ml extract three times daily, reduces cramps, irritation, and inflammation.

Marshmallow, slippery elm—mucilaginous, soothe intestinal tract.

Homeopathy

Take remedy according to symptoms:

Aconite

Apis mellifica

Argentum nitricum

Arsenicum album

Bryonia

Calcarea carbonica

Chamomilla

China

Colchicum

Colocynthis

Gelsemium

Ipecacuanha

Mercurius solubilis

Natrum sulphuricum

Nux vomica

Phosphorus

Podophyllum

Pulsatilla

Sulfur

Veratrum album

Aromatherapy

Lavender, neroli—relieve stress.

Eucalyptus, chamomile—antispasmodics.

Myrrh—has antibacterial and antiviral properties.

Ayurvedic medicine

Triphala

Cassia pods

Henbane

Coriander

Chinese medicine

Herbal remedies are prescribed.

Skullcap root, golden thread, kapok flowers, dandelion root—for acute diarrhea.

Psoralea fruit, codonopsis root, astragalus—for chronic diarrhea.

Acupuncture—aids recovery from bowel infection.

Bodywork

Acupressure

Reflexology

Mindbody therapy

Biofeedback

Diverticulitis

Diverticulitis is an inflammation of abnormal pouches called diverticula on the walls of the lower intestine which results in cramps, bloating, and pain in the lower left side of the abdomen, and constipation, or both constipation and diarrhea. The cause is lack of fiber in the diet, consequently, the sigmoid part of the colon has to exert so much pressure to propel the feces that the walls of the intestine herniate. If the pouches become infected or if there is an obstruction, antibiotics or surgery may be necessary. Many individuals have diverticula that do not become inflamed. The solution is to eat high fiber foods, although in the acute stage, vegetables may not be tolerated. Drink plenty of fluids.

Foods

Whole foods

Whole grains

Whole wheat

Bran cereals

Unprocessed wheat bran

Oat bran

Fresh fruits

Fresh vegetables

Prunes

Ground flaxseed or psyllium seed—1 to 3 T.

Juices

Apple

Beet

Cabbage

Carrot

Celery

Lemon

Pineapple

Papaya

Prune

Herbal therapy

Aloe vera—gel, take after meals, soothes intestinal tract.

Chamomile—tincture or tea, an anti-inflammatory, soothing to the digestive tract.

Slippery elm—powder, one to two cups tea daily, soothes irritated intestinal walls.

Peppermint—tea or enteric-coated oil of peppermint capsules, an anti-inflammatory and antispasmodic.

Wild yam—reduces pain and inflammation.

Homeopathy

Take remedy according to symptoms:

Belladonna

Bryonia

Colocynthis

Chinese medicine

Acupuncture

Bodywork

Massage

Acupressure

Chiropractic

Consult a qualified practitioner.

Mindbody therapy

Biofeedback

Ear Infection

Inflammation and infection of the middle ear, called *otitis media,* is a result of blockage of the Eustachian tubes that run from the back of the throat to the middle ear. Fluid gathers and pressure builds up, causing pain. Symptoms are a throbbing pain and sometimes fever. If there is a sudden sharp pain and pus drains from the ear, the eardrum has been perforated. Ear infection can be of a bacterial, viral, or fungal nature. It can also be the result of a structural obstruction or an allergic reaction to food, air, pollen, mold, or dust.

In a study, 86% of the children affected with ear infections were relieved of the condition when foods they were allergic to were removed from the diet, taking several months for the infection to clear totally. Most common offenders are milk, wheat, eggs, peanuts, and soy products. Allergies cause an inflammation and swelling of the middle ear, which allows fluid to become trapped and infection to fester.

Craniosacral manipulation by an osteopath has cured middle ear infection caused by restriction of the respiratory apparatus. While fluid is not able to drain because of the restriction, it stagnates and bacteria is allowed to breed. For more information contact: the Cranial Academy, 8606 Allisonville Road, Suite 130, Indianapolis, Indiana 46250, 317-595-0411. Breast-feeding has shown to prevent middle ear infection;[41] the longer the infant is nursed the greater the protection. The reason is likely due to antibodies in the milk.

Nutrients

Vitamin C—500 mg to 1 g, for infection, supports the immune system.

Bioflavonoids—work synergistically with vitamin C.

Herbal therapy

Mullein or garlic oil—warm and drop into ear and keep in with cotton. *Do not place oil in ear if eardrum is ruptured.* Take garlic oil in capsules orally.

Echinacea—1 to 2 ml tincture or 0.5 to 1 g dried root or 2 to 4 ml extract three times daily with ear drops, an antibiotic, supports the immune system.

Goldenseal—tea or tincture three times daily, an antibiotic.

Peppermint tea—relieves pain, an antiseptic.

Homeopathy

Take remedy according to symptoms:

Aconitum napellus

Belladonna

Chamomilla

Ferrum phosphoricum

Hepar sulphuris calcareum

Magnesia phosphorica

Mercurius solubilis

Pulsatilla

Silicea

Aromatherapy

Rosemary, peppermint—mix and massage area around ear, along lymph nodes, and unto neck.

Lavender—place several drops in ear with Qtip.

Tea tree, lavender—use in vaporizer, have antiseptic properties.

Ayurvedic medicine

Treatments are given to drain the lymphatic fluids.

Garlic

Vitamin C

Chinese medicine

Gentian, honeysuckle, forsythia—powders, combine and add to juice or applesauce, have antibiotic properties.

Chiropractic

Spinal manipulation

Bodywork

Massage—of ear area, helps keep Eustachian tubes open.

Eczema

Eczema is an inflammation of the skin with persistent itching and often weeping blisters that then dry into scabs or crusts. Also known as atopic dermatitis, the disease is caused by allergies and in some cases is hereditary. Stress may also be a factor. Individuals with eczema may not be able to properly metabolize fatty acids. Symptoms of the disease have improved when heavy coffee drinkers have stopped drinking the beverage. Determine any allergy and remove from diet or environment.

Nutrients

Evening primrose or black currant oil—500 mg twice daily, reduces symptoms; children under 12—250 mg twice daily; evening primrose oil can also be applied topically.

EPA/DHA—540 and 360 mg, respectively, or 1 T flaxseed oil, for individuals when primrose oil proves ineffective.

Vitamin C—can reduce symptoms.

Bioflavonoids—work synergistically with vitamin C.

Zinc—45 to 60 mg, if deficient.

Foods

Organic whole foods

Dandelion greens

Purslane

Fatty fish

Albacore tuna

Mackerel

Herring

Salmon

Sardines

Juices

Beet

Black currant

Carrot

Cucumber

Red grape

Parsley

Spinach

Wheatgrass

Herbal therapy

Licorice root—1 to 2 g or 2 to 4 ml extract or 2 to 5 ml tincture three times daily, take orally or apply cream topically, glycyrrhizin component reduces inflammation and itching.

Chamomile or calendula—cream, apply topically, have anti-inflammatory properties.

Chickweed—cream, apply topically, relieves itching.

Aloe vera—gel, apply topically.

Witch hazel—apply topically.

Red clover—relieves symptoms.

Green tea—200 to 300 mg extract or cups of tea drunk throughout the day, has antiallergenic properties.

Homeopathy

Take remedy according to symptoms:

Antimonium crudum

Arsenicum album

Arum triphyllum

Calcarea carbonica

Calendula

Dulcamara

Graphites

Hepar sulphuris calcareum

Mezereum

Petroleum

Rhus toxicodendron

Sulfur

Aromatherapy

Lavender, 1 ml, palmrosa 1 ml, calophyllum 10 ml, rose hip seed oil 30 ml—in base of carrier oil 1:1, for dry eczema; apply topically three to four times daily, relieve itching and regenerate skin tissue.

Thyme, thujonal type 1 ml, eucalyptus citriodora 1 ml, calophyllum 10 ml, rose hip seed oil 30 ml—in base of carrier oil 1:1, for weeping eczema; apply topically three to four times daily.

Lavender, bergamot, geranium—very diluted with carrier oil, by professional therapist, reduce inflammation and itching.

Ayurvedic medicine

Kutki 200 mg, manjista 300 mg, turmeric 200 mg, neem 200 mg—mix and take 1 tsp twice daily after meals.

Neem oil—apply topically.

Cassia pods

Aloe vera

Chinese medicine

Herbal preparations prescribed improve symptoms.

Wormwood

Peony root

Chinese gentian

Dittany bark, puncture vine fruit—for itching.

Acupuncture

Bodywork

Acupressure

Shiatsu

Reflexology

Mindbody therapy

Meditation

Yoga

Biofeedback

Imaging

Hypnotherapy

Epilepsy

Epilepsy is a dysfunction of the electrical activity in the brain. Seizures may involve loss of consciousness or be of a milder form with symptoms such as momentary loss of awareness, rapid heart beat, sweating, and high blood pressure. The illness is not always, but can be, inherited. Children in a study who had both migraine headaches and epileptic seizures had no seizures or had fewer when foods they were allergic to were eliminated from the diet. The common offenders are cow's milk and cheese, citrus fruits, eggs, wheat, corn, pork, tomatoes, and chocolate.

The dose of anticonvulsant drugs may be able to be lessened only after pursuing other alternatives and doing so gradually over many weeks. Drug therapy may always be necessary but at a level that has lesser side effects. The intention of adjunct or alternative therapy is to moderate brain activity. Eliminate stimulants that activate brain activity such as coffee, alcohol, tea, tobacco, colas, and chocolate.

Nutrients

Calcium, magnesium—1 g each before bedtime and half the dose 12 hours later,[42] in citrate, gluconate, or chelated form, moderates the nervous system.

Herbal therapy

Valerian—tincture, one dropperful in water three to four times daily, a mild relaxant and depressant.

Scullcap—1 tsp tincture three times daily for petit mal.

Homeopathy

Take remedy according to symptoms after seizure has expired:

Aconite

Belladonna

Chamomilla

Ignatia

Zinc

Aromatherapy

Rosemary—small doses may be helpful, *use only under the supervision of a aromatherapist.*

Ayurvedic medicine

Saraswati churna 200 mg, brahmi 300 mg, jatamansi 200 mg, punarnava 300 mg—mix and take ¼ tsp twice daily after meals.

Chinese medicine

Sweet flag root

Bamboo juice

Chiropractic

Consult a qualified practitioner.

Bodywork

Massage

Shiatsu

Deep tissue massage

Movement therapy

Reflexology

Mindbody therapy

Biofeedback—learn to produce slower brain waves through controlling the autonomic nervous system.

Hypnotherapy

Eye Problems

Cataracts

In cataracts damage to the protein of the lens of the eye clouds the lens and impairs vision. Oxidation of the lens from exposure to the sun and other sources in the environment is partly responsible for the destruction and nothing can reverse the situation once it has developed. Nutrient deficiencies, selenium, for example, may contribute to cataract formation. Symptoms are blurred or hazy vision, seeing spots, or the feeling of a film over the eye. Vitamin C supplementation may help improve vision.

Glutathione, an antioxidant, is found to be especially lacking in cataracts as well as vitamin C, vitamin E, and folic acid. Vitamin A and the carotenoids are important for eye health, lutein a carotenoid is found in the lens. Foods containing these antioxidants are fruits and vegetables, spinach and other green leafy vegetables, broccoli, asparagus, legumes, avocados, oranges, dark berries, plums, and cherries. The herb bilberry is high in antioxidants, 240 to 480 mg of extract daily are recommended to protect the lens and retina, as are rosemary, turmeric, and ginger. Homeopathy remedies include Calcarea carbonica, Calcarea fluorica, Causticum, Natrum muriaticum, phosphorus, and Silicea. Take remedy according to symptom. Chinese medicine includes wolfberry, chrysanthemum, and rumania.

Conjunctivitis

This condition is an inflammation of the membrane that lines the eye, also known as pinkeye. *Blepharitis* is an inflammation of the eyelid. The cause may be a bacterial infection, a virus, or it may be an allergic reaction. A cool compress can be placed on the eye; or bathe the eye in tepid boiled water to which a little salt has been added. An eyewash made from an infusion of calendula, eyebright, or chamomile, kept sterile, can reduce swelling and redness; add goldenseal if there is an infection. Use echinacea, eyebright, sage, and goldenseal as tea. A warm aromatherapy compress with a few drops of lavender, chamomile, or rose oil can soothe the area and help heal the infection. Green myrtle oil is an anti-inflammatory and can be mixed with water and sprayed into the eye or onto a closed eye and then blink several times. Homeopathy remedies include Apis mellifica, Argentum nitricum, Euphrasia, Hepar sulphuris calcareum, Mercurius solubilis, Natrum muriaticum, Pulsatilla, and sulfur. Take remedy according to symptoms. Chinese medicine includes violet, chyrsanthemum flowers, and bamboo leaves—boil, strain, cool, and use as eyewash.

Glaucoma

Glaucoma is pressure within the eyeball that damages nerve fibers of the optic nerve. Increased pressure evolves when the passage that allows fluid into the eye becomes clogged. The cause is unknown although in some cases there may be an underlying condition. Allergies can exacerbate the situation. Vitamin C, 2 to 5 g, can reduce elevated pressure, as well as rutin at 20 mg three times daily. In studies, 250 mg magnesium has lowered pressure. Cranial osteopathy is helpful in dispersing fluid within the head which relieves pressure in the eyes. The homeopathic remedy belladonna is effective for chronic simple glaucoma. Diets high in fatty fish and fresh fruits and vegetables are recommended for prevention of glaucoma.

Macular Degeneration

A degeneration of the macula, which is a portion of the retina in the back of the eye. It is the leading cause of blindness. The cause of the disease is oxidation from the sun and other environmental agents; smoking is also linked to the condition. Antioxidants protect the eye from free radical damage; the carotenoids are important for eye health especially lutein and zeaxanthin which are concentrated in the macula. Zinc is needed for the synthesis of enzymes that are necessary for retinal cell function.

Nutrients recommended for macular degeneration are vitamin C 1 g, bioflavonoids, vitamin E 400 IU with mixed tocopherols, selenium 200 mcg, and the carotenoid complex. Foods containing antioxidants and carotenoids include fresh fruits and vegetables, spinach, kale, carrots, asparagus, dark berries, sweet potatoes, dried fruits, garlic, ginger, and Brazil nuts. Oyster, crab, turkey, and pumpkin seeds are good sources of zinc. Gingko biloba 120 to 240 mg extract, has been shown to help macular degeneration in the early stages. Bilberry, 40 to 80 mg extract three times daily, has a high concentration of bioflavonoids called anthocyanosides that act as antioxidants. They also strengthen the capillaries of the retina reducing any possibility of hemorrhage.[43]

Night Blindness

Night blindness is an inability to see well in dim or dark light. It is an indication of vitamin A deficiency, a nutrient necessary for the production of visual purple. Nutrients recommended are vitamin A, the carotenoid complex, and zinc, if there is a deficiency. The herb bilberry is high in bioflavonoids and aids in the regeneration of visual purple.

Other alternative medicine and therapies that aid in the prevention and improvement of eye problems are Ayurvedic medicine, Chinese medicine including acupuncture, chiropractic, craniosacral therapy, shiatsu, movement therapies that help alleviate the physical and emotional stress that is induced by vision problems, Qigong, reflexology, and yoga.

Fibrocystic Breast Disease

Most premenopausal women experience fibrocystic breast disease characterized by tenderness, sometimes painful breasts, and small lumps that can be felt. It may be part of PMS and is associated with an excess of estrogen. If the lump is tender or painful, it is likely a cyst and not a tumor. Avoiding coffee and any foods or drugs containing caffeine can reduce symptoms significantly; allow 6 months for results. Eat a low-fat diet and eliminate dairy, meats, eggs, and poultry unless they are certified hormone free. Aerobic exercises have shown to alleviate breast tenderness. Natural progesterone applied topically days 15 to 25 of the menstrual cycle can result in the disappearance of the cysts.

Nutrients

Vitamin E—200 to 600 IU with mixed tocopherols, for 3 months, can reduce symptoms.

Vitamin B_6—25 to 50 mg three times daily, may reduce symptoms.

Evening primrose oil—may reduce symptoms.

Foods

Fresh fruits

Fresh vegetables

Dark leafy greens

Sea vegetables

Parsley

Shiitake mushrooms

Onions

Fatty fish

Salmon

Albacore tuna

Herring

Mackerel

Sardines

Soy products

Whole grains

Low-fat yogurt

Nuts

Seeds

Extra virgin olive oil

Cold pressed walnut oil

Cold pressed organic canola oil

Garlic

Herbal therapy

Chasteberry—alleviates tenderness.

Dandelion—for cysts.

Parsley—for swelling.

Mullein—helps reduce pain.

Echinacea—supports the immune system.

Homeopathy

Take remedy according to symptoms:

Carbo animalis

Phytolacca

Silica

Mindbody therapy

Meditation

Biofeedback

Hypnotherapy

Fibromyalgia

Similar to chronic fatigue syndrome, fibromyalgia involves bodily aches and pains with fatigue as a secondary symptom accompanied by insomnia and depression. The cause is unknown but stress may be a factor. Exercise is very important in reducing the symptoms. Individuals with the disease often have low serotonin levels. Herbs that are beneficial for chronic fatigue syndrome may also help fibromyalgia.

Nutrients

Magnesium—300- to 600-mg citrate or aspartate and malic acid 1200 to 2400 mg taken together may lessen muscle pain.

Vitamin E—100 to 300 IU with mixed tocopherols, can reduce symptoms.

SAMe—800 mg, reduces pain and depression.

5-HTP—50 to 100 mg three times daily, from the plant Griffonia simplicifoli, increases synthesis of serotonin, decreases pain, improves sleep quality; can be combined with magnesium and 300 mg St. John's wort for maximum effectiveness.

Foods

Fresh fruits

Fresh vegetables

Whole grains

Fatty fish

Salmon

Albacore tuna

Sardines

Herring

Mackerel

Nuts

Seeds

Extra virgin olive oil

Ginger

Turmeric

Herbal therapy

Licorice root—2 g three times daily for 8 weeks.

Ginseng—1 to 2 g, take following time span of licorice root.

Black cohosh—has anti-inflammatory properties.

Homeopathy

Take remedy according to symptoms:

Arnica montana

Bryonia

Calcarea carbonica

Causticum

Cimicifuga

Kalmia latifolia

Ranunculus bulbosus

Rhus toxicodendron

Ruta graveolens

Aromatherapy

Camphor—massage, has a warming effect and promotes healing.

Ayurvedic medicine

Boswellia—two capsules twice daily, has anti-inflammatory properties.

Chinese medicine

Acupuncture—very effective in relieving pain and other symptoms.

Chiropractic

Spinal manipulation—helpful for some individuals.

Bodywork

Massage—stimulates circulation and easing pain in stiff areas.

Deep tissue manipulation

Movement therapies

Polarity therapy

Mindbody therapy

Meditation—reduces stress.

Yoga—stretching asanas relaxes muscles and relieves symptoms.

Biofeedback

Imagery

Hypnotherapy—reduces muscle pain, fatigue, and insomnia.

Gallbladder Disease

Gallstones and *inflammation* of the gallbladder, which rarely happens without the presence of gallstones, are most common in women. Pain felt in the upper-right quarter of the abdomen, then often moving to the back, is frequently the result of a stone blocking the bile duct. Stones are formed when there is an excess of cholesterol in the bile or a deficiency of substances such as lecithin needed to disperse the fat.

Gallstones are primarily composed of cholesterol that crystalizes and hardens into stones ranging from the size of tiny seeds to one inch in diameter. They are formed usually as a result of too much saturated fat and cholesterol in the diet, and it is recommended that consumption of saturated fats be reduced and cholesterol containing foods kept at 300 mg daily.

Too much sugar and too little fiber in the diet have been shown in studies to promote gallbladder attacks. Coffee, regular or decaffeinated, stimulates gallbladder contractions and can bring on an attack. Skipping meals can cause a gallbladder attack because the gallbladder needs to be active in producing bile acids which keep cholesterol dissolved. Some individuals may be deficient in HCl (stomach hydrochloric acid). Obesity and constipation are risks for forming stones. Food allergies have been shown to precipitate gallbladder inflammation but not stones; eggs, onions, and pork are the most common offenders.

Nutrients

Phosphatidyl choline—300 to 2000 mg, extract from lecithin, protects against stone formation by increasing lecithin content of bile.

Vitamin C—2 g in divided doses, shown in studies to reduce cholesterol stone formation.

Foods

Fresh fruits

Oranges

Apples

Pears

Cherries

Fresh vegetables

Beets

Spinach

Artichokes

Parsley

Radish

Watercress

Whole grains

Oat bran

Flaxseeds

Corn

Beans

Soybeans

Lentils

Peas

Almonds

Low-fat yogurt

Turmeric

Extra virgin olive oil—shown to discourage stone formation.

Juices

Apple

Beet

Carrot

Citrus

Cucumber

Grape

Pear

Herbal therapy

Turmeric—100 to 200 mg curcumin three times daily increases solubility of bile preventing gallstone formation.[44]

Milk thistle—600 mg extract, keeps bile soluble.

Celandine—reduces symptoms.

Peppermint—tea or several drops oil mixed in water or 1 to 2 capsules enteric-coated peppermint, drink with meal, can help symptoms, helps dissolve gallstones.

Chamomile

Homeopathy

Take remedy according to symptoms:

Berberis vulgaris

Calcarea carbonica

Chelidonium majus

China

Colocynthis

Dioscorea

Lycopodium

Nux vomica

Podophyllum

Aromatherapy

Lavender, rosemary—massage over gallbladder area, help relieve pain.

Ayurvedic medicine

Kalanchoe

Chinese medicine

Lysimachia, pyrrosia leaf, rhubarb—can help dissolve small stones.

Acupuncture—reduces inflammation.

Mindbody therapy

Yoga

Gingivitis

Gingivitis is an inflammation of the gums and *periodentitis* is the inflammation of the gums and surrounding tissues that can eventually result in loss of bone support. Symptoms are gums that are red, swollen, and bleed easily. They often recede and bad breath may be present. A good diet and proper oral hygiene are essential in preventing gum disease. Sugar significantly increases plaque formation while adversely affecting white blood cell function. Toothpaste or mouthwash containing sanguinarine, an alkaloid from the herb bloodroot, helps prevent plaque formation and has anti-inflammatory and antimicrobial properties. Centella extract, 30 mg twice daily, a triterpenoid from gota kola, has effective wound healing properties especially effective for severe gum disease and after surgery.

TMJ (temporomandibular joint syndrome) can also cause a loss of bone support. Ear and jaw pain and difficulty in opening the mouth are symptoms, often a result of underlying muscle tension. *Bruxism,* or grinding of teeth, is usually a part of the syndrome. Calcium, 1 g, and magnesium, 350 mg, taken twice daily can relax muscles. Acupuncture, biofeedback, imagery, and craniosacral osteopathy are therapies that can bring relief.

Nutrients

Coenzyme Q_{10}—50 to 100 mg, reduces symptoms.

Vitamin C—100 to 300 mg, if deficient, more effective when taken with bioflavonoids.

Bioflavonoids—300 mg, as effective as vitamin C.

Calcium—500 mg twice daily, reduces bleeding and inflammation, helps loose teeth.

Folic acid—0.1% solution as mouthwash, rinse for 1 to 5 minutes, reduces inflammation and bleeding.

Carotenoid complex—safer than vitamin A with equal effectiveness; deficiency can cause plaque formation and infection.

Zinc—60 mg if deficient; severity of gum disease associated with low zinc levels; can be used as mouthwash, 5% zinc solution, twice daily.

Vitamin E—400 to 800 IU, beneficial for severe peridontal disease.

Foods

Whole foods

Whole grains

Fresh vegetables

Dark green leafy vegetables

Fresh fruits

Citrus fruits

Dark berries

Grapes

Peanuts

Low-fat dairy

Fish

Juices

Carrot

Cantaloupe

Citrus

Dark berries

Herbal therapy

Chamomile, echinacea, or myrrh—tincture or infusion as mouthwash, have anti-inflammatory and antibacterial properties.

Goldenseal—as mouthwash, has antibacterial properties.

Aloe vera—gel, mix 1 T in water as mouthwash or apply directly to sore gums; soothes inflammation and heals tissues.

Green tea—200 to 300 mg extract twice daily or several cups of tea drunk throughout day, contains flavonoids and has polyphenol content, inhibits plaque formation.

Homeopathy

Take remedy according to symptoms:

Calendula

Chamomilla

Kreosotum

Mercurius solubilis

Natrum muriaticum

Phosphorus

Silicea

For abcesses:

Belladonna

Hepar sulfuris

Mercurius solubilis

Silicea

Aromatherapy

Niaouli—rub into gums, an antiseptic, reduces inflammation; use as floss to cleanse between teeth.

Myrrh—as mouthwash, has anti-inflammatory properties.

Peppermint, anise, thyme or sage—a few drops in glass of water as a disinfectant mouthwash.

Ayurvedic medicine

Coconut oil, goldenseal, or myrrh—massage bleeding gums.

Amla—5 g powder in one cup water daily.

Chinese medicine

Acupuncture—effective treatment for gingivitis.

Gout

Gout is a painful condition affecting the joints, especially in the toes, and is caused by the deposition of urate crystals. There is either an overproduction of uric acid or an inefficiency in eliminating it from the body. The acidic compound results from the breakdown of proteins, specifically purines. Foods that are high in purines should be restricted or avoided in the diet; they include organ meats, meats, sardines, mackerel, anchovies, herring, chicken, dried beans and peas, turkey, shellfish, and yeast. Caffeine can raise uric acid levels; limiting alcohol consumption can reduce the number of attacks. Drinking a lot of water aids the excretion of uric acid. Being overweight exacerbates the condition and a slow weight-loss program should be followed.

Nutrients

Vitamin C—500 to 1000 mg in divided doses, increases excretion of uric acid; amounts of 3 g may increase uric acid production in some individuals.

Quercetin—200 to 400 mg between meals, inhibits the enzyme xanthine oxidase from producing uric acid, has anti-inflammatory properties.

Foods

Fresh fruits

Cherries

Strawberries

Dark berries

Pineapple

Avocado

Fresh vegetables

Celery

Asparagus

Dandelion greens

Whole grains

Ginger

Turmeric

Garlic

Cayenne

Juices

Beet

Cabbage

Carrot

Celery

Cherry

Cucumber

Dark berry

Watermelon

Herbal therapy

Devil's claw—1 to 2 g dried powdered root three times daily or 4 to 5 ml tincture three times daily, relieves joint pain and reduces uric acid levels.

Celery seed—extract, 2 to 4 tablets daily, reduces uric acid levels.

Chiso—contains xanthine oxidase inhibitors that help prevent synthesis of uric acid.[45]

Feverfew, turmeric—have anti-inflammatory properties.

Cayenne—reduces pain.

White willow bark—relieves pain, a precursor of aspirin.

Homeopathy

Take remedy according to symptoms:

Arnica montana

Belladonna

Berberis vulgaris

Bryonia

Calcarea fluorica

Colchicum autumnale

Ledum palustre

Lycopodium

Pulsatilla

Rhododendron

Rhus toxicodendron

Sulfur

Urtica

Aromatherapy

Rosemary, chamomile—mix in carrier oil and massage; place several drops in warm water and soak affected area.

Lavender, frankincense—mix with carrier oil and massage affected area.

Ayurvedic medicine

Consult a qualified practitioner.

Chinese medicine

Cinnamon

Aconite root

Angelica root

Wild ginger

Acupuncture

Bodywork

Deep tissue massage

Reflexology

Mindbody therapy

Meditation

Yoga

Imagery

Headache

Most headaches, characterized by a dull pain, are tension or stress related. Other sources may be a musculoskeletal problem in the upper back and neck that can be helped with craniosacral therapy by an osteopath; or pressure from the sinuses. A headache on awakening may be an indication of high blood pressure. About 10% of headaches are called *migraines*—throbbing in nature, genetic in origin, they are the result of constriction and dilation of blood vessels in the brain. Severe headaches that appear suddenly or that increase in severity may be caused by an underlying condition and should be checked by a physician.

Allergies, especially to certain foods, and food sensitivies are suspected of being the major causes of migraines, in children as well as adults. The effect from the allergen may not be felt for days following ingestion. Hormonal fluctuations and stress can also be factors in the illness. Migraines will usually appear when there are simultaneous triggers or when there is an excess of one, such as eating too much of an allergic food.

Foods contain elements that effect changes in the blood vessels which precipitate migraines in predisposed individuals. These compounds are found in foods such as cow's milk, chocolate, red wine and other alcoholic beverages, aged and hard cheeses, citrus fruits, cured meats and fish, yeast products, nuts, figs, dates, raisins, onions, aspartame, MSG, and caffeine. Smoking and birth control pills can contribute to headaches. Saturated fats contain chemicals that stimulate the production of substances that can cause migraines.

Nutrients

5-HTP—200 to 600 mg, increases serotonin and endorphin levels which are pain killers, from an herbal plant, as effective as pharmaceuticals for migraines without the side effects, most effective when taken for longer periods of time. Headache sufferers often have low serotonin levels.

Vitamin B_2—400 mg, may relieve symptoms.

Magnesium—350 mg, may relieve and reduce migraines especially in young women and individuals with low tissue or low ionized magnesium serum levels, take with vitamin B_6, 50 mg, which increases intracellular accumulation of magnesium; intravenous injection, 1 to 3 g, is effective for acute migraine and cluster and tension headaches.

Calcium—800 mg, may relieve symptoms, take with vitamin D.

Vitamin D—400 IU

SAMe—may relieve symptoms.

Evening primrose oil—6 to 8 capsules, has anti-inflammatory properties, relieves pain.

Foods

Whole organic foods

Fresh fruits

Fresh vegetables

Onions

Whole grains

Rye

Legumes

Soybeans

Fatty fish

Salmon

Mackerel

Sardines

Albacore tuna

Black sesame seeds

Basil

Cilantro

Garlic

Ginger
Turmeric
Cayenne

Juices

Beet
Carrot
Celery
Cucumber
Parsley
Spinach
Watercress

Herbal therapy

Feverfew—125 mg leaf extract or 50 mg freeze-dried capsules daily, taken consistently can prevent or decrease frequency of migraines.[46]

Ginger—⅓ tsp powdered four times a day, or 2 to 3 ml tincture three times a day or 2½ tsp fresh, prevents and alleviates pain and inflammation, blocks prostaglandin synthesis in the same way aspirin does.[47]

Gingko biloba—increases blood circulation to the brain.

Willow bark, lemon balm aka melissa—relieves pain.

Homeopathy

Take according to symptoms:
Aconite
Apis
Belladonna
Bryonia
Cimicifuga
Cyclamen
Gelsemium
Hypericum
Ignatia amara
Iris versicolor
Kali bichromicum
Lachesis
Natrum muriaticum

Nux vomica
Pulsatilla
Ruta
Sanguinaria canadensis
Sepia
Silicea
Spigelia

Aromatherapy

Melissa, mandarin petitgrain, Roman chamomile, lemon verbena, ylang ylang, clary sage—any one or combination as massage oil; acts on the central nervous system calming nerves, dilating blood vessels, and lowering blood pressure.

Ayurvedic medicine

Brahmi—an herbal preparation.
Asnayilwadi thaila oil—use externally, can help relieve headaches.

Chinese medicine

Ginger
Ginseng
Acupuncture

Chiropractic

Consult a qualified practitioner.

Bodywork

Deep tissue massage
Movement therapies
Shiatsu
Polarity therapy
Reflexology

Mindbody therapy

Meditation
Yoga—relieves tension and stress.
Biofeedback—improves control over autonomic body functions specifically tension and the dilation of blood vessels.
Imagery

Heart Attack

A common predictor of heart attack is *angina,* a pain in the chest usually experienced upon exertion or after eating. The pain occurs because there is not sufficient blood reaching the heart due to atherosclerosis or a narrowing of the arteries. The actual cause of most heart attacks is the formation of a blood clot in a coronary artery that has been narrowed by atherosclerosis. The clot blocks the supply of blood carried by the artery and that portion of the heart subsequently dies.

What happens mechanically at the time of death from a heart attack is *ventricular fibrillation,* an erratic heartbeat that interrupts delivery of oxygenated blood to the brain. The determining factor of whether the death of a portion of the heart muscle actually results in the whole heart expiring may depend on the condition of the autonomic nervous system that governs involuntary actions like breathing, digestion, and heartbeat. If the autonomic nervous system is in sympathetic mode, which has a contractility effect, as opposed to the parasympathetic, which is relaxing, fibrillation is more likely to happen. In some cases, death from heart attack is due to an *artery spasm.* Artery spasms occur when the sympathetic nervous system is dominant and the adrenals are overactive. Heart *arrythmias* or irregular heartbeats can be the result of an activated sympathetic system as well.

Genetic predisposition can play a role in heart disease but no matter what condition the arteries are in, heart disease can be halted and reversed through changes in diet and lifestyle. Stress not only raises serum cholesterol but increases the activity of the sympathetic nervous system and the adrenal glands. Smoking affects the sympathetic nervous system in the same way and damages the arteries by constricting the blood vessels, which inhibits blood circulation and the oxygenation of tissues. Excessive caffeine puts the sympathetic system and the adrenals into overdrive and should be avoided in sensitive individuals, or limited to two cups daily. Obesity puts added strain on heart muscles and high blood pressure stresses the arteries.

The diet should include the right kinds of fat and other foods to keep the arteries from developing atherosclerosis and to dissolve any plaque that has already formed. Omega-3 fats, found in fatty deep cold-water fish and in some vegetable sources, the highest concentrations being in walnuts, flaxseed, rapeseed (source of canola oil), and purslane, a green leafy vegetable, inhibit blood clotting, encourage activity of the parasympathetic nervous system, increase blood flow, protect against heart arrythmias, dissolve clots, lower blood triglycerides, raise HDL cholesterol, and have anti-inflammatory properties. Antioxidants and other compounds found in fruits and vegetables prevent plaque from building up on the arterial walls, reduce blood pressure, and strengthen heart muscles. Excellent blood thinners that prevent clotting are the omega-3 fatty acids, vitamin E, and garlic, onions, and cayenne. Exercise is vitally important in maintaining the integrity of the arteries and heart muscles as well as facilitating the circulation of oxygenated blood.

Nutrients

Vitamin E—400 to 800 IU with mixed tocopherols, an antioxidant and blood thinner.

Vitamin C, bioflavonoids—500 to 100 mg in divided doses, aid tissue elasticity and arterial integrity.

Flaxseed oil—1 T, an omega-3 fatty acid.

Coenzyme Q_{10}—60 mg three times daily, improves oxygen utilization at the cellular level, allows exercise to be performed without problems.[48]

Carnitine—1 g twice daily, an amino acid, aids heart muscle metabolism[49] and the transport of fats.

Arginine—an amino acid, stimulates dilation of blood vessels; enables exercise after angina; reduces platelet aggregation.[50]

Bromelain—a blood thinner and anti-inflammatory, decreases pain from angina; derived from pineapple.

Foods

Fatty fish

Salmon

Mackerel

Sardines
Herring
Albacore tuna
Anchovies
Sea bass
Fresh fruits
Apple
Pineapple
Fresh vegetables
Green leafy vegetables
Spinach
Asparagus
Carrots
Shiitake mushrooms
Oyster mushrooms
Onions
Nuts
Brazil nuts
Walnuts
Seeds
Whole grains
Brown rice
Corn
Legumes
Soybeans
Soymilk
Peanuts
Garlic
Cayenne
Ginger
Turmeric
Extra virgin olive oil
Cold pressed organic canola oil
Ground flaxseeds—1 to 2 T.

Juices

Beet
Carrot
Celery
Cucumber

Dark berries
Grapes
Pineapple
Tomato

Herbal therapy

Hawthorne—1 tsp tincture in warm water four times daily or 1 to 2 capsules freeze-dried extract four times daily, increases blood flow, contains anthocyanidins which strengthen and protect blood vessels from damage; improves heart function.[51]

Gingko biloba—improves circulation.

Ginseng—lowers cholesterol, normalizes blood pressure.

Motherwort—prevents palpitations.

Cayenne—a blood thinner.

Garlic—an antioxidant, helps dissolve clots, lowers cholesterol and blood pressure.

Ginger—lowers cholesterol.

Turmeric—lowers cholesterol.

Homeopathy

As preventive—Cactus and Crataegus, act on heart muscle, arteries, blood pressure, and circulation.

Take remedy according to symptoms:
Aconitum napellus
Arnica montana
Cactus grandiflorus
Digitalis
Glonoinum
Lachesis lanceolatus
Latrodectus mactans
Lilium
Naja
Oxalicum acidum
Rhus toxicodendron

Aromatherapy

Ylang Ylang—massage, for heart palpitations; a relaxant.

Lavender, peppermint, rosemary—strengthen heart muscle.

Ayurvedic medicine

Treatments prescribed are effective in treating heart disease.

Guggul—reduces cholesterol.

Chinese medicine

Herbal preparations prescribed are effective in treating heart disease.

Tree ear—mushroom available in dried form, has anticoagulant effect.

Kudzu—for angina.

Acupuncture

Chiropractic

Improves cardiovascular function.

Bodywork

Massage

Shiatsu

Movement therapies

Qigong—lowers blood pressure.

T'ai chi

Reflexology—reduces high blood pressure.

Mindbody therapy

Meditation

Biofeedback—regulates autonomic nervous system.

Imagery

Hypnotherapy—modifies pain and anxiety.

Heartburn

Heartburn or acid reflux occurs when hydrochloric acid and pepsin from the stomach seep into the lower part of the esophagus, irritating the lining which is not suited for the strong acids. Sometimes the pain is mistaken for a heart attack. Acids are allowed to pass into the esophagus because of the relaxation of the esophageal sphincter, a small ring-shaped muscle that opens to let food into the stomach but closes tightly to keep contents in. This muscle can become weakened. A *hiatal hernia* can develop in this area, which also causes acid reflux.

Eating too fast or too much puts pressure on the sphincter muscle, weakening it, as does too much body weight. Eating the wrong foods or food combinations can cause heartburn. Foods that can act as muscle relaxants causing the sphincter muscle to open inappropriately are chocolate, fatty foods, and alcohol. Foods that increase the acidity of the stomach are coffee, beer, milk, and colas. Coffee, citrus foods, hot spicy foods, and tomatoes can irritate an already sensitive esophagus. Anxiety and stress can interfere with digestion. It is best to eat 3 hours before lying down. Lying on the left side eases symptoms because the esophagus enters the stomach on the right. Drinking water at the first sign of pain can dilute irritating acids.

Foods

Fresh fruits

Pineapple

Papaya

Kiwi

Fresh vegetables

Parsley

Ginger

Garlic

Fennel

Dill

Juices

Carrot

Celery

Herbal therapy

Chamomile—3 to 4 cups daily between meals, soothes inflamed and irritated mucous membranes of the digestive tract.

Peppermint—relieves heartburn.

Licorice—two tablets or ⅛ tsp powder of DGL (an active component) extract before or between meals, reduces production of stomach acid;[52] protects and soothes lining of the stomach and duodenum.

Gentian—take 30 minutes before meals, relieves or prevents heartburn.

Aloe vera—gel, soothes stomach membranes.

Homeopathy

Take remedy according to symptoms:

Ammonium carbonicum

Conium maculatum

Kali carbonicum

Lobelia

Natrum phosphoricum

Sulfur

Chinese medicine

Acupuncture

Chiropractic

Manipulation of the lower thoracic area of the spine clearing blood and nerve pathways to digestive organs.

Bodywork

Massage

Qigong—relieves stress.

T'ai chi

Reflexology

Mindbody therapy

Yoga

Biofeedback

Hemorrhoids

Hemorrhoids are distended, enlarged veins around the anus, internally or externally. Repeated straining causes them to swell, itch, and become painful. If they rupture, they bleed a bright red. Pregnancy, sitting or standing for long periods, constipation, diarrhea, weak veins, heavy lifting, and irritating foods like coffee, alcohol, and hot spices can cause the condition. A sitz bath, sitting in warm tub water for 15 minutes several times a day, is helpful.

Nutrients

Vitamin C, bioflavonoids—500 to 1000 mg in divided doses, strengthen capillary walls.

Foods

Whole foods

Whole grains

Buckwheat

Fresh fruits

Citrus fruits

Blackberries

Blueberries

Cherries

Persimmons

Fresh vegetables

Dark green leafy vegetables

Purslane

Legumes

Lentils

Juices

Carrot

Celery

Parsley

Spinach

Watercress

Herbal therapy

Witch hazel—use as compress, an astringent, eases itching and soothes irritation.

Aloe vera—apply directly to area, an astringent, contains healing properties.

Butcher's broom—100 mg three times daily, contains chemicals called ruscogenins which are anti-inflammatory and have a tightening effect on blood vessels; prevents hemorrhoids from developing.

Calendula—salve, apply topically, eases pain and itching.

Goldenseal, bayberry, yarrow, spearmint, or mullein—tea, ease itching and irritation.

Pilewort aka collinsonia—tea or apply topically.

Homeopathy

Take remedy according to symptoms:

Aesculus hippocastanum

Aloe socotrina

Arnica montana

Berberis vulgaris

Calcarea fluorica

Graphites

Hamamelis virginiana

Ignatia amara

Nux vomica

Pulsatilla

Ratanhia

Sepia

Sulfur

Aromatherapy

Niaouli—apply topically, tightens tissues. *Do not use during pregnancy; has estrogenlike compounds.*

Cypress, juniper, lavender, lemon, or rosemary—mix in carrier oil and apply topically.

Ayurvedic medicine

Preparation available in health food stores.

Aloe vera—as juice, drink ½ cup three times daily.

Triphala guggulu—200 mg twice daily after meals.

Abhayarishta

Dadimadi ghritha

Chinese medicine

Acupuncture

Bodywork

Qigong
Reflexology

Mindbody therapy

Yoga
Imagery

Hepatitis

Hepatitis can be acute and short in duration or chronic and long-lasting. Liver cells are either inflamed and damaged or they die, leaving a malfunctioning liver. Viruses are the most common cause of hepatitis, indicated by alphabetical letters; other causes are alcohol, exposure to industrial chemicals, fumes, and drugs, recreational or pharmaceutical, including acetaminophens like Tylenol. Symptoms include fatigue, fever, nausea, vomiting, loss of appetite, and possibly dark urine and a yellowing of the skin called *jaundice*. *Hepatitis A* can be transmitted by poor hygiene and through food. *Hepatitis B* and *C* are transmitted by sexual contact and blood.

The objective of treatment for any liver disease including *cirrhosis* is allowing the liver to regenerate itself as it is an organ that has great capability to do so. To minimize stress on the liver, the diet should be low in protein and fat and contain plenty of fresh fruits and vegetables. Drink lots of water and take specific herbs that have been shown to contain protective and regenerative properties. Alcohol, tobacco, and most drugs are metabolized by the liver and should be avoided. Getting sufficient rest is important and taking steam baths or saunas will help in the detoxification process.

Nutrients

Phosphatidyl choline—3 g, reduces liver damage.[53]

Thymus extracts—200 mg three times daily crude extracts or 40 mg purified proteins three times daily, helps repair liver damage and increase immune cell numbers.[54] *Take only under the supervision of a physician.*

Catechin—500 to 750 mg three times daily; can improve viral hepatitis; a bioflavonoid.

Vitamin C—2 g, may prevent infective hepatitis during blood transfusions and treat viral hepatitis; for acute cases, 50 to 100 g intravenously daily.

Bioflavonoids—work synergistically with vitamin C.

Vitamin E—1200 IU with mixed tocopherols, can repair liver damage.

Beta-carotene

Vitamin B complex

Foods

Fresh fruits

Grapes

Grapefruit

Plums

Fresh vegetables

Dandelion greens

Enoki mushrooms

Water chestnuts

Whole grains

Barley

Legumes

Low-fat yogurt

Ginger

Turmeric

Garlic

Coriander

Juices

Beet

Carrot

Wheatgrass

Fruits

Vegetables

Herbal therapy

Dandelion—tea, capsules, or tinctures, detoxifies and rejuvenates liver cells.

Milk thistle—extract, regenerates and protects liver cells from injury;[55] silymarin, a flavonoid, is the active compound; treatment should contain 140 to 210 mg silymarin three times daily.

Licorice—1 to 2 g powdered root or 2 to 4 ml extract three times daily, protects liver cells from injury.

Homeopathy

Take remedy according to symptoms:

Bryonia

Chelidonium

Hydrastis

Lachesis

Lycopodium

Magnesia muriatica

Mercurius

Natrum sulphuricum

Nux vomica

Phosphorus

Sulfur

Aromatherapy

Thyme (thujanol type)—regenerates liver cells.

Peppermint—regenerates the liver.

Greenland moss—detoxifies and regenerates the liver.

Carrot seed—stimulates regeneration of liver cells due it its sesquiterpene alcohol carotol (50%) content.

Basil—for viral hepatitis.

Clove—dilute 1 drop to 20 ml solution, has antiviral and antibacterial properties; external use only.

Ayurvedic medicine

Treatments prescribed are effective for acute and chronic hepatitis.

Aloe gel, shatavari, Chyavan prush—for chronic hepatitis.

Kutki 200 mg, guduchi 300 mg, shanka pushpi 400 mg—take two times daily after meals, for hepatitis B.

Chinese medicine

Schisandra—extract or berries, contains ligands that regenerate liver tissues.

Gardenia fruit, oriental wormwood—for hepatitis A.

Ginseng, peony root, mulberry, licorice, astragalus—for hepatitis B.

Bodywork

Qigong

Mindbody therapy

Imagery

Herpes

The herpes simplex virus causes sores in and outside of the mouth, in the genital areas, as well as other parts of the body. A sign of eruption is a tingling sensation followed by blisters that eventually crust over and disappear. The virus lives in nerve cells, protected from immune-system defenses, and remains dormant most of the time for life. The virus is contracted by skin to skin contact. Triggers that can cause an outbreak are fatigue, viral infections, sunlight, menstruation, and stress. In some people, foods high in the amino acid arginine can bring about an eruption; the highest amounts are found in chocolate, nuts, and gelatin. To test for sensitivity to arginine, eat a handful of nuts or chocolate and see if there is a reaction overnight.

Shingles or herpes zoster, which is the same virus that causes chicken pox, is characterized by a painful rash usually on one side of the body. Nerve pain, called *postherpetic neuralgia,* may persist after the rash has disappeared and can be helped by 1200 to 1600 IU vitamin E orally and 30 IU applied topically; and by intramuscular injections of Vitamin B_{12}. Intramuscular injections of 100 mg three times weekly of adenosine monophosphate, a naturally occurring compound in the body, can accelerate healing of shingles, reduce pain, and may prevent postherpetic neuralgia. Capsaicin containing cream from red pepper applied topically can help relieve pain.

Nutrients

Lysine—500 mg, twice daily, reduces symptoms and recurrence.

Vitamin E—apply topically, reduces pain.

Zinc sulfate—0.025% solution, apply topically three times daily, dries blisters and prevents viral replication.

Vitamin C and bioflavonoids—600 mg three times daily, reduce blister formation and symptoms, take at first sign of appearance.

Foods

Fish

Chicken

Turkey

Eggs

Low-fat dairy

Fresh fruits

Fresh vegetables

Dandelion greens

Dulse

Potatoes

Rye

Legumes

Cayenne

Garlic

Juices

Beet

Apple

Carrot

Celery

Cranberry

Grape

Pear

Prune

Strawberry

Herbal therapy

Tea tree oil—has antiviral properties, dries up blisters, and reduces recurrence.

Melissa aka lemon balm—infusion or cream, apply topically several times daily, speeds healing.

Echinacea—tincture three times daily, has antiviral properties, supports immune system.

St. John's wort—cream or infusion, contains hypericin which has antiviral activity.

Licorice—glycyrrhizin-containing gel, apply three to four times daily, inhibits viral replication; also helpful for shingles.

Homeopathy

Take remedy according to symptoms:

Apis mellifica

Arsenicum album

Borax

Dulcamara

Graphites

Hepar sulphuris calcareum

Mercurius solubilis

Natrum muriaticum

Petroleum

Rhus toxicodendron

Sepia

Aromatherapy

Melissa—contains antiviral components, dries up blisters.

Tea tree—has antiviral properties, dries up blisters and reduces recurrence.

Geranium 1 part, melissa 1 part, lavender 1 part, tea tree 10 parts—apply to lesions three times daily.

Ayurvedic medicine

Shatavari 500 mg, guwelsattva 200 mg, kamadudha 200 mg, neem 300 mg—mix and take 2 tsp twice daily.

Tikta ghee—apply topically.

Chinese medicine

Acupuncture—relieves pain.

Mindbody therapy

Meditation—reduces stress.

Biofeedback

Imagery

Hypertension—High Blood Pressure

When pressure exerted by blood on the walls of the arteries is greater than normal, blood pressure rises. Usually, blood pressure falls when at rest. It rises in response to strenuous physical activity, stress, or a perceived danger in which the sympathetic nervous system dominates, arteries constrict, and more blood is sent to the brain increasing blood pressure. This heightened state of the sympathetic system does not seem to retreat in individuals with hypertension and damage to the heart, kidney, arteries, and other organs becomes inevitable.

Blood pressure is considered high at a reading of 140/90. There are no symptoms of the illness and it is recommended individuals over 40 be checked. Hypertension can be controlled by permanent diet and lifestyle changes; this includes reducing stress, maintaining proper weight (not more than 5 lb overweight), and eating foods containing compounds that reduce blood pressure such as celery, garlic, and fresh fruits and vegetables. Having a home monitor is helpful. Smoking, alcohol, refined sugar, food allergies, and high-sodium foods can contribute to hypertension. Some people may need extra calcium to stabilize blood pressure. Some individuals are salt sensitive which causes a rise in their blood pressure. Daily exercises and various stress reduction techniques lower systolic and diastolic blood pressure.

Nutrients

Calcium—800 to 1000 mg in citrate form, lowers blood pressure, especially effective in salt sensitive individuals.

Magnesium—350 mg, lowers blood pressure, especially in individuals taking potassium depleting diuretics.

Coenzyme Q_{10}—50 mg twice daily, significantly reduces blood pressure.[56]

Selenium—may be especially beneficial for women at risk of hypertension.

Vitamin C—1 g, may be helpful in reducing blood pressure.

Taurine—6 g, may lower blood pressure by reducing adrenaline levels.

Arginine—2 g three times daily, may help in reducing blood pressure.

Foods

Fresh fruits—contain potassium which lowers blood pressure

Banana

Melons

Citrus fruits

Fresh vegetables

Green leafy vegetables

Dandelion greens

Kelp

Arame

Potatoes

Celery

Tomatoes

Onions

Fatty fish

Salmon

Albacore tuna

Anchovies

Sardines

Mackerel

Herring

Seafood

Whole grains

Legumes

Lentils

Soymilk

Nuts

Low-fat dairy products

Extra virgin olive oil

Garlic

Oregano

Black pepper

Ginger

Basil

Tarragon

Saffron

Cayenne

Juices

Beet

Carrot

Celery

Cucumber

Parsley

Spinach

Herbal therapy

Garlic—600 to 900 mg extract, prevents and reduces blood pressure; eat one raw clove daily.

Hawthorne—100 to 250 mg extract three times daily, normalizes blood pressure.

Homeopathy

Take remedy according to symptoms:

Argentum nitricum

Aurum metallicum

Belladonna

Calcarea carbonica

Glonoinum

Lachesis

Natrum muriaticum

Nux vomica

Phosphorus

Plumbum

Sanguinaria canadensis

Aromatherapy

Marjoram, lavender, geranium, sandalwood, rose, clary sage—reduce blood pressure by relaxing tension.

Ayurvedic medicine

Treatments are given according to metabolic type.

Convolvolus pluricaulis

Ashwaganda

Respirine—an extract from rauwolfia, *use only under the supervision of a physician.*

Chinese medicine

Herbal treatments prescribed are effective in reducing blood pressure.

Acupuncture

Chiropractic

Consult a qualified practitioner.

Bodywork

Massage

Deep tissue manipulation

Shiatsu

Movement therapies

Qigong—lowers blood pressure.

T'ai chi—improves heart rate and blood pressure.

Reflexology

Mindbody therapy

Meditation—reduces blood pressure.

Yoga—relaxes autonomic nervous system.

Biofeedback—learn to monitor blood pressure and recognize relaxed state, controlling sympathetic nervous system.

Imagery—reduces stress and heart rate.

Hypnotherapy—decreases blood pressure by affecting the sympathetic nervous system.

Infection

Whether microorganisms, usually viral or bacterial, cause infection depends on the condition of the *immune system* which is made up of the lymph nodes, thymus gland, bone marrow, spleen, tonsils, appendix, and white blood cells. Swollen lymph nodes, night sweats, and fevers of unknown origin may indicate a hidden infection, and a physician should be consulted. Infection of the gums is often not evident so dental checkups and good oral hygiene are important.

Although genetics and stress play a role, diet has a great influence on the strength of the immune system. Certain components in food increase the potency and concentration of white bloods cells that are the body's primary line of defense against foreign elements. White blood cells, which search and destroy bacteria, viruses and even cancer tumors, include T-cells that produce the chemicals interferon and interleukin, B-cells that produce antibodies, and cells called natural killer cells.

Immune suppressors are an excess of saturated fats, polyunsaturated fats such as safflower, sunflower, corn, and soybean oils, which are often used in cooking and found in many processed foods, and refined sugar, all of which inhibit the activity of white blood cells. Carotenoids and antioxidants in fruits and vegetables, garlic, and yogurt (must contain live cultures) are major immune boosters by, for example, enhancing the potency of T-cells and increasing the blood concentration of natural killer cells and the production of antibodies.

Tonsilitis is an infection of the tonsils which are part of the immune system. At the first sign of the illness, gargle with one-half warm water and one-half hydrogen peroxide four times daily as a disinfectant. Follow herbal remedies and diet for infections, especially using garlic and echinacea.

Inflammations are a normal response of the body to infection. The immune, hormone, and circulatory systems begin working to heal the affected area. Hormones called prostaglandins respond to inflammations. Prostaglandins are made from fatty acids and some of them can exacerbate the inflammation while others can reduce it. Polyunsaturated and trans-fatty acids stiumlate production of inflammatory prostaglandins. Gamma linolenic acids (GLA) found in black currant, borage, and evening primrose oils, and in fatty fish, produce anti-inflammatory prostaglandins. Ginger, turmeric, and the herb boswellia are also anti-inflammatories.

To heal *wounds* before infection sets in, the nutrients vitamin A, vitamin C (1 to 3 g), zinc (150 mg), vitamin E, vitamin B complex, and bromelain (from pineapple) are beneficial. Herbal anti-inflammatories are calendula, St. John's wort, and chamomile. Apply topically comfrey, witch hazel, horsetail, or aloe vera.

Nutrients

Vitamin A—a deficiency creates environment for infection.

Beta carotene—25,000 to 100,000 IU, can be taken instead of vitamin A.

Vitamin C—1 to 3 g, has antiviral properties, can reduce symptoms and length of infection.

Bioflavonoids—1 g in divided doses, work synergistically with vitamin C.

Vitamin E—200 IU with mixed tocopherols, enhances immune cell activity.

Zinc—15 to 25 mg, aids the production of antibodies and T-cells; especially helpful for recurrent infections.

Multivitamin and mineral—for the elderly.

Propolis—tincture, apply topically and take orally, product from bees, an antiseptic and has healing properties.

Foods

Fresh fruits

Figs

Plums

Fresh vegetables

Spinach

Cabbage

Carrots

Kale

Maitake mushrooms

Enoki mushrooms

Shiitake mushrooms

Onions

Water chestnuts

Sweet potatoes

Pumpkin

Low-fat yogurt

Fatty fish

Salmon

Albacore tuna

Herring

Sardines

Mackerel

Seafood

Shellfish

Oysters

Raw honey

Extra virgin olive oil

Cold pressed organic canola oil

Cold pressed flaxseed oil

Ginger

Raw garlic

Dill

Horseradish

Basil

Ground flaxseeds—1 to 2 T

Juices

Apple

Berry

Carrot

Grape

Orange

Citrus

Fruits

Vegetables

Leafy green vegetables

Herbal therapy

Echinacea—0.5 to 1 g dried root or 2 to 4 ml tincture or extract three times daily, boosts the immune system.

Astragalus—1 to 2 g dried root or 2 to 4 ml tincture or extract three times daily, elevates antibody levels.

Pau d'arco—has antifungal properties.

Goldenseal—has antibacterial properties.

Juniper, melissa, eucalyptus, licorice—have antiviral properties.

Homeopathy

Take remedy according to symptoms:

Aconitum napellus

Belladonna

Bryonia

Calcarea carbonica

Calendula

Ferrum phosphoricum

Graphites

Hepar sulphuris calcareum

Mercurius solubilis

Silicea

Sulfur

Aromatherapy

Tea tree, eucalyptus, thyme—massage, have anti-viral properties; stimulates immune system.

Cedarwood—for fungal infections.

Frankincense—strengthens immune system.

Ayurvedic medicine

Ashwagandha—stimulates immune system.

Chinese medicine

Schisandra

Forsythia

Honeysuckle

Acupuncture—stimulation of acupoints supports the immune system.

Bodywork

Qigong—boosts immune system by encouraging flow of qi, reduces stress.

T'ai chi

Reflexology

Mindbody therapy

Biofeedback—reduces stress.

Imagery

Insomnia

Insomnia may be caused by anxiety, stress, depression, too much caffeine, overeating, numerous health conditions, and the use of stimulating drugs. Food allergies can cause insomnia and *narcolepsy,* a condition in which an individual falls asleep suddenly, at any time, and anywhere. Eating carbohydrates 30 minutes before bedtime increases production of serotonin, a neurotransmitter that can reduce anxiety and promote sleep. For some individuals, warm milk has a sedative effect. As we age, the body requires less sleep. Natural progesterone may be helpful for PMS and menopause-related sleeplessness as a hormone imbalance can cause irritability and sleep disturbances. Exercise in the late afternoon or early evening can promote better sleep. Melatonin is only effective if there is a deficiency or body levels are low.

Restless leg syndrome and *sleep apnea,* a condition in which there is intermittent cessation of breathing during sleep that may be caused by a problem in the central nervous system affecting the diaphragm or a blockage in the upper airway, can benefit by weight loss if overweight and by regular exercise. Caffeine, drugs, and alcohol should be avoided and stress reduced. Food allergies or a deficiency of iron or folic acid may be a factor in restless leg syndrome; taking 200 to 800 IU vitamin E can alleviate symptoms of the condition by increasing blood circulation to the legs; 80 mg gingko biloba extract three times daily may be beneficial. Rhus toxicodendron or causticum are homeopathic remedies that can be beneficial for restless leg syndrome; and for sleep apnea, lachesis, or homeopathic opium.

Nutrients

Calcium—600 to 1000 mg, take with magnesium in the gluconate, chelate, or citrate forms for best absorption 45 minutes before bedtime, a neuromuscular relaxant.

Magnesium—250 to 400 mg, take with calcium.

5-HTP—100 to 300 mg, take near bedtime preferably with a carbohydrate such as fruit or juice, decreases time to fall asleep, decreases awakenings, increases REM and deep sleep, more effective than tryptophan, from an herbal plant.

Foods

Fresh fruits

Bananas

Figs

Dates

Fresh vegetables

Lettuce

Whole grains

Legumes

Peanuts

Walnuts

Cashews

Almonds

Sunflower seeds

Turkey

Low-fat milk

Low-fat yogurt

Fatty fish

Albacore tuna

Salmon

Herring

Sardines

Mackerel

Basil

Juices

Carrot

Celery

Lettuce

Spinach

Herbal therapy

Valerian—150 to 400 mg or 4 to 6 ml tincture or 1 to 2 ml extract, 30 minutes before bedtime, facilitates sleep and induces deep sleep; also effective when taken with melissa (80 mg), also known as lemon balm; is not habit forming, does not produce hangover side effects like drugs and melatonin;[57] *do not take if pregnant or if taking antidepressants or sedatives.*

Hops—2 capsules freeze-dried extract, a sedative and relaxant.

Chamomile, passionflower, skullcap—contain mild sedative properties. Passionflower, 6 to 8 ml tincture, 2 to 4 ml extract, or 300 to 450 mg, can be taken with 5-HTP.

Homeopathy

Take remedy according to symptoms:

Aconitum napellus

Arnica montana

Arsenicum album

Calcarea phosphorica

Chamomilla

Cocculus

Coffea cruda

Ignatia amara

Kali phosphoricum

Lycopodium

Muriaticum acidum

Nux vomica

Pulsatilla

Rhus toxicodendron

Silicea

Sulfur

Zincum metallicum

Aromatherapy

Melissa—a sedative.

Lavender—contains calming properties; inhaling oil can be as effective as tranquilizers.

Bergamot—relieves tension.

Chamomile, jasmine, rose—have a calming effect and alleviate anxiety.

Ayurvedic medicine

Treatments are applied according to metabolic type.

Brahmi—a mild sedative.

Henbane

Chinese medicine

Herbal preparations are prescribed to relieve insomnia.

Hoelen

Fleeceflower stem

Wild jujube

Acupuncture—effective in promoting sleep possibly due to the production of endorphins.

Chiropractic

Consult a qualified practitioner.

Bodywork

Massage

Shiatsu

Qigong

T'ai chi

Polarity therapy

Reflexology

Mindbody therapy

Meditation

Yoga

Biofeedback

Imagery

Hypnotherapy—methods are taught to induce sleep.

Irritable Bowel Syndrome

Irritable bowel syndrome, also known as spastic colon, is a condition in which the intestinal muscles go into spasm. It can be caused by food sensitivities, caffeine, and other stimulants including alcohol, tobacco, and drugs; malabsorption of sugars—the lactose in milk, high fructose content in fruit juices and dried fruit, and sorbitol and xylitol used in dietetic products; or as the result of a bacterial imbalance in the colon.

Symptoms include alternating diarrhea and constipation, distended colon, gas, pain, nausea, and loss of appetite. Stress can exacerbate the condition. The most common food offenders are wheat and corn cereals, dairy, coffee, tea, chocolate, citrus fruits, onions, and potatoes. Eating a high fiber diet is recommended to help alleviate symptoms.

Nutrients

Acidophilus—as liquid, take with meals.

Psyllium seeds—three times daily, regulates bowel activity.

Evening primrose oil—400 mg, prior to and during menstruation.

Foods

Whole grains

Fresh fruits

Fresh vegetables

Legumes

Cilantro

Anise

Ginger

Juices

Carrot

Cabbage

Celery

Parsley

Herbal therapy

Peppermint oil—90 mg or 0.2 to 0.4 ml enteric-coated capsules two or three times daily between meals, to bypass stomach acids, three times daily between meals, reduces symptoms;[58] can be combined with 50 mg caraway seed oil in enteric-coated capsules three times daily.

Chamomile—3 to 5 ml extract three times daily between meals, a carminitive (gas-relieving).

Fennel, wormwood—carminitives.

Slippery elm, marshmallow—soothes lining of digestive tract.

Homeopathy

Asafoetida—3×

Take remedy according to symptoms:

Aloe

Argentum nitricum

Carbo vegetabilis

Colchicum

Colocynthis

Lilium tigrinum

Lycopodiium

Mercurius solubilis

Natrum carbonicum

Nux vomica

Podophyllum

Sulfur

Aromatherapy

Peppermint—1 to 2 drops three or four times daily.

Chamomile, lavender—massage abdomen, have antispasmodic properties.

Ayurvedic medicine

Treatments prescribed are effective in treating the condition.

Coriander

Hollyhock

Pancha karma

Chinese medicine

Rhubarb

Dandelion

Magnolia

Angelica

Bodywork

Acupressure

Qigong

T'ai chi

Mindbody therapy

Meditation

Yoga

Biofeedback

Imagery

Hypnotherapy

Kidney Stones

Kidney stones are hardened crystalized deposits that form from an excess of minerals and oxalates that concentrate in the urine, grow, and can block the flow of urine through the kidneys. Symptoms include pain in the lower back or pelvic area and possibly blood in the urine. It is often a hereditary condition and can also be caused by infection or from medications.

Testing the kind of stones passed determines which foods need to be restricted in the diet. Most often the stones are made up of calcium and oxalates. Excessive calcium excretion may be due to a parathyroid abnormality but is more likely caused by an excess of protein in the diet. It is recommended that daily protein intake from meat, chicken, and fish be limited to 7 or 8 ounces.

Oxalates are found in many foods, but according to a study only a few, other than protein, actually raise urinary oxalate levels—spinach, rhubarb, beet greens, chocolate, tea, wheat bran, nuts, almonds, peanuts, and strawberries.

Calcium should not be restricted in the diet; lower calcium intake actually increases the risk of stone formation. Calcium binds with oxalates in the gut and prevents their absorption and consequently leads to the formation of stones. Sodium stimulates excretion of calcium and should be restricted to 2500 mg daily. Caffeine increases calcium excretion. High sugar drinks and citrus juices are risks for stone formation.

Drinking water throughout the day is very important in keeping the mineral content of the urine in dilution; 16 ounces every 4 hours is recommended. A high fiber diet reduces urinary excretion of calcium; however, some individuals do not absorb calcium well and eating too much fiber can result in an overall calcium deficiency.

Nutrients

Magnesium—200 to 400 mg, in citrate form with meals, lowers risk of stone formation.[59]

Vitamin B_6—10 to 50 mg, reduces elevated urinary oxalates.

Glucosamine sulfate—60 mg, can reduce urinary oxalate levels.

Chondroitin sulfate—60 mg, can reduce urinary oxalate levels.

Foods

Fresh fruits

Avocado

Banana

Cranberries

Black cherries

Kiwi

Fresh vegetables

Green leafy vegetables

Potato

Asparagus

Parsley

Radish

Whole grains

Brown rice

Barley

Oats

Corn

Legumes

Peanuts

Sesame seeds

Cashews

Almonds

Cumin

Coriander

Fennel

Juices

Lemonade—4 oz lemon juice to 2 qt water daily, sweeten lightly

Beet

Carrot

Cranberry

Cucumber

Kiwi

Watermelon

Herbal therapy

Couchgrass, stinging nettle, lovage, horsetail, parsley, Java tea—diuretics, help prevent stone formation.

Khella, gravel root—relaxes the ureters allowing stones to pass.

Homeopathy

Take remedy according to symptoms:

Berberis

Lycopodium

Magnesia phosphorica

Nux vomica

Sarsaparilla

Tabacum

Aromatherapy

Juniper, fennel, geranium, lemon—mix with carrier oil and massage bladder area, add drops to bath.

Ayurvedic medicine

Barley soup with ¼ tsp punarnava three times daily.

Chinese medicine

Ginseng

Water plantain

Cinnamon twigs

Poria

Ephedra

Acupuncture

Bodywork

Acupressure

Qigong—reduces tension, massages kidney, improves circulation.

T'ai chi

Reflexology

Lupus—Systemic Lupus Erythematosus, SLE

Lupus is an autoimmune disease, which means the immune system is confused and attacks the body's own tissues. Damage from lupus may affect the kidneys, lungs, and vascular system. The illness can cause arthritis and is characterized by a red rash, painful and sore joints, weakness, and fatigue. *Discoid lupus erythematosus* is a milder form of the disease.

The type of fat in the diet is important; saturated fats and polyunsaturated fats including sunflower, corn, and safflower oils are inflammatory and can exacerbate the condition. In studies, improvement has been shown when omega-3 fatty acids are included in the diet. Alfalfa seeds and sprouts aggravate the disease and food allergies may precipitate an inflammation.

Nutrients

Flaxseed oil—source of omega-3 fatty acids.

Black currant oil—500 mg twice daily, has anti-inflammatory properties.

Foods

Whole foods

Fatty fish

Sardines

Salmon

Mackerel

Albacore tuna herring

Extra virgin olive oil

Cold pressed organic canola oil

Fresh fruits

Fresh vegetables

Walnuts

Pistachios

Macadamia nuts

Brazil nuts

Pumpkin seeds

Garlic

Ground flaxseeds—1 to 2 T, sprinkle over foods.

Juices

Carrot

Celery

Herbal therapy

Feverfew—for arthritic symptoms.

Ayurvedic medicine

Consult a qualified practitioner.

Chinese medicine

Herbal combinations prescribed are effective in improving lupus.

Bodywork

Deep tissue massage

Qigong

Reflexology

Mindbody therapy

Meditation

Biofeedback

Imagery

Hypnotherapy

Menopause

Menopause is a natural life transition for women and usually occurs between the ages of 45 and 55. Hormonal changes result in a decline of estrogen and some women experience symptoms such as hot flashes, mood swings, and vaginal dryness. These changes may begin 4 to 6 years before the cessation of menstruation.

Certain foods contain plant estrogens that are helpful in balancing hormone levels in the body. Phytoestrogens are similar in structure to estrogen and can alleviate and prevent menopausal symptoms. Soybeans, for example, contain natural estrogens called isoflavones that help prevent osteoporosis, heart disease, and estrogen-related cancers such as breast cancer. In a study, soybeans and flaxseed were tested and found to increase estrogenic activity in postmenopausal women; when they stopped eating the foods, estrogen cell activity also dropped. One cup of soybeans contains 300 mg isoflavones which equals the estrogenic effect in one Premarin (a synthetic hormone) tablet.

For those taking hormone replacements, natural forms are available. It is recommended that the hormone progesterone accompany estrogen.

Low-dose estrogen creams are effective for vaginal dryness. Antihistamines, diuretics, caffeine, and alcohol have a tendency to dry mucous membranes including those in the vagina. Regular exercise reduces hot flashes and other menopausal symptoms.

Nutrients

Vitamin E—800 IU with mixed tocopherols, reduces symptoms; also apply topically for vaginal dryness.

Vitamin C—1 g, take with bioflavonoids.

Bioflavonoids—help to alleviate hot flashes.

Boron—3 mg, increases estrogen blood levels.

Gamma-oryzanol—300 mg, relieves hot flashes and other menopausal symptoms, from rice bran oil.

Foods

Soybeans

Soy milk

Tofu

Soy nuts

Tempeh

Miso

Whole grains

Brown rice

Flaxseeds

Fresh fruits

Apples

Srawberries

Pears

Grapes

Dates

Figs

Pomegranates

Raisins

Peaches

Fresh vegetables

Tomatoes

Asparagus

Broccoli

Beets

Parsley

Legumes

Peanuts

Potatoes

Seeds

Nuts

Almonds

Hazelnuts

Honey

Dill

Cumin

Cinnamon

Coriander

Fennel

Juices

Apple

Beet

Celery

Carrot

Grape

Parsley

Peach

Pear

Spinach

Herbal therapy

Chasteberry aka Vitex—1 to 2 g powdered berries or 4 ml extract three times daily, regulates hormone levels; reduces hot flashes and mood swings.

Black cohosh—1 to 2 g powdered rhizome or 3 to 4 ml extract or 4 to 6 ml tincture twice daily; relieves hot flashes and other menopausal symptoms.

Dong quai—1 to 2 g powdered root, 4 ml tincture, or 1 ml extract three times daily reduces symptoms including hot flashes.

Licorice, red clover—have estrogenic activity; licorice—1 to 2 g powdered root or 4 ml extract three times daily.

Skullcap—reduces anxiety.

Motherwort—for palpitations and anxiety.

Ginkgo biloba—40 mg extract, increases blood flow, helpful for cold hands and feet that often accompanies menopause.

Homeopathy

Take remedy according to symptoms:

Belladonna

Calcarea carbonica

Glonoinum

Graphites

Ignatia amara

Lachesis

Lilium tigrinum

Natrum muriaticum

Pulsatilla

Sepia

Staphysagria

Sulfur

Aromatherapy

Clary sage—has estrogenlike components, eases symptoms.

Rose—stabilizes nervous system, helps irritability and mood swings.

Ylang Ylang—a relaxant.

Ayurvedic medicine

Menopause is a vata imbalance and a natural transition that should not be a cause for disease if doshas are in balance.

Cinnamon—especially effective during menopause.

Calamus root

Celery seeds

Aloe vera—taken internally helps hot flashes, nightsweats, and swelling.

Coriander—acts as a diuretic, has a cooling effect.

Chinese medicine

Herbal preparations prescribed are effective in relieving symptoms.

Shan Zhu Yu, ginseng—for hot flashes and sweating.

Chinese senega—for insomnia, depression, and irritability.

Angelica, peony root, thorowax root—relieve symptoms.

Acupuncture

Bodywork

Acupressure

Qigong—exercises are relaxing and relieve tension.

T'ai chi

Reflexology

Mindbody therapy

Meditation—relieves tension.

Yoga

Menstrual Problems

Dysmenorrhea is a condition of painful menstruation and there are two classifications: primary, which occurs soon after menstruation begins and declines with age and after childbirth; and secondary, which develops later in life and is the result of endometriosis or other pelvic diseases. The development of cramps, when the uterus goes into spasm, is caused by high levels of hormonelike fatty acids called prostaglandins.

Endometriosis develops when cells from the lining of the uterus migrate outside the uterus. These cells still respond to the monthly hormonal cycles and release blood during menses. However, the blood has nowhere to go and so the area becomes inflamed and painful. *Uterine fibroids* are benign muscle tumors produced when estrogen activity is high as they depend on estrogen for growth. They appear in premenopausal women and shrink at menopause and in the absence of estrogen replacement therapy. They do not turn malignant. Birth control pills add to estrogen levels in the body. Symptoms of uterine fibroids include a feeling of fullness, frequent urination, and heavy and cramping menstruation.

Menorrhagia is heavy menstruation and should be tested to determine if there is any underlying condition. If none, there may be an iron deficiency because of excessive blood loss. If deficient, iron supplements help decrease excess blood flow. Vitamin A deficiency, intrauterine devices, and hypothyroidism are other possible causes of the condition.

Amenorrhea is irregular or absent menstruation. A major cause is too little fat in the diet. Estrogen regulates the menstrual cycle, and the hormone is partly made from fat and cholesterol, so sufficient fat is needed to keep menses on a regular schedule. Extra virgin olive oil is a good source of the right kind of fat. Fluid retention is a normal and benign reaction to the hormonal activity during the menstrual cycle and can be alleviated by limiting salt intake and getting exercise. It is recommended that saturated fats found in meats, eggs, and full-fat dairy products be limited or avoided in the diet as they are inflammatory and can exacerbate menstrual problems.

Nutrients

Vitamin A—50,000 IU, normalizes blood loss.

Vitamin C—200 mg, take with bioflavonoids three times daily, protects blood vessels and reduces blood loss.

Bioflavonoids—200 mg, work synergistically with vitamin C.

Vitamin E—800 IU with mixed tocopherols, relieves symptoms.

Niacin—200 mg, reduces cramps; take 100 mg every 2 to 3 hours during cramping.

Calcium—800 to 1000 mg, antispasmodic, relieves cramps; take 250 to 500 mg every four hours during cramping.

Magnesium—300 mg, relieves cramps, take with calcium; take 100 mg every 4 hours during cramping.

Pyconogenol—200 mg, from the bioflavonoid group, relieves cramping.

Black currant oil—500 mg, reduces cramping.

Foods

Fatty fish

Salmon

Sardines

Mackerel

Herring

Albacore tuna

Fresh fruits

Pineapple

Berries

Fresh vegetables

Asparagus

Carrots

Eggplant

Whole grains

Ground flaxseeds

Seeds

Nuts

Legumes

Soybeans

Extra virgin olive oil

Cold pressed organic canola oil

Ginger

Basil

Cinnamon

Juices

Fruits

Vegetables

Berries

Pineapple

Herbal therapy

Black cohosh—2 to 4 ml tincture three times daily, eases cramps; take for no longer than 6 months.

Blue cohosh—1 to 2 ml tincture three times daily; eases cramps; also for amenorrhea, uterine fibroids, endometriosis.

Dong quai—eases cramps.

Chasteberry (Vitex)—2 capsules or 40 drops, relieves cramps, balances hormonal system; also for amenorrhea, uterine fibroids, endometriosis.

Crampbark—relieves cramps.

Yarrow—antispasmodic, diuretic, relieves cramps, reduces inflammation; also for menorrhagia, endometriosis.

Uva Ursi—reduces symptoms by constricting blood vessels in the lining of the uterus.

Cinnamon, Shephard's purse—for menorrhagia.

Red clover—contains phytoestrogens that balance hormone levels, relieves cramps.

Strawberry, raspberry—anti-inflammatory, reduce cramps.

Ginger, white willow bark—pain reliever.

Dandelion leaf—diuretic, for fluid retention; also for menorrhagia.

Squaw vine—for menorrhagia.

Homeopathy

Take remedy according to symptoms:

Aconite

Belladonna

Bovista

Caulophyllum thalictroides

Chamomilla

China

Cimicifuga

Cocculus

Colocynthis

Ignatia

Ipecac

Lachesis

Lilium tigrinum

Magnesia phosphorica

Nux vomica

Pulsatilla

Sabina

Sepia

Veratrum album

Aromatherapy

Anise—for amenorrhea, contains estrogenlike properties.

Clary sage—for amenorrhea, has estrogenlike qualities due to the sclareol content.

Roman chamomile—antispasmodic, for cramps.

Rosemary, camphor type—relieves cramps.

Geranium, rose, or cypress—for menorrhagia, massage, or put drops in bath.

Ayurvedic medicine

Treatments given according to metabolic type.

Shatavari, manjistha—in equal portions for menorrhagia.

Aloe vera—can help induce menstruation.

Basil

Caraway—for cramps.

Cedar

Celery seeds—for amenorrhia.

Chinese medicine

Herbal treatments are prescribed.

Ginger

Ginseng

Cinnamon

Cornelian Asiatic cherry—for menorrhagia.

Acupuncture

Chiropractic

Consult a qualified practitioner.

Bodywork

Massage

Acupressure

Shiatsu—pressure is applied to meridians that can relieve menstrual difficulties.

Qigong

Reflexology

Mindbody therapy

Yoga—relieves stress, balances hormone levels, toning of pelvic area.

Biofeedback

Imagery

Hypnotherapy

Multiple Sclerosis

Multiple sclerosis is an inflammation of the myelin sheaths that surround and protect nerve fibers causing nerve electrical transmissions to become dysfunctional. The cause is not known but the two most prominent theories are a virus or autoimmunity in which the immune system mistakenly attacks the sheaths. Stress, environmental toxins, and food sensitivities can exacerbate the condition. Symptoms vary and include muscle weakness, loss of coordination, loss of vision and bowel and bladder control, and paralysis. The illness can stabilize or go into remission. In studies, a low-fat diet has been shown to improve symptoms significantly. The Swank diet is recommended. Regular exercise is beneficial. Some individuals have experienced benefits from apithery, a treatment involving bee venom which has anti-inflammatory properties.

Nutrients

Black currant oil—500 mg, contains gamma-linolenic acid (GLA), an anti-inflammatory; evening primrose oil is an alternative.

Vitamin B complex—50 to 100 mg

Vitamin B_{12}—if low levels are found in the serum, red blood cells and cerebral spinal fluid, 2 mg for deficiency, up to 60 mg therapeutically, methylcobalamin form.

Carotenoid complex

Vitamin C

Bioflavonoids

Vitamin E—400 to 800 IU

Multivitamin and mineral

Magnesium—350 to 400 mg

Selenium—100 to 300 mcg

Soy lecithin—5 g granules

Coenzyme Q_{10}—100 mg

Foods

Organic whole foods

Fatty fish

Salmon

Sardines

Albacore tuna

Herring

Mackerel

Fresh vegetables

Spinach

Purslane

Fresh fruits

Pineapple

Blueberries

Whole grains

Legumes

Garbanzos

Nuts

Seeds

Extra virgin olive oil

Cold pressed organic canola oil

Ginger

Turmeric

Juices

Fruits

Vegetables

Herbal therapy

Padma 28—2 pills three times daily, increases muscle strength and improves other symptoms.

Homeopathy

Take remedy according to symptoms:

Agaricus

Kali phosphoricum

Phosphorus

Tarantula

Aromatherapy

Lemon verbena—an anti-inflammatory.

Juniper, rosemary—mix with carrier oil and use for massage.

Ayurvedic medicine

Ashwagandha

Chinese medicine

Acupuncture

Bodywork

Massage

Deep tissue massage

Mindbody therapy

Meditation

Yoga

Biofeedback

Imagery

Hypnotherapy

Osteoporosis

Loss of calcium from bone causes osteoporosis and is found most frequently in postmenopausal women and men in their 70s. Symptoms are low back pain, stooped posture, loss of height, and increased risk of fracture. Heredity, exercise, and diet are the most important factors in the condition. After the age of around 30, calcium no longer builds bone or adds to bone mass. However, sufficient dietary calcium is still necessary to maintain bone mass and retard bone loss. After menopause women need to eat sufficient amounts of estrogenic foods such as soy to prevent further bone loss. Weight-bearing exercises such as walking, weight lifting, yoga, and T'ai chi help build bone density.

Excess protein in the diet leaches calcium out of the bones; salt, caffeine (over 2 or 3 cups daily), carbonated soft drinks, smoking, and excessive exercise also cause calcium excretion. Magnesium, vitamin D, boron (found in fruits and nuts), manganese, and zinc are necessary for calcium bone metabolism. Isoflavones from soy protein in the amount of 90 mg daily has been found to increase bone density. It is recommended that optimal intake of calcium be 1500 mg daily, although it will not prevent a genetic predisposition to the disease.

Nutrients

Calcium—800 to 1000 mg, if diet only provides 500 to 700 mg; citrate, lactate, aspartate are the most absorbable forms.

Magnesium—250 to 350 mg, deficiency often found in osteoporosis patients, can improve bone density.

Vitamin D—220 IU, take with calcium for maximum effectiveness.

Boron—3 mg

Manganese—10 to 20 mg

Zinc—10 to 30 mg

Copper—2 mg, helps prevent bone loss; balances zinc.

Vitamin K—1 mg, for postmenopausal women, prevents calcium loss and increases bone density.[61]

Silicon—increases bone mineral density.

Strontium—1 to 3 mg, reduces bone pain and increases bone mass.

Foods

Whole grains

Oats

Fresh fruits

Pineapple

Apples

Pears

Grapes

Raisins

Dates

Peaches

Fresh vegetables

Green leafy vegetables

Broccoli

Cabbage

Dandelion greens

Kale

Avocado

Spinach

Asparagus

Onions

Parsley

Legumes

Soy products

Low-fat dairy

Fatty fish

Salmon

Herring

Mackerel

Albacore tuna

Sardines

Seafood

Eggs

Honey

Garlic

Black pepper

Ginger

Juices

Apple

Beet

Berry

Carrot

Celery

Green leafy vegetables

Lemon

Parsley

Pineapple

Herbal therapy

Horsetail—contains silicon, helps maintain bone mass.

Black cohosh—improves bone density, has estrogenic activity.

Licorice—has estrogen and progesterone effects.

Dong quai, false unicorn, fennel—have estrogenic activity.

Homeopathy

Take remedy according to symptom:

Calcarea carbonica

Calcarea fluorica

Calcarea phosphorica

Phosphorus

Silicea

Symphytum officinale

Ayurvedic medicine

Black sesame seeds, shatavari, ginger—mix and eat one ounce daily.

Amla

Chinese medicine

Herbal preparations are prescribed.

Acupuncture

Chiropractic

For back pain.

Bodywork

T'ai chi

Reflexology

Mindbody Therapy

Yoga

Overweight

Overweight is caused most often by overeating and underexercising. An individual is considered overweight if 20% over ideal weight. A medical examine is advisable to determine if there is any underlying health condition. Excessive weight can increase the risk of heart disease, high blood pressure, some forms of cancer, diabetes, osteoarthritis, and gallstones. Eating high-fiber foods, complex carbohydrates, low-fat foods, and exercising on a regular basis is a healthful way to lose weight. Changing food habits and keeping excess weight off will be easier to maintain if a weight reduction program is undertaken on a gradual basis.

Nutrients

5-HTP—600 to 900 mg, can reduce appetite and promote loss of weight,[60] a precursor to serotonin.

CoEnzyme Q_{10}—100 to 300 mg if deficient, may increase weight loss along with a low-calorie diet.

Chromium—200 to 400 mcg, picolinate form, can facilitate weight loss in some individuals by increasing insulin sensitivity which helps stabilize blood sugar levels and stimulates thermogenesis or burning of calories.

Foods

Whole foods

Whole grains

Fresh fruits

Fresh vegetables

Seaweed

Low- or nonfat dairy products

Fatty fish

Salmon

Albacore tuna

Sardines

Herring

Seafood

Skinless poultry

Legumes

Extra virgin olive oil

Cold pressed organic canola oil

Cayenne

Ginger

Garlic

Black pepper

Hot mustard

Fenugreek—spices that raise metabolic rate

Juices

Beet

Celery

Citrus

Carrot

Grape

Parsley

Pineapple

Spinach

Watercress

Herbal therapy

Ephedra—20 to 30 mg ephedrine, ephedrine content stimulates metabolism; can have side effects including insomnia, irritability, and hyperactivity, tolerance level varies between individuals; promotes fat loss but preserves lean body mass; *use under medical supervision only.*

Yohimbine—stimulates the burning of fat; especially effective for lower-body fat; has same side effects as ephedra plus hypertension and heart palpitations; *use under medical supervision only.*

Aromatherapy

Fennel

Juniper

Rosemary

Ayurvedic medicine

Guggul—lowers cholesterol, helps burn fat.

Garcinia cambozia—suppresses appetite, aids digestion.

Boswellia—increases metabolic rate.

Chinese medicine

Acupuncture—auricular acupuncture, in which needles are placed in the ear, points are pressed when there is a food craving.

Bodywork

Massage

Mindbody therapy

Meditation—reduces stress.

Yoga—relaxing; helps gain control over the mind.

Imagery

Hypnotherapy

Metropolitan Life Height and Weight Chart

Men				
Height		**Small Frame**	**Medium Frame**	**Large Frame**
Feet	**Inches**			
5	2	128–134	131–141	138–150
5	3	130–136	133–143	140–153
5	4	132–138	135–145	142–156
5	5	134–140	137–148	144–160
5	6	136–142	139–151	146–164
5	7	138–145	142–154	149–168

Metropolitan Life Height and Weight Chart *(Continued)*

Men

Height		Small	Medium	Large
Feet	Inches	Frame	Frame	Frame
5	8	140–148	145–157	152–172
5	9	142–151	148–160	155–176
5	10	144–154	151–163	158–180
5	11	146–157	154–166	161–184
6	0	149–160	157–170	164–188
6	1	152–164	160–174	168–192
6	2	155–168	164–178	172–197
6	3	158–172	167–182	176–202
6	4	162–176	171–187	181–207

*Weights at ages 25 to 59 based on lowest mortality. Weight in pounds according to frame (in indoor clothing weighing 5 lb, shoes with 1-in heels).

Women

Height		Small	Medium	Large
Feet	Inches	Frame	Frame	Frame
4	10	102–111	109–121	118–131
4	11	103–113	111–123	120–134
5	0	104–115	113–126	122–137
5	1	106–118	115–129	125–140
5	2	108–121	118–132	128–143
5	3	111–124	121–135	131–147
5	4	114–127	124–138	134–151
5	5	117–130	127–141	137–155
5	6	120–133	130–144	140–159
5	7	123–136	133–147	143–163
5	8	126–139	136–150	146–167
5	9	129–142	139–153	149–170
5	10	132–145	142–156	152–173
5	11	135–148	145–159	155–176
6	0	138–151	148–162	158–179

*Weights at ages 25 to 59 based on lowest mortality. Weight in pounds according to frame (in indoor clothing weighing 3 lb, shoes with 1-in heels).

Pregnancy

Pregnancy lasts 40 weeks from the last day of menstruation. Changes in hormonal levels cause symptoms such as nausea in the first trimester, digestion problems and constipation in the second, and, in the third trimester, the growth of the fetus may result in back pain and swelling of the legs. *Varicose veins,* which can develop in susceptible individuals, may be due to an inherited weakness in the structure of the veins. Blood gathers in pools causing the vein to bulge. Topical application of a cream used in Europe that contains horsechestnut or escin, has shown to be beneficial in affecting venous circulation. A drop in the hormone levels of estrogen and progesterone can cause depression and weepiness after birth.

A nutrient-dense diet and avoiding certain substances before conception and throughout pregnancy can help bring about the birth of a healthy baby. For example, intake of 0.4 mg folic acid has been found to be necessary one month before conception to prevent neural birth defects that occur in the first 28 days of pregnancy. The vitamin should be continued during the first trimester. In the last trimester sufficient amounts of omega-3 fatty acids should be included in the diet. Good sources are fatty fish and fortified eggs. Calcium needs are doubled during pregnancy and the diet should include 1500 mg. Calcium also helps prevent preeclampsia and premature births.

Alcohol, drugs, including some prescription drugs, cigarettes, and excessive caffeine (more than 2 to 3 cups coffee) should be avoided to minimize the risk of conditions such as low birth weight, sudden-death syndrome, retarded growth, hyperactivity, attention deficit disorder, and emotional problems of the child. It is important to get sufficient rest, sleep, nonjarring exercise, and to reduce stress. Exercises that strengthen the abdominal muscles ease pain in the lower back.

Nutrients

Folic acid—400 mcg

Iron—on consultation with a physician; large amounts can cause a zinc deficiency.

Vitamin B$_6$—10 to 25 mg three times daily, for morning sickness.

Vitamin C—25 to 500 mg daily, for morning sickness.

Vitamin K—5 mg, take with vitamin C for morning sickness.

Foods

Whole organic foods

Whole grains

Whole wheat

Amaranth

Fresh fruits

Fresh vegetables

Green leafy vegetables

Low-fat dairy

Fortified eggs

Fatty fish

Salmon

Albacore tuna

Herring

Sardines

Mackerel

Legumes

Soybeans

Lentils

Nuts

Walnuts

Seeds

Pumpkin seeds

Extra virgin olive oil

Cold pressed organic canola oil

Ginger

Herbal therapy

Raspberry—relaxes the uterus, most commonly used pregnancy herb, eases discomforts of pregnancy including morning sickness; good for breastfeeding; helps prevent miscarriage.

Partridge berry—use for 3 weeks prior to, and during, delivery, eases discomforts.

Crampbark—soothes uterus, helps prevent miscarriage.

Dandelion, nettles—tone and nourish.

Vitex—15 drops three times daily, promotes lactation.

Sage—dries up milk production when breastfeeding is no longer desired.

Ginger—250 mg four times daily or 1.5 to 3 ml tincture three times daily, for morning sickness.

Homeopathy

For pregnancy and delivery, take remedy according to symptoms:

Arnica montana

Calcarea phosphorica

Carbo vegetabilis

Caulophyllum thalictroides

Cimicifuga

Ferrum metallicum

Ferrum phosphoricum

Nux vomica

Pulsatilla

Sepia

For varicose veins:

Arnica montana

Calcarea carbonica

Carbo vegetabilis

Hamamelis virginiana

Lycopodium

Pulsatilla

Zincum metallicum

For postpartum depression:

Arsenicum album

Aurum metallicum

Calcarea carbonica

Cimicifuga

Ignatia amara

Natrum muriaticum

Phosphorus

Pulsatilla

Sepia

For morning sickness:

Asarum

Colchicum autumnale

Ipecacuanha

Kreosotum

Lacticum acidum

Nux vomica

Pulsatilla

Sepia

Tabacum

Aromatherapy

Lavender, geranium, neroli—massage or by diffuser, have relaxing and calming properties.

Clary sage, jasmine—ease depression and anxiety.

Chamomile—massage abdomen and lower back, eases pain.

Mandarin 4 ml, rosehip seed oil 20 ml, and hazelnut oil 200 ml—prevent stretch marks.

Ayurvedic medicine

Clove—tones uterine muscles.

Aloe vera—apply topically for stretch marks.

Chinese medicine

Acupuncture—alleviates morning sickness and pain during labor.

Chiropractic

Consult a qualified practitioner.

Bodywork

Massage

Movement therapies

Acupressure

Mindbody therapy

Yoga

Imagery

Hypnotherapy

Premenstrual Syndrome (PMS)

PMS is characterized by symptoms including mood swings, irritability, insomnia, joint pain, tender breasts, headache, and bloating and starts approximately 2 weeks before menstruation begins. The cause is likely a hormonal imbalance, too much estrogen being produced by the body as opposed to the amount of progesterone. In studies, eating complex carbohydrates such as bread, potatoes, pasta, rice and oats throughout the day has relieved symptoms due either to the release of serotonin, a neurotransmitter that elevates mood, or to the stabilization of blood sugar levels. Caffeine-sensitive individuals have experienced relief when the beverage has been eliminated from the diet. Estrogenic foods such as soy and other legumes stabilize hormone levels by interfering with and limiting the uptake of estrogen that the body produces. Regular exercise has been shown to reduce symptoms of PMS.

Nutrients

Vitamin B_6—50 to 200 mg, relieves symptoms.

Vitamin B complex

Evening primrose oil or black currant oil—500 mg twice daily throughout the month increasing during symptoms if necessary.

Magnesium—200 to 400 mg, may help reduce symptoms.

Calcium—1000 to 1300 mg, prevents mood swings and other symptoms.

Vitamin A—10,000 to 25,000 IU

Vitamin E—200 to 300 IU with mixed tocopherols, may reduce symptoms.

Foods

Fresh fruits

Fresh vegetables

Carrots

Dandelion greens

Whole grains

Legumes

Soybeans

Lima beans

Black beans

Peanuts

Nuts

Seeds

Fatty fish

Salmon

Sardines

Mackerel

Albacore tuna

Extra virgin olive oil

Cold pressed organic canola oil

Herbal therapy

Vitex aka chasteberry—2 ml extract or 175 to 225 mg, decreases estrogen to balance progesterone; in a study was as effective as vitamin B_6.[62]

Dong quai—1 to 2 g powdered root, 4 ml tincture, or 1 ml extract three times daily, relieves PMS symptoms, normalizes hormone balance; known as the "female ginseng."

Scullcap, valerian—sedative and tranquilizing effect, relieve tension and irritability.

Dandelion—a diuretic, for water retention.

Crampbark, raspberry—for cramps.

Homeopathy

Take remedy according to symptoms:

Bovista

Calcarea carbonica

Caulophyllum thalictroides

Chamomilla

Cimicifuga

Kreosotum

Lachesis

Lilium tigrinum

Lycopodium

Natrum muriaticum

Nux vomica

Pulsatilla

Sepia

Veratrum album

Aromatherapy

Geranium—apply topically to relieve pain in breasts.

Clary sage—has estrogenlike properties, eases PMS symptoms.

Neroli, jasmine, ylang ylang—use as full body massage, beginning several days before symptoms begin.

Juniper—for water retention.

Auyurvedic medicine

Treatments are prescribed according to metabolic type and to balance the doshas.

Angelica

Chinese medicine

Herbal preparations are prescribed.

Angelica

Peony

Hoelen

Skullcap

Acupuncture

Chiropractic

Consult a qualified practitioner.

Bodywork

Massage

Deep tissue manipulation

Movement therapies

Acupressure

Shiatsu

Reflexology

Mindbody therapy

Meditation—relaxing and reduces tension.

Yoga

Biofeedback

Imagery

Hypnotherapy

Prostate Problems

Prostate problems include inflammation, enlargement, or cancer of the prostate gland which surrounds the urethra, the tube through which urine flows. An inflammation of the gland is called *prostitis* resulting in pain during urination and ejaculation, frequent urination and possibly low back pain. The causes include infection, too much or too little ejaculation, jarring exercises such as horseback and bicycle riding, and food irritants like caffeine, alcohol, tobacco, and red pepper. Drinking plenty of water is important in keeping a flow of urine and in preventing dehydration, which can be in effect even though not thirsty, and is a condition that is very stressful for the prostate.

Enlargement of the prostate, called *benign prostatic hyperplasia* (BPH), usually occurs in men over 50 and causes difficulty in urination because enlargement squeezes the urethra it surrounds and interferes with urine flow. BPH is due to an excess of testosterone in the gland. Symptoms are night and frequent urination and a diminishing in force and continuity of the urine stream. It is recommended that foods irritating to the prostate be avoided such as caffeine, tobacco, alcohol, and hot spices. Herbal remedies have shown to be just as effective as prescription drugs without the side effects. Incidences of *prostate tumors* have been associated with diets high in saturated fats.

Impotence is often a psychological problem more than a physical one. Drugs, tobacco, diabetes, and atherosclerosis can affect blood circulation which influences erectile ability. The herb yohimbe has been shown to improve erectile and ejaculatory activity. Hypnotherapy may also be beneficial. Ginseng and the Ayurvedic herb ashwaganda can enhance sexual energy.

Nutrients

Zinc picolinate—30 to 60 mg, for prostitis and BHP.

Vitamin C—2 mg, three times daily, for prostitis.

Flaxseed oil or evening primrose oil—1 to 3 tsp, improves urinary flow and reduces swelling of BPH.

Glycine, alanine, glutamic acid—200 mg each, help maintain urinary flow and reduce swelling for BPH, are amino acids.

Beta sitosterol—60 to 130 mg, improves urinary flow and other symptoms of BPH,[63] a plant sterol found in foods such as soybeans, brown rice, and whole wheat.

Foods

Pumpkin seeds—one handful daily, has more glycine, alanine, and glutamic acid than used in the above study, also contains zinc

Whole grains

Ground flaxseeds

Whole wheat

Brown rice

Corn

Legumes

Peanuts

Soybeans—reduce risk of cancer due to the phytoestrogen content

Cooked tomatoes—contain lypocene, a carotenoid, prevent cancer of the prostate

Seeds

Sunflower seeds

Nuts

Almonds

Walnuts

Brazil nuts

Fresh fruits

Fresh vegetables

Garlic

Extra virgin olive oil

Cold pressed organic canola oil

Cold pressed soybean oil

Juices

Beet

Carrot

Celery

Cucumber

Pumpkin

Radish

Herbal therapy

Saw palmetto—160 mg extract twice daily, inhibits an enzyme that converts testosterone to its more active form that stimulates the proliferation of cells in the prostate, promotes shrinkage of gland and improves urinary function.[64]

Licorice—prevents testosterone conversion reducing enlargement of gland.

Pygeum—50 mg twice daily, relieves BPH symptoms[65] due to three compounds: a diuretic, an anti-inflammatory, and a cholesterol reducer that can collect in the gland.

Nettle—2 to 3 tsp extract or 2 to 4 ml tincture three times daily, improves urinary flow.

Flower pollen—60 to 125 mg two or three times daily, used in Europe for prostatitis and BPH, reduces symptoms.

Homeopathy

Take remedy according to symptoms for BPH:

Apis mellifica

Causticum

Chimaphila unbellata

Clematis

Lycopodium

Pulsatilla

Sabal serrulata

Staphysagria

Thuja

Ayurvedic medicine

Treatments are prescribed.

Chinese medicine

Herbal remedies are prescribed.

Acupuncture

Bodywork

Acupressure

Shiatsu

Qigong

T'ai chi

Reflexology

Mindbody therapy

Yoga

Psoriasis

Psoriasis is an acceleration in the growth of skin cells that results in patches of dry scaly itchy skin. The cause is unknown although it tends to run in families. Stress is often a trigger and gluten in foods or alcohol can precipitate the condition in some individuals. A sluggish liver may also be a factor. Getting sunlight is a common and effective remedy to alleviate symptoms. Antioxidants neutralize free radicals that play a role in inflammatory diseases like psoriasis.

In studies, fish oil, in amounts equivalent to 5 oz of fatty fish daily, has significantly alleviated symptoms.[66] The oil in fish contains anti-inflammatory properties. Saturated fats and omega-6 fatty acids should be limited in the diet as they have an inflammatory effect on the body. Bathing in oatmeal (fill cheesecloth and tie to faucet) or sea salt can relieve symptoms.

Nutrients

Vitamin C—1 g, an antioxidant.

Bioflavonoids—work synergistically with vitamin C.

Vitamin E—400 IU with mixed tocopherols, an antioxidant.

Flaxseed oil—1 to 3 T, can relieve symptoms, has anti-inflammatory properties.

Vitamin A—50,000 IU, if deficient.

Zinc—30 mg, if deficient.

Foods

Whole foods

Fatty fish

Salmon

Mackerel

Sardines

Albacore tuna

Fresh fruits

Figs

Olives

Fresh vegetables

Sauerkraut

Onion

Carrots

Celery

Parsley

Ground flaxseeds

Low-fat yogurt

Extra virgin olive oil

Cold pressed organic canola oil

Fennel

Garlic

Juices

Fruit—citrus fruits may aggravate symptoms in some individuals.

Apple

Beet

Carrot

Cucumber

Grape

Herbal therapy

Angelica—contains psoralens that inhibit cell division.

Capsaicin—cream, apply topically, alleviates redness, scaling, pain and itching, from red pepper.

Chamomile—cream, has anti-inflammatory properties, alleviates symptoms.

Milk thistle—2 capsules twice daily, cleanses liver, an anti-inflammatory.

Oregon grape—an antioxidant, slows cell proliferation; can also be used topically.

Burdock root—2 to 4 ml or 1 to 2 g three times daily, blood purifier.

Licorice—glycyrrhetinic acid-containing cream, has effect similar to that of topical hydrocortisone.

Homeopathy

Take remedy according to symptoms:

Arsenicum album

Calcarea carbonica

Graphites

Mercurius solubilis

Mezereum

Petroleum

Psorinum

Rhus toxicodendron

Sepia

Staphysagria

Sulfur

Aromatherapy

Bergamot—use as massage or in vaporizer.

Lavender, chamomille—use as massage, creams, or in bath.

Ayurvedic medicine

Effective treatments are prescribed.

Chinese medicine

Dittany bark, puncture vine fruit—can help itching.

Acupuncture—stimulation of appropriate points relieves symptoms.

Bodywork

Acupressure

Reflexology

Mindbody therapy

Meditation—reduces stress.

Yoga

Biofeedback

Imagery

Hypnotherapy—learn relaxation techniques.

Raynaud's Disease

Raynaud's disease is a constriction of the blood vessels of the extremities which go into spasm and turn white or bluish in response to cold. It is a painful condition due to the diminished blood supply and affects most often the fingers but sometimes the toes, ears, nose, and cheeks. *Raynaud's phenomenon* has similar symptoms and responds to the same remedies but the cause involves connective tissue.

Nicotine constricts the flow of blood and should be avoided; birth control pills can also affect circulation. Keep the affected areas warm and if there is no response to warmth, consult a physician.

Nutrients

Inositol hexaniacinate—3 to 4 g or 200 mg niacin, improves circulation and decreases spasms.

Evening primrose oil—1 to 4 g, reduces the number and severity of attacks; inhibits action of prostaglandins that play a role in blood vessel constriction.

L-carnitine—1 g three times daily, reduces spasms.

Foods

Fatty fish
Salmon
Mackerel
Albacore tuna
Sardines
Herring
Fresh fruits
Apples
Figs
Fresh vegetables
Leafy green vegetables
Legumes
Soybeans
Nuts
Seeds
Whole grains
Eggs
Seafood
Low-fat dairy
Ginger

Garlic
Cayenne
Mustard

Juices

Fruits
Vegetables

Herbal therapy

Ginkgo biloba—60 to 240 mg extract, improves blood circulation.

Garlic—400 to 500 mg, 2 to 4 ml tincture, or one clove raw garlic, improves blood circulation.

Indian snakeroot—contains the compound reserpine which dilates blood vessels.

Homeopathy

Take remedy according to symptoms:

Arsenicum album
Cactus
Carbo vegetabilis
Chelidonium
Hepar sulphuris calcareum
Lachesis
Secale
Sepia
Veratrum album

Aromatherapy

Black pepper, lemon, rosemary, peppermint—massage into affected areas for warmth and increased circulation.

Ayurvedic medicine

Mustard and sesame seed oils—warm and massage hands.

Chinese medicine

Dong quai
Peony
Chinese angelica
Cinnamon twigs
Acupuncture

Chiropractic

Spinal and neck manipulation improves blood circulation to extremities.

Bodywork

Massage—improves circulation and relaxes.

Qigong

Mindbody therapy

Biofeedback—application of methods to warm hands and feet.

Imagery

Stress

Stress is inherent in our way of life and is part of the human condition. What is important is how we react to it. Reacting with anger, fear, depression, and anxiety without release of the tension can result in illness, either directly or indirectly. Symptoms include muscle tension, high blood pressure, psychological problems, digestive disorders, a weakened immune system, cancer, and heart disease.

When the mind perceives a threat, whether real or imagined, the brain instantly and automatically evaluates the situation. Then the subconscious begins to prepare the body for a response. The sympathetic system causes the blood to flow to the muscles, the muscles and blood vessels constrict, and the body is flooded with hormones from the pituitary and adrenal glands. Heart rate increases and oxygen consumption accelerates. Production of digestive juices is reduced and blood sugar levels increase as the liver releases glucose into the bloodstream. This process becomes harmful when it remains a perpetual state with few periods of full relaxation or full release of the tension. After years pass, many illnesses can develop, including an artery spasm that can result in a heart attack.

Stress is caused mainly by emotional or psychological situations. The mind affects the body and vice versa; if the mind is agitated or worried, the body will be tense. If the body is tense, the mind will be in a high state of vigilance. Eventually, resources like hormones and chemicals become depleted, the body gets tired of adapting to the stressful situation, organs become exhausted and functioning collapses. Only when the mind and body are in a state of calm can energies be directed toward repair, maintenance, and strengthening of the body and the immune system.

Physical exercise oxygenates body tissues, dissipates stress hormones, and relieves tension. Hormones called endorphins are produced and give a sense of well-being. The result of regular exercise is a slower heart rate, lowered blood pressure, a normal functioning respiratory system, and relaxed muscles.

During stress, breathing becomes shallow and rapid. Because oxygen is necessary for the metabolism of every cell in the body, it affects the functioning of the autonomic nervous system which regulates automatic functions like heart rate, respiration, and digestion. Proper breath control stabilizes and strengthens the tone of the nervous system.

Deep breathing uses the full capacity of the diaphragm, a muscle located below the lungs that contracts when breathing in and allows the lungs to expand with air. Shallow breathing only involves the upper lobes of the lungs. This leaves over a million alveoli, the tiny sacs that absorb oxygen which is then transported by the hemoglobin of the blood to all the cells of the body, empty. The consequence is that the cellular structure does not receive enough oxygen to carry out its work.

There are various deep breathing methods but basically the idea is to take a slow deep breath through the nostrils, hold to the count of 7, then exhale through the mouth to the count of 8 or 10 and repeat three more times. This can be practiced several times a day.

Nutrients

Vitamin B complex—50 mg, regulates nerves.

Magnesium—200 to 300 mg, a muscle relaxant.

Vitamin C—500 to 1000 mg in divided doses, urinary excretion of the vitamin increases during stress.

Foods

Whole foods

Fresh fruits

Fresh vegetables

Shiitake mushrooms

Potatoes

Onions

Yam

Whole grains

Pasta

Oats

Legumes

Low-fat dairy

Low-fat yogurt

Fatty fish

Salmon

Sardines

Mackerel

Albacore tuna

Seafood

Extra virgin olive oil

Cold pressed organic canola oil

Honey

Garlic

Juices

Fruits

Vegetables

Carrot

Lettuce

Herbal therapy

Passion flower—1 dropperful tincture three or four times daily or freeze-dried caps, reduces stress.

Chamomile, spearmint—have mild relaxant properties, reduce stress.

Valerian—a sedative, helps promote sleep.

Ginseng—1 to 2 g root or 100 mg extract, tones and strengthens organs of body.

Homeopathy

Take remedy according to symptoms:

Aconitum napellus

Argentum nitricum

Arsenicum album

Calcarea carbonica

Gelsemium

Ignatia amara

Kali phosphoricum

Lycopodium

Natrum muriaticum

Phosphorus

Pulsatilla

Silicea

Aromatherapy

Mandarin 1 ml, mandarin petitgrain 1 ml, lemon verbena 1 ml—for anxiety and stress.

Roman chamomile 1 ml, clary sage 1 ml, spikenard 1 ml, carrier oil 10 ml—for extreme stress.

Lavender, rose, rosemary, bergamot—have sedative and relaxing properties.

Ayurvedic medicine

Treatment varies according to body type.

Chinese medicine

Herbal preparations are prescribed.

Astragalus

Ginseng

Acupuncture

Bodywork

Massage

Deep tissue manipulation

Movement therapies—the muscles are interrelated with the nervous and psychological systems.

Qigong

T'ai chi

Acupressure

Shiatsu

Reflexology

Mindbody therapy

Meditation—lowers blood pressure, and heart and respiratory rates.

Yoga

Biofeedback—becoming aware of and control of the autonomic nervous system.

Imagery—establishes the connection between the visual cortex of the brain and the autonomic nervous system.

Hypnotherapy—learn methods of relaxation.

Stroke

Eighty percent of strokes are caused by a clot in an artery of the brain that cuts off blood and oxygen supply. The cells around the clot are damaged or die, and the body organ that is controlled by that particular part of the brain is affected. The remaining 20% of strokes result from hemorrhages, due to a defective clotting mechanism. The blood vessels rupture and blood spills into the brain. *Transient ischemic attacks* or TIAs are mini strokes that usually clear within minutes but could indicate a more serious attack in the future. Symptoms of stroke include sudden numbness, blurred vision, weakness or paralysis, loss of speech, dizziness, and headache.

Risk factors for strokes are diabetes, high blood pressure, atherosclerosis, high serum cholesterol, lack of exercise, smoking, and taking birth control pills. Too much salt in the diet, even if it does not raise blood pressure, has been shown to induce strokes. Excessive alcohol consumption can cause strokes. Eating fatty fish can reduce clotting potential. The oils in fish make the structures of cellular membranes more pliable enabling easier passage of blood; saturated fats have the opposite effect, making them more rigid.

Nutrients

Vitamin B complex—prevents platelets from aggregating.

Evening primrose, borage, or black currant oil—anticoagulants, lower blood pressure.

Foods

Fresh fruits

Dark berries

Avocado

Dried apricots

Pineapple

Fresh vegetables

Leafy green vegetables

Spinach

Carrots

Sweet potatoes

Pumpkin

Potatoes

Onions

Fatty fish

Salmon

Herring

Mackerel

Sardines

Albacore tuna

Seafood

Whole grains

Legumes

Nuts

Seeds

Low-fat dairy

Ginger

Garlic

Turmeric

Juices

Fruits

Vegetables

Dark berry

Pineapple

Herbal therapy

Ginkgo biloba—60 to 240 mg extract; increases blood flow to the brain; reduces fragility of the capillaries.

Willowbark, meadowsweet, wintergreen—an anticoagulant, has aspirinlike properties.

Bilberry—contains compounds that help prevent blood clots, breaks down plaque.[67]

Garlic—an anticoagulant, reduces blood pressure.

Ginger—an anticoagulant, as a tea, grate 1 to 2 tsp.

Aromatherapy

Lavender, rosemary—for paralysis, massage spinal column and affected area.

Ayurvedic medicine

Treatments are prescribed for rehabilitation after paralysis.

Chinese medicine

Peony

Wolfberry

Acupuncture—helps recover mental and physical function.

Bodywork

Massage—improves circulation to affected limbs.

Movement therapies

Qigong

T'ai chi—rebalances flow of qi.

Reflexology

Mindbody therapy

Meditation—reduces stress after stroke.

Yoga

Biofeedback—helps rehabilitate and improve body functions after stroke.

Imagery

Ulcers

Ulcers usually form in the duodenum, the upper part of the small intestine; a peptic ulcer is in the stomach as well as the duodenum and is so called because of the involvement of pepsin, a digestive enzyme. Ulcers are sores that can bleed. They form when there is too much acid for the mucosal lining to tolerate. They are often caused by an infection of the bacteria, Helicobacter pylori; food allergies are also a possibility. It is believed that this bacteria releases acids into the area and may also be the cause of *gastritis*. Antibiotics are necessary for its eradication.

Stress, coffee, alcohol, aspirin, tobacco, sugar, 7 Up, colas, and milk can increase the amount of acid in the stomach; smoking hinders the healing process; and salt is a stomach and intestinal irritant. Stress can also affect the strength of the immune system and its ability to prevent illness. A high fiber diet helps heal and prevent ulcers. Eating smaller frequent meals is recommended until the ulcer heals.

Nutrients

Vitamin A—20,000 IU, heals mucosal tissue of the lining of the stomach and duodenum.

Zinc—25 to 30 mg, speeds healing of ulcers; beneficial for healing bedsores.

Foods

Bananas—stimulate the proliferation of mucosal cells that form a barrier between the lining and acid

Fresh fruits

Pineapple

Blueberries

Papaya

Fresh vegetables

Dark green leafy vegetables

Potatoes

Enoki mushrooms

Whole grains

Brown rice

Corn

Legumes—especially red and white beans

Seafood

Raw honey

Garlic

Turmeric

Thyme

Cinnamon

Cardamom

Cloves

Ginger

Juices

Cabbage—one quart daily, strengthens lining of the stomach, increases mucus activity, an antibiotic that destroys the Helicobacter bacteria, contains compounds found in antiulcer drugs, heals ulcers in a period from 2 days to 3 weeks

Fruits

Vegetables

Carrot

Celery

Kale

Potato

Wheatgrass

Nutrients

Bioflavonoids—500 mg three times daily, studies show several flavonoids can inhibit H. pylori and can prevent ulcer formation, the flavone compound has effect similar to that of bismuth citrate.

Bismuth subcitrate—240 mg twice daily before meals, obtain from a compounding pharmacy, a natural mineral that acts as an antacid and inhibits H. pylori bacteria; more effective than Pepto Bismol.

Herbal therapy

Licorice—DGL extract, 2 chewable tablets or 250 to 500 mg 15 minutes before meals, protects and heals lining of the stomach and duodenum, inhibits H. pylori.

Peppermint—soothes lining of stomach and intestine.

Aloe vera—1 tsp juice after meals, has healing properties.

Cayenne—capsules, capsaicin content helps heal ulcers.

Green tea—high in antibacterial and antioxidant compounds.

Garlic—tincture, prevents damage from ulcers by stimulating production of protective substances, has antibacterial activity.

Calendula—has anti-inflammatory and healing properties.

Chamomile—3 to 5 ml tincture or 2 to 3 cups tea daily; soothes irritation of mucous membranes.

Thyme, cinnamon—tinctures, have antibacterial activity.

Ginger—contains anti-inflammatory compounds; eat honey-candied ginger, honey has antibacterial compounds.

Bilberry—stimulates production of mucus.

Meadowsweet—contains compounds that help heal and prevent ulcers.

Comfrey—topical treatments for skin ulcers; beneficial for bedsores, or decubitus ulcers, and for diabetic ulcers.

Homeopathy

Take remedy according to symptoms:

Arsenicum album

Belladonna

Calendula

Hamamelis

Lathesis

Nux vomica

Silicea

Aromatherapy

Chamomile, frankincense, geranium, marjoram—massage abdomen area, help relieve ulcer symptoms.

Ayurvedic medicine

Pitta type most likely to suffer ulcers; herbal remedies are prescribed.

Licorice—½ tsp powder three times daily.

Coconut—milk and fruit.

Ashwagandha

Cinnamon, cardamom, cloves—¼ tsp ground mixture.

Bitter orange

Coriander

Kalanchoe

Chinese medicine

Dandelion

Ginseng

Corydalis tuber

Acupuncture—reduces acid in stomach.

Bodywork

Shiatsu

Movement therapies—relieves strain on digestive system.

Qigong

Reflexology

Mindbody therapy

Meditation

Yoga

Biofeedback

Imagery

Vaginitis

Vaginitis is an inflammation of the lining of the vagina. It is caused by a hormonal imbalance during postmenopause or postpartum; by irritations from allergies or irritating substances and chemicals; or by bacteria, candidiasis, or yeast infection, and trichomoniasis. The symptoms include itching, pain, and a white discharge. It is recommended sugar and possibly fruit juices be avoided in the diet as yeast thrives in that particular environment. Boric acid and gentian violet have shown to be as effective as prescribed antibiotics.

Nutrients

Vitamin A—improves the integrity of vaginal mucous membranes.

Vitamin C

Bioflavonoids

Vitamin E—orally, applied topically may relieve itching.

Lactobacillus—dissolve in water and use as a douche.

Foods

Yogurt—1 cup daily, reduces and prevents infections, must contain live cultures

Whole foods

Fresh fruits

Fresh vegetables

Shiitake mushrooms

Whole grains

Legumes

Soybeans and ground flaxseeds—for hormonal imbalance

Garlic

Cinnamon—for candidiasis

Herbal therapy

Tea tree—terpinen-4-ol component effective against infections; as cream or douche as effective as pharmaceutical antifungals; 2 to 3 drops in 1 T yogurt, soak tampon and insert into vagina daily for six nights; mix with vitamin E oil, place in capsule and insert into vagina daily for 6 weeks.

Garlic—juice or capsules, allicin component kills infectious organisms; take orally or mix with warm water and douche.

Goldenseal—contains antibiotic compounds berberine and hydrastine.

Apple cider vinegar—douche, 2 T in one quart water, helps reestablish vaginal acidity which is an environment that destroys infections.

Boric acid—600 mg capsules twice daily, insert into vagina, for chronic cases use for 4 months, has antibiotic properties; burning sensation may occur if acid leaks from vagina—reduce dosage.

Gentian violet—soak tampon, effective against Candida albicans, has antibiotic properties; will stain clothes a purple color.

Echinacea—an antibacterial, supports immune system, take tea or tincture daily.

Homeopathy

Take remedy according to symptoms:

Arsenicum album

Borax

Graphites

Hydrastis

Pulsatilla

Sepia

Aromatherapy

Tea tree—very effective for candidiasis and trichomoniasis.

Thyme, thujanol type—effective against infections, stimulates immune system.

Malaleuca alternifolia—controls vaginal infections.

Foods

oods are the raw material that provide energy for the 60 trillion cells that make up the human body. Each cell is a miniuniverse and the integrity of billions of its chemical reactions that take place every minute depends a great deal on food and specifically the kinds of food that are consumed. Substances in food have an influence on nearly every health condition. They can act as sedatives, tranquilizers, analgesics, decongestants, diuretics, antidepressants, anti-inflammatories, and anticoagulants. Food compounds can stimulate chemical reactions that produce natural killer cells and interferon to fight cancer, infections, viruses, and bacteria. They contain components that can regulate cholesterol, lower blood pressure, relieve ulcers, dissolve blood clots, and stimulate the immune system. They have phytoestrogens that help the body regulate the hormone estrogen. Plant estrogens are weaker and more benign as they occupy estrogen receptor sites on the cells and replace the more potent and aggressive hormones that the body makes and the more harmful estrogens circulating in the body from environmental sources.

Elements in food can also cause or exacerbate numerous health conditions including depression, mental confusion, anxiety, inflamed joints, clogged arteries, a malfunctioning cell metabolism, and they can interfere with nerve impulse transmission and muscle function. For example, hormonelike substances called eicosanoids, which include prostaglandins, leukotrienes, and thromboxanes, that control blood clotting and inflammation and affect autoimmune disorders, are made from fatty acids. Two kinds of eicosanoids are omega-6 and omega-3. Omega-6s are the fatty acids from saturated fats found in meats and dairy products, transfats like margarine, and polyunsaturated fats used in salads and cooking and present in processed foods. These particular fatty acids produce eicosanoids that are inflammatory. They aggravate certain diseases like asthma and arthritis, affect the stickiness of blood platelets forming blood clots, and accelerate the proliferation of cells, a factor in cancer. They are an influence in illness such as diabetes, rheumatoid arthritis, multiple sclerosis, psoriasis, high blood pressure, migraines, and atherosclerosis.

On the other hand, omega-3s found in fatty fish and some plants produce eicosanoids that reduce inflammation, relax smooth muscle of the blood vessels, and prevent blood platelets from clumping together. The body needs both kinds of fatty acids for various body processes including injury repair, cell growth, proper immune response, and blood clotting. What is important is that the ratio of omega-6s be less than omega-3s. Because most diets contain the reverse, eating 1 to 3 ounces of fatty fish daily or the equivalent amount two or three times a week plus reducing omega-6s will help establish a proper balance. Extra virgin olive oil and cold pressed organic canola oil, because of their inherent properties, are the preferable oils to use in salads and cooking.

Substances in food can cause food intolerances or sensitivities in some people. Unlike allergies, intolerances create reactions that are more subtle and delayed. In fact, several hours to days may pass before a reaction is noticed. Headaches, depression, fatigue, irritable bowel syndrome, rheumatoid arthritis, and mental problems are some of the health conditions that can result. The actual intolerance does not involve the blood or immune system and so it may not be detected by conventional allergy tests. It is recommended that a suspected food be eliminated from the diet for one week, then be reintroduced, while monitoring the effects throughout the process.

Organically grown produce and foodstuffs are preferable because pesticides and fungicides are poisonous and are cumulative. The chemicals from a wide range of foods accumulate in the body. Not only can residues remain on the exterior of the plant, but because spraying can be systemic, the chemical is absorbed through the roots and becomes incorporated into the tissues and flesh. In addition, waxes that are often used on selected produce may contain fungicides. One study has shown that organic foods are higher in nutritive value than those grown conventionally.[68]

Getting nutrients from whole foods in a varied diet is preferable to taking supplements as a substitute in maintaining optimal health. There are nutrients and phytochemicals yet to be discovered in foods that likely play a crucial role. Nutrients work synergistically and isolating them can result in a lessening pharmacological effect. For example, foods containing 40 mg of vitamin C and 10 IU of vitamin E neutralize as many free radicals as 500 mg vitamin C and 800 IU vitamin E. The gamma tocopherol, one of a family of tocopherols, scavenges nitrogen oxides, a class of free radicals that damage DNA, but the alpha-tocopherol, used in supplements, has no effect.[69] Large amounts of alpha can also cause a depletion of gamma in the body. The array of carotenoids are just as important as beta carotene;

lycopene, the red color in tomatoes, for instance, has 10 times more antioxidant activity. EPA and DHA, the beneficial components of fish oil, may not be as effective as eating the whole fish.

The internal equilibrium of nutrients in the body can easily be disturbed by arbitrarily ingesting supplements, especially high doses. A deficiency of nutrients has adverse health effects. With adequate amounts of nutrients the body functions properly, but when too much of a nutrient is ingested or if supplements are taken when the body does not need them, certain results can occur including an inhibiting rather than an enhancing effect and causing a deficiency of other nutrients. Excess nutrients can remain unmetabolized, accumulate in the body and interfere with the utilization, metabolism, absorption, and activity of other nutrients and physiological functions. Hormonal and glandular supplements are questionable because the long-term effects are not fully understood. For example, supplemental DHEA, an adrenal hormone that declines naturally with age, can increase insulin resistance, cause the growth of unwanted hair, decrease levels of HDL cholesterol, raise the risk of heart attack, and exacerbate some cancers. Melatonin, a brain hormone, can induce depression, aggravate allergies, constrict blood vessels, suppress fertility and sex drive, and cause hypothermia and retinal damage. Glandulars are extracts from animal adrenal, pituitary, thymus, and reproductive glands. It is advisable to take these supplements only under the supervision of a physician.

Protein supplements are usually unnecessary except for specific amino acids when diagnosed as deficient. People in general may be eating too much protein. It is not stored in the body and an excess is converted to carbohydrate, a process that taxes the kidneys and that causes a loss of calcium in the urine. Nutritional yeast is a good food source of the B complex vitamins and trace minerals. Wheat germ is a good food source of vitamin E but turns rancid relatively quickly and should be used within a reasonable amount of time and kept refrigerated. Acidophilus in liquid, capsule, or freeze-dried form contains friendly bacteria and can be taken after meals. It is especially necessary for individuals taking antibiotics, which destroy beneficial intestinal organisms.

Because there is no magic pill for any health condition, including aging, the best preventive and healing strategy is to eat a varied nutrient-dense diet, exercise on a regular basis, and have a systematic procedure for reducing stress.

Food Groups

Fruits and Vegetables

The deeper the color of fruits and vegetables, the higher the antioxidant activity. Oxygen renegades are the target of antioxidants. When an oxygen molecule loses an electron, it becomes what is called a free radical and begins searching for a replacement. In trying to steal an electron from other healthy cells, free radicals cause damage to healthy cells and create scores of new free radicals. Free radicals cause mutations in DNA, the genetic material in the cells, and not only destroy healthy cells but turn the fats in many cells rancid, which disrupts cell metabolism. After years of these silent assaults in the body, individuals can develop a chronic disease or illnesses ranging from atherosclerosis to cancer, and experience an acceleration in the aging process.

Environmental pollutants and chemicals, drugs, cigarette smoke, pesticides, and radiation are some of the sources that cause cells to oxidate, and antioxidants are the antidote. They can kill, deter, and hinder the destructive elements and even repair cellular damage. Fresh fruits and vegetables have abundant amounts of antioxidants as well as other health-protecting phytochemicals, vitamins, minerals, and fiber.

Fresh or frozen vegetables and fruits are better than canned or processed in nutritive value; onions and garlic are best eaten raw although onions can also be cooked. The cruciferous family of vegetables are rich in phytochemicals that have anticancer and pathogenic activity but should be lightly cooked as they contain compounds that can be toxic when eaten raw on a regular basis. They include cabbage, broccoli, Brussels sprouts, kale, collards, mustard greens, kohlrabi, daikon, radish, turnip, and rutabaga. Raw beet greens, spinach, and chard contain oxalic acid which removes iron and calcium from the body and so should be lightly cooked as should mushrooms which contain carcinogenic compounds that are destroyed by heat. Green skins on potatoes are poisonous and should be removed before cooking; and celery that has brown spots indicating a fungus should not be consumed.

Some less familiar leafy vegetables that are very nutritious are Swiss chard, a large, crinkly or flat leafy vegetable, red or white in color. Sauté or lightly steam both the stems and leaf. Kale, a good source of calcium, is green and tightly curled and can be lightly steamed or cooked longer if the leaves are older. Collards have large blue-green leaves and can be prepared in the same way as kale. Arugula is a peppery bitter green and is astringent in quality, which is good for digestion. Young leaves or blossoms can be mixed in salads, larger leaves added to stir fries or soups. Beet greens contain calcium, magnesium, and iron, and vitamins A, B complex, and C. Because they contain oxalic acid, they should be lightly steamed or sautéed. Eat raw beet greens sparingly. Dandelion greens are high in vitamins A and C and contain more calcium than broccoli. They can be used raw in salads or lightly steamed. Sauté the roots. Both leaves and roots, fresh or dried, can be made into a tea. Mustard greens have a curly shape and are best sautéed and also can be added to soups and stews.

Legumes

Legumes are peas, lentils, peanuts, carob, and beans, including soybean products like soy milk, tofu, and tempeh. They grow in pods on vines; peanuts grow underground. Legumes are high in protein, 25 to 38%, which is more than eggs and many meats, have no cholesterol or saturated fat, and contain numerous vitamins and minerals including calcium, iron, zinc, potassium, and the B vitamins. Soybeans are a complete protein and when the other legumes are combined with grains, they also constitute a complete protein. Legumes contain omega-3 fatty acids, complex carbohydrates which have a low glycemic index, and fiber. They contain phytochemicals that have anticancer activity and that reduce serum cholesterol. They are beneficial for the heart, liver, kidneys, pancreas, lungs, and intestinal tract. Some beans are more difficult than others to digest due to the fact that the human body is unable to fully break down the complex carbohydrate. A suggestion is to find the beans that are best tolerated, garbanzo, black, aduki, and anasazi beans, for example. Black soybeans are easier to digest than the lighter colored varieties. Soymilk can be substituted for dairy milk as a beverage or in any recipe cup for cup; soy yogurt for dairy yogurt or sour cream, and tofu for cream cheese.

Legumes, including their sprouts and also alfalfa sprouts, should not be eaten raw as they contain toxins that are destroyed when heated. Beans can be stored for several years but as they age, they become tougher and take longer to cook. Soaking beans helps to release the more indigestible starch and phytic acid, which has a binding action on minerals making them inaccessible to the body. Depending on the kind, soak beans for 2 to 24 hours; for the longer times, refrigerate during soaking. Strain, rinse, and cover with fresh water. Boil uncovered for 10 minutes then cover and simmer until soft and tender. Add acidic ingredients like tomatoes and lemon after beans have softened.

Grains

Grains are valuable for their starch content and vitamins, minerals, and fiber as well as some protein. (See illustration.) Refining and processing reduces nutrient values and raises their glycemic index. Complex carbohydrates stabilize blood sugar levels. Grains include wheat, rye, oats, rice, millet, buckwheat, bulgur, couscous, amaranth, barley, kamut, spelt, tef, quinoa, and wild rice. Substitute ⅞ to 1 cup whole-wheat flour for 1 cup white flour in bread recipes, and the same for whole-wheat pastry flour in quick breads, cookies, and cakes. Whole grains can become rancid so store in airtight containers in a cool place or in the refrigerator.

TOTAL NUTRIENTS IN THE KERNEL OF WHEAT

Germ is 2½% of Kernel	Bran is 14% of Kernel	Endosperm is 83% of Kernel
Of the whole kernel the germ contains:	Of the whole kernel the bran contains:	Of the whole kernel the endosperm contains:
64% Thiamine	73% Pyridoxine	70–75% Protein
26% Riboflavin	50% Pantothenic acid	43% Pantothenic acid
21% Pyridoxine	42% Riboflavin	32% Riboflavin
8% Protein	33% Thiamine	12% Niacin
7% Pantothenic acid	19% Protein	6% Pyridoxine
2% Niacin		3% Thiamine

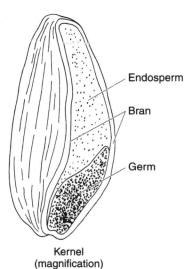

Endosperm
Bran
Germ

Kernel
(magnification)

Other nutrients found in the whole wheat grain are:

Calcium	Chlorine
Iron	Sodium
Phosphorus	Silicon
Magnesium	Boron
Potassium	Barium
Manganese	Silver
Copper	Inositol
Sulfur	Folic Acid
Iodine	Choline
Fluorine	Vitamin E

And other trace materials

The more unfamiliar grains include *blue corn* which is sweeter than yellow corn and has a higher content of protein and manganese. It can be substituted for yellow corn in any recipe. *Bulgur* is whole wheat berries that are steamed and cracked. Bulgur is easier to chew, has a lighter texture, and needs less cooking than cracked wheat. Bulgur is the main ingredient in tabouli. *Couscous,* a tiny bead like pasta, is made from wheat and is easily prepared by simmering in water for one minute and letting stand covered for 10 minutes. The grain is available as whole wheat or refined. *Amaranth* is an ancient grain that has a high protein content and contains a variety of components including calcium, magnesium, and silicon. It is categorized by botanists as a C_4 plant meaning it is superior in the process of photosynthesis, which makes it a very nutritious food. Amaranth can be cooked as a side dish, added to soups and stews, or popped like popcorn. The amount of amaranth in packaged products and cereals is usually not very significant.

Kamut means wheat in Egyptian and can be used in breads, baked goods, and pasta. It has a flavorful, buttery taste and can often be tolerated by individuals who are allergic to regular wheat. *Quinoa* can be used as a cereal, has the highest protein content of any grain, an amino acid profile similar to milk, more calcium than milk, and contains other nutrients including B vitamins and vitamin E. Prepare as a side dish, a substitute for rice in any recipe, or add to soups. *Spelt* is an ancient red wheat and is best used in cereals and breads. Easily assimilated by the body, it may be tolerated by individuals allergic to common wheat. *Tef* is a sweet grain originally from Ethiopia. It has a high mineral content and can be used as a side dish or as flour in baked goods and quick breads. Substitute part wheat flour for tef in recipes.

Barley, whole, also known as Scotch barley, is nutritious and chewy and can be eaten alone or combined with brown rice or beans, or as a base for soup. Pearl barley is refined losing fiber and nutrient content. *Basmati* is a long grain Himalayan rice with a nutty, buttery flavor. White basmati lacks the fiber and nutrient value of brown basmati. Texmati and calmati are basmati hybrids. *Buckwheat* is gluten-free and suitable for cereal/grain induced allergies. It has a high essential amino acid profile and is a good source of the bioflavonoid, rutin. Buckwheat groats can be used as a hot cereal or as a side dish and formed into croquettes or patties. Buckwheat flour is used in pancakes, crepes, and waffles, and can be partly substituted (10%) for wheat flour in baked goods, breads, and pasta. Japanese soba are buckwheat noodles.

Nuts and Seeds

Nuts and seeds contain fat, protein, B complex vitamins, vitamin E, iron, magnesium, and other minerals. Some are high in omega-3 fatty acids. To improve digestibility, they can be soaked overnight or toasted lightly before eating. As they are easily susceptible to rancidity, shelled nuts and seeds bought whole and stored in the refrigerator are the safest. Sliced, roasted, blanched, and pieces of nuts and seeds are suspect because they have been exposed to air and light. Whole nuts with a protective covering like almonds and hazelnuts are better preserved. Nuts in the shell keep well up to a year in a dry cool place.

Meats and Poultry

Meats are the most concentrated form of protein. The fat is saturated and contains cholesterol which is incorporated throughout the meat and unable to be removed. Meats supply complete protein, B complex vitamins, iron, potassium, and other minerals. Organ meats are usually richer in vitamins and minerals than muscle meats. Luncheon meats, frankfurters and sausages are often high in fats and may contain nitrites that can be converted to cancer-causing nitrosamines in the stomach.

Most of the saturated fat and cholesterol in poultry is in the skin and therefore can be removed. Duck and goose have more fat in the meat than chicken or turkey. Poultry is a good source of complete protein, B complex vitamins, and iron. Animals raised for food commercially are given drugs, hormones and other toxic chemicals to increase weight or sale viability, which can affect human health. It is more healthful to choose meats and poultry that have been raised free range and without hormones or drugs.

Seafood

Fish are the best source of omega-3 fatty acids especially fatty fish such as salmon, mackerel, albacore tuna, herring, and sardines. They are also a complete protein and contain valuable trace minerals. Coastal waters are usually more polluted and therefore some fish species and shellfish are especially vulnerable in picking up the toxins. Wild fish are preferable to farmed fish which are often fed drugs to prevent diseases as a result of overcrowding. Fresh fish spoils easily and should be eaten within 2 days.

Eggs

Egg whites are an excellent source of complete protein and although the yolk has a cholesterol content, lecithin and choline are also present and these are fat emulsifiers. The yolk also contains vitamins A, B_2, niacin, biotin, D and E, and the minerals copper, iron, sulfur, and phosphorus, as well as unsaturated fatty acids. Some eggs are available that are fortified with omega-3 fatty acids. Raw egg white should not be consumed in great quantities because it contains a protein, avidin, that interferes with the absorption of biotin. Eggs should be obtained from free range chickens that are raised hormone and drug free.

Dairy Products

Dairy products are a good source of calcium and complete protein. *Yogurt* has special properties, antibiotic in nature, that stimulate the immune system and the production of interferon which activates natural killer cells that fight viruses and cancer tumors; and it contains cultures that promote healthy intestinal bacteria that ward off numerous pathogens and diseases.

The lactose in yogurt, cheese, and buttermilk has already been broken down and may be tolerated by those individuals who cannot metabolize lactose; lactose intolerance causes bloating and flatulence. Goat's milk may be easier to digest for some individuals than cow's milk. Because milk contains saturated fat and cholesterol, especially concentrated in cheese, it is recommended that low-fat or nonfat products be consumed. The protein in milk can adversely affect some individuals by aggravating health conditions such as asthma, sinusitis, and bronchitis. It can also irritate an already overactive immune system in cases of allergies and other autoimmune disorders. Milk products that are not organic may contain residues of drugs and hormones that have been fed to dairy cows.

Seaweed

Seaweed or sea vegetables are rich in minerals that are absorbed from seawater. They are a good source of iodine. *Dulse* is reddish purple in color and mildly tangy and salty in flavor. Tear or cut in pieces and add to salads or vegetable and grain dishes. Toast in the oven for 2 minutes at 350 degrees and use as a bacon substitute. *Hiziki* is dark brown or black and contains more minerals than other seaweeds. It is available dried in long strands that can be sautéed or simmered with vegetables. *Kelp* is available in powder or pill forms. It can also be toasted for 2 minutes in a 350-degree oven and eaten as a snack or rehydrated and sautéed. It complements vegetables, grains, legumes, and seafood.

Wakame is a tenderizing seaweed that increases the digestibility of foods it is cooked with. Add to legume and vegetable dishes, toast to crisp and crumble over foods or rehydrate and cook until soft. *Kombu* can be used in almost all foods or toasted as a snack. When rehydrated it becomes mucilaginous. *Nori* is dark and crisp and available in sheets or flakes. It is used to wrap sushi and rice and can be added to soups and as a condiment for salads, vegetables, and grains. *Arame* has a mild, sweet taste and can be sautéed, combined with vegetables, or rehydrated and added to salads. *Agar* is a gelling agent that can be a substitute for commercial gelatin which is made from the bones, cartilage, and hides of horses, pigs, and cattle. Agar is soothing to the digestive tract and adds bulk to the food. It is available in powdered, granular, flaked, and bar form.

Fermented Foods

Fermented foods are predigested by bacteria, yeast, and molds that change the composition of the food. As part of a daily diet, they encourage the production of beneficial bacteria in the intestine that are necessary for complete and proper digestion, a strong immune system, and as an aid to the production of anticancer compounds. Fermented foods include yogurt with live active cultures, kefir, miso, tempeh, soy sauce, umeboshi, amasake, kombucha, natto, and apple cider and brown rice vinegars. *Miso* is a fermented paste made from soybeans. It can be used as a bouillon and as a replacement for salt, soy sauce, and worcestershire sauce. Simmer for no longer than 1 minute to preserve the microorganisms. *Natto* is fermented soybeans and can be used as a condiment with rice, pasta, and other grains or added to soups. *Tempeh* is fermented soybeans and has a meaty taste that can substitute for burgers and meat in other dishes. It can be fried, grilled, baked, broiled, or steamed. *Umeboshi* is fermented plums and used as a seasoning to replace salt and vinegar. *Amasake* is made from fermented sweet rice and available as a beverage in the refrigerated sections of food markets.

Sweeteners

Honey is made from the nectar of flowers and the subsequent enzymatic action in the stomach of bees. It is 75% glucose and fructose. Raw, minimally filtered honey, contains the most nutrients. Substitute ½ to ¾ cup honey for 1 cup sugar. *Maple syrup* is the sap from the sugar maple tree that is boiled to reduce water content and is 65% sucrose. It can be used in place of honey or sugar in recipes. Substitute ½ to ⅔ cup maple syrup for 1 cup of sugar. *Maple sugar* is evaporated maple syrup and can be used in place of refined sugar. *Molasses* is a by-product of the refining of sugar cane and is rich in minerals. It is 35 to 75% sucrose. Blackstrap is 35% sucrose and the most nutrient-dense. Molasses is used as a sweetener in baked goods, specifically rye bread, ginger cakes, cookies, baked beans, and as a syrup.

Unrefined evaporated cane juice, known as *rapadura*, is the juice of sugar cane and contains vitamins, minerals, and other nutrients. It is 82% sucrose. Use it as a substitute for refined sugar which is 99% sucrose. So-called cane juices and cane sugars in various forms that are found in commercial products are not the same and no better than refined sugar. *Barley malt* is an extract from roasted barley sprouts and its sugars are 65% maltose. It is less sweet than honey and works well in most baked goods. It is the preferred sweetener of many bakeries. *Brown rice syrup* is a mild sweetener, not as suitable for baked goods as other sweeteners, but good for toppings on, for example, pancakes and waffles. The sugars are mostly maltose. *Date sugar* is dehydrated and coarsely ground dates in which most nutrients remain intact. It is 65% fructose and sucrose. Substitute ⅔ cup date sugar for 1 cup white sugar. Sprinkle on top of foods and on baked goods after they have been removed from the oven. Date sugar can also be dissolved in hot water and used like honey or maple syrup. *Stevia* is an herb that is 30 times sweeter than sugar and has no calories. Two drops of extract sweetens 1 cup of liquid. Use to sweeten beverages and desserts.

Fruits are a good source of sweeteners. Juices can be added to breads, cookies, and muffins. Soaked dried fruits and dates can be ground, blended, or mashed into a paste or butter and substituted for other sweeteners in a recipe. Mashed bananas, pureed apples, and applesauce add sweetness and moistness to quickbreads, muffins, and cookies. Fruits can be used as cake fillings, frostings, and toppings. Soaked dried fruits, mashed bananas, or berries can be cooked with arrowroot to a gel and spread on cakes, tarts, or other desserts.

Raw or *turbinado sugar* is highly processed like white sugar except for the final filtration. It is 96% sucrose. *Corn syrup* is corn sugar in a liquid state, highly refined, mostly glucose. *Fructose*, the sugar in fruits and honey, when commercially processed, is highly refined from corn and not much better in nutrient value than refined white sugar. *Brown sugar* is refined sugar either burnt or with added molasses and is 98% sucrose. *Aspartame*, also known as Nutrasweet and Equal, is a combination of the amino acids phenylalanine and aspartic acids made from petrochemicals. Excessive amounts of phenylalanine can cause fetal brain damage and because it changes into aldehyde in the body, can adversely affect liver cells. Aspartame has been implicated in menstrual disorders, headaches, dizziness, seizures, and behavioral problems in children and an increased risk of cancer.[70]

Food Lists

Following are lists of the pharmacological activity of plants, rich food sources of nutrients, including fatty acids, and the glycemic index of various foods. More information can be obtained from the U.S. Department of Agriculture and NAPR-ALERT or Natural Products Alert, a database of over 100,000 studies at the University of Illinois in Chicago.

Pharmacological Activity

Analgesic activity

chili peppers
cinnamon
clove
coffee
garlic
ginger
licorice
onion
peppermint

Antibacterial activity

apple
banana
basil
beet
blueberry
cabbage
carrot
cashew
celery
chili pepper
chives
coconut

cranberry
cumin
daikon
dill
flaxseed
garlic
ginger
honey
horseradish
licorice
lime
nori
nutmeg
olive
onion
papaya
plum
purslane
radish
sage
seaweed
tea, black, green, oolong
umeboshi
watermelon
yogurt

Anticancer activity

asparagus
barley
basil
berries
broccoli
Brussels sprouts
cabbage
cantaloupe
carrot
cauliflower
celery
chili pepper
chives
citrus fruits
cucumber
daikon
eggplant
fennel
fenugreek
flaxseed
garlic
ginger

lentils
licorice
melons
mints
miso
mushrooms, enoki, shiitake, maitake
mustard greens
oats
olive oil
onions
oregano
papaya
parsley
parsnips
peppers
potatoes
rice, brown
rosemary
rutabagas
sage
seafood
soybeans
tarragon
tea, black, green, oolong
thyme
tomatoes
turmeric
turnips
whole wheat
winter squash

Anticoagulant activity

amaranth
cinnamon
cumin
fish oil
garlic
ginger
grape
melons
mushroom, tree ear
onion
Swiss chard
tea
watermelon

Antioxidant activity

apricots
asparagus

avocado
basil
berries
Brazil nut
broccoli
Brussels sprouts
cabbage
carrot
cauliflower
chili peppers
clove
collards
cumin
fish
garlic
ginger
grapefruit, pink
grapes, red
kale
licorice
marjoram
nutmeg
oats
olive oil, extra virgin
onion, red, yellow
orange
peanut
peppers
peppermint
pumpkin
sage
sesame seeds
spearmint
spinach
sweet potatoes
tomatoes
vegetables, green leafy
watermelon

Antiviral activity

apples
barley
black currant
blueberry
chives
coffee
collards
cranberry
dandelion

dill
flaxseed
garlic
ginger
gooseberry
grapes
grapefruit
lemon
mushroom, shiitake
onion
orange
peach
pineapple
plums
raspberry
sage
seaweed
spearmint
strawberry
tea, black, green, oolong

Cholesterol-lowering activity

almonds
apple
avocado
barley
beans, dry
carrots
garlic
grapefruit
mushrooms, shiitake
oats
olive oil
rice, brown
soybeans
walnuts

Salicylate activity

almonds
apples
blueberries
cherries
currants
curry powder
dates
licorice
oranges
paprika
peppers

persimmons
pineapple
prunes
raspberries
tea, black, green, oolong

Sedative activity

anise
celery seed
clove
cumin
fennel
garlic
ginger
honey
marjoram
onion
parsley
sage
spearmint

Rich Sources of Nutrients

Protein

amaranth
dairy products
eggs
fish
grains, whole
legumes
meats
poultry
quinoa
soybeans

Carbohydrates

fruits
grains, whole
legumes
sugars
vegetables

Vitamin A

blueberries
chilis, red
corn
dairy products
eggs

fruits, yellow
liver
prunes
tomatoes
vegetables, dark green
vegetables, yellow

Vitamin B₁

eggs
fish
grains, whole
legumes
meat
molasses, blackstrap
nuts
organ meats
poultry
yeast, nutritional

Vitamin B₂

dairy products
eggs
fish
grains, whole
legumes
meat
meats, organ
molasses, blackstrap
nuts
vegetables, leafy green
yeast, nutritional

Niacin

dairy products
fish
grains, whole
legumes
meat
meats, organ
peanuts
poultry
yeast, brewers

Vitamin B₆

banana
fish
grains, whole
legumes
meats

meats, organ
molasses, blackstrap
potatoes
poultry
vegetables, green leafy
wheat germ
yeast, brewers

Vitamin B₁₂

dairy products
eggs
fish
meat
meats, organ

Folic acid

asparagus
avocado
beans
broccoli
Brussels sprouts
bulgur
dairy products
fruits, citrus
grains, whole
liver
meat
meats, organ
okra
oyster
raspberries
salmon
sunflower seeds
vegetables, leafy green
vegetables, root
wheat germ
whole wheat
yeast, brewers

Pantothenic acid

dairy products
eggs
fish
fruits
grains, whole
legumes
meat
meats, organ
nuts

royal jelly
salmon
vegetables
wheat germ
yeast

Biotin

banana
dairy products
eggs
fish, saltwater
grains, whole
legumes
liver
meat
mushrooms
oats
peanuts
poultry
rice, brown
soybeans
yeast, brewers

Choline

cabbage
cauliflower
eggs
fish
grains, whole
legumes
meat
meats, organ
oats
soybeans
vegetables
wheat germ
yeast, brewers

Inositol

beans
cantaloupe
dairy products
fruits, citrus
grains, whole
legumes
liver
meat
molasses
nuts

oranges
raisins
wheat, whole
yeast, brewers

PABA

dairy products
grains, whole
meats
meats, organ
molasses
mushrooms
poultry
vegetables, green leafy
wheat germ

Vitamin C

acerola berries
beans, sprouted
berries
broccoli
Brussels sprouts
cantaloupe
cauliflower
currants
fruits, citrus
grains, sprouted
guava
kale
kiwi
papaya
parsley
peas, green
peppers, red, green
rose hips
squash
strawberry
tomatoes
vegetables, green leafy

Vitamin D

butter
cod-liver oil
eggs
fatty fish
meats, organ
sunlight
vitamin D fortified foods

Vitamin E

avocado
eggs
grains, whole
legumes
meats, organ
molasses
nuts
seeds
vegetables, leafy green
vegetable oils
wheat germ oil

Vitamin K

leafy green vegetables
eggs
polyunsaturated oils
soybeans
blackstrap molasses
cauliflower
broccoli
Brussels sprouts
cabbage
liver
oats
whole wheat
rye
dairy products
kelp

Bioflavonoids

citrus fruits—white segments
fruits
black currants
buckwheat
onions
apples
black tea
soybeans
blueberries

Carotenoids

dark green vegetables
yellow/orange vegetables
tomatoes
watermelon
guava
apricots
peaches
cantaloupe
pumpkin
pink grapefruit
mango

Calcium

dairy products
mackerel w/bones
sardines w/bones
salmon w/bones
green leafy vegetables
dried figs
tofu
turnip greens
kale
broccoli
okra
soybeans
beans
sesame seeds
whole grains
quinoa
almonds
Brazil nuts
hazelnuts
hiziki
molasses
amaranth

Chromium

brewers yeast
whole grains
dairy products
meat
liver
mushrooms
beets
grapes
honey
raisins
clams
black pepper

Copper

oysters
nuts
seafood
legumes
whole grains

potatoes
green vegetables
meat
organ meats
raisins
almonds
blackstrap molasses

Iodine

seafood
iodized salt
seaweed

Iron

oysters
meat
organ meats
poultry
fish
dried fruit
blackstrap molasses
apricots
raisins
leafy green vegetables
eggs
cherries
whole grains
legumes
oysters
dulse
hiziki

Magnesium

nuts
whole grains
beans
dark green vegetables
fish
meat
kiwi
dairy products
molasses

Manganese

nuts
whole wheat
whole grains
leafy green vegetables

pineapple
blueberries
seeds
legumes
eggs
tea
avocado
seaweed

Molybdenum

legumes
dark leafy green vegetables
whole grains
dairy products
organ meats

Potassium

blackstrap molasses
fruits
avocado
banana
legumes
green leafy vegetables
vegetables
potatoes
tomatoes
dairy products
whole grains
dried fruits
almonds
peanuts
sunflower seeds
fish
meats
poultry

Selenium

Brazil nuts
sesame seeds
brewers yeast
whole grains
tuna
wheat germ
fish
herring
oysters
clams
organ meats

Silicon

cucumbers
grains, whole
vegetables, root

Sulfur

beans
Brussels sprouts
cabbage
dairy products
eggs
fish
garlic
horseradish
kale
meats
onions
peppers, hot
turnips
wheat germ

Vanadium

corn
dill
fish
meat
mushrooms
olives
parsley
radish
soybeans
whole grains

Zinc

brewers yeast
crab
dulse
eggs
fish
herring
kelp
meat
mushrooms
organ meats
oysters
peas, black-eyed
pecans
poultry

pumpkin seeds
sardines
sunflower seeds
soybeans
turkey
wheat germ
whole grains

Fats

Saturated fatty acids
  animal fat
  beef
  butter
  coconut oil
  fatty meats
  lamb
  palm kernel oil
  palm oil
  pork
  veal
  vegetable shortening
Monounsaturated fatty acids
  avocado
  canola oil
  cashews
  macadamia nuts
  olive oil
  peanut oil
  peanuts
  pistachios
  pumpkin seeds
  walnut oil
  walnuts
  peanut oil
Polyunsaturated fatty acids
  corn oil
  cottonseed oil
  fish
  flaxseed oil
  flaxseeds
  grapeseed oil
  safflower oil
  sunflower oil
  sunflower seeds
  sesame oil
  sesame seeds
  soybean oil
  soybeans

walnuts
walnut oil
Omega-6 fatty acids
   black currant oil
   borage oil
   corn oil
   cottonseed oil
   evening primrose oil
   grapeseed oil
   meats
   nuts
   peanut oil
   poultry
   safflower oil
   seeds
   sesame oil
   soybean oil
   sunflower oil
Omega-3 fatty acids
   canola oil
   chia seeds
   fish oils
   flaxseed oil
   flaxseeds
   greens, dark leafy
   hemp oil
   hemp seeds
   pumpkin seeds
   purslane
   soybean oil
   soybeans
   walnuts
   walnut oil
   roe
   mackerel
   anchovies
   herring
   salmon
   sardines
   whitefish
   tuna, albacore
   turbot
   shark
   bluefish
   bass, striped
   tuna
   lake trout
   Atlantic sturgeon

Percent of Fatty Acids

	%SFA	%MUFA	%PUFA	%Other
Beef fat	51	44	4	1
Butter	54	30	4	12
Canola oil	6	62	31	1
Chicken fat	30	47	22	1
Coconut oil	77	6	2	15
Corn oil	13	25	62	
Cottonseed oil	27	19	54	
Flaxseed oil	9	18	73	
Lard	41	47	12	
Margarine	18	48	29	5
Olive oil, extra virgin	14	77	9	
Palm oil	51	39	10	
Peanut oil	13	49	33	5
Safflower oil	10	13	76	1
Sesame oil	13	46	41	
Soybean oil	15	24	61	
Sunflower oil	11	20	69	
Vegetable shortening	26	43	25	6
Walnut oil	16	28	56	

Glycemic Index (GI)

The glycemic index is an indicator of the effect carbohydrates (starches and sugars) have after ingestion on sugar levels in the blood. Carbohydrates that quickly turn into glucose or sugar have a high glycemic index and cause a rapid rise in blood glucose. The pancreas responds by releasing the hormone insulin into the bloodstream to control the elevation of glucose. The pancreas can eventually become exhausted from overstimulation which can result in adult onset diabetes in genetically susceptible individuals. High blood insulin levels are also associated with heart disease and hypertension. Carbohydrates that break down during digestion and absorption more slowly have a low glycemic index, and release sugars into the bloodstream at a gradual and prolonged pace. Less insulin is necessary for regulation, relieving the pancreas of overwork.

There are a number of factors that determine glycemic index values. Amylose starches, because their molecules are in rows and close together, are more difficult for enzymes to break down. Amylopectic starches branch out and are therefore more accessible to enzymatic action. Foods contain both starches, but one is more predominant. Another factor is whether a food is refined or left in its original state. The encasement of whole foods, beans, and seeds in fiber acts as a barrier protecting the starch granules in the interior from rapid enzymatic action, which will slow the rate of digestion, absorption, and conversion to glucose.

The smaller the size of the starch granule, the easier it is for enzymes to facilitate conversion to glucose. Steel roller mills commonly used today grind grains to a much finer degree than grains that are stoneground. The more refined, the less fiber present in the finished product, the faster the food will be digested and absorbed, and the faster the rise in blood glucose. The same food that is processed in different ways will result in differing GI values.

Foods that contain fat and those of an acidic nature like oranges, lemons, vinegar, and sourdough breads, delay the emptying time of the stomach resulting in slower digestion and absorption of a meal. Because fat takes longer for the the stomach to digest, potato chips or french fries, for example, have a lower glycemic index than baked potatoes. Table sugar, because it is not pure glucose but contains two molecules, one glucose and one fructose, takes longer to digest than some starches. Nuts and meats contain little or no carbohydrate and, when combined with starches and sugars, will slow down digestion and absorption. Combining low GI and high GI foods at the same meal will moderate blood sugar levels.

Low glycemic index foods such as whole grains, pasta (because of the large particle size of semolina or whole grains), beans, vegetables, fruit, and low-fat yogurt can help regulate blood sugar levels for diabetics due to the slow digestion rate and consequent gradual release of sugar into the bloodstream. For overweight individuals, low-GI foods tend to contain fewer calories, and because of the prolonged release of sugar into the blood, hunger pangs are abated for longer periods of time. Individudals lacking sustained energy throughout the day can benefit by the gradual and sustained release of energy produced from low-GI foods.

The glycemic index of a food is calculated from an approximate average of a group of individuals tested and often from an average of tests that have been conducted in a number of different countries. Most studies use pure glucose as the reference food giving it a GI of 100. All foods are measured in equivalent amounts of 50 g of *carbohydrate*. This should be kept in mind when reading GI values because, for example, carrots have a high glycemic index but 50 g of carbohydrate grams is far above the normal amount (11 g in one cup) eaten at one time. Blood sugar responses are not consistent, varying in an individual from day to day as well as from one person to another, which can be quite significant, as much as double the effect.

Low GI—below 55

High GI—over 70

Breads	
English muffins	70
Pretzels	83
Pumpernickel, whole grain	51
Rye	76
Sourdough	52
White	70
Wholewheat	67
Wholewheat, pita	57
Wholewheat, stoneground	53
Dairy	
Ice cream	61
Ice cream, lowfat	50
Ice milk	50
Milk, nonfat	32

Milk, whole	23
Yogurt, lowfat	33
Yogurt, nonfat	14

Fruits

Apple	36
Apple, dried	29
Apricot	57
Apple juice, unsweetened	40
Apricot, dried	31
Banana	55
Cantaloupe	65
Cherries	22
Dates	103
Grapefruit	25
Grapefruit juice	48
Grapes	46
Kiwi	52
Mango	55
Orange	44
Orange juice	46
Papaya	58
Peach	42
Pear	38
Pineapple	66
Pineapple juice	46
Plum	39
Raisins	56
Watermelon	7

Grains

Barley	25
Buckwheat groats	54
Bulgur	48
Cheerios	74
Cornflakes	84
Kelloggs All Bran	51
Kelloggs Raisin Bran	73
Muesli	56

Oat Bran	55
Oatmeal	49
Pasta	
Couscous	65
Spaghetti	
White	41
Wholewheat	37
Popcorn	55
Post Grapenuts	67
Post Shredded Wheat	67
Rice	
Basmati	58
Brown	55
Parboiled	48
Rice bran	19
Rice cakes	82
White, short grain	72
Taco shells	68
Wheat, shredded	67

Legumes

Baked beans	48
Black beans	30
Garbanzos	33
Kidney beans	27
Lentils	29
Navy beans	38
Peanuts	14
Pinto beans	39
Soybeans	17
Soymilk	31
Split peas	32
Split pea soup	60

Sugars

Fructose	23
Glucose	100
Honey	58
Lactose	46

Maltose	85		Pumpkin	75
Sucrose	65		Sweet corn	55
Vegetables			Sweet potato	54
Beets	69		Yam	51
Carrots	90		**Miscellaneous**	
Green peas	48		Chocolate	49
Parsnips	90		Coca Cola	63
Potato			Crackers, soda	74
Baked	93		Graham crackers	74
French fries	75		Jam, strawberry	51
New	62		Jelly beans	80
Potato chips	54		Snickers bar	41

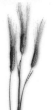

Diet and Food Composition

Weights and Measures

Metric Conversions

1 teaspoon	= 5 milliliters (ml)
1 tablespoon	= 15 milliliters
1 ounce	= 30 milliliters
1 cup	= 235 milliliters or ¼ liter
1 quart	= 0.95 liter
1 gallon	= 3.8 liters

Weights

1 microgram	= 1/1,000,000 gram
1000 micrograms	= 1 milligram
1 milligram	= 1/1000 gram
1000 milligrams	= 1 gram
1.00 ounce	= 28.35 grams
3.57 ounces	= 100.00 grams
0.25 pound	= 113.00 grams
0.50 pound	= 227.00 grams
1.00 pound	= 16.00 ounces
1.00 pound	= 453.00 grams

Capacity Measurements

1 quart	= 4 cups
1 pint	= 2 cups
1 cup	= ½ pint
1 cup	= 8 fluid ounces
1 cup	= 16 tablespoons
2 tablespoons	= 1 fluid ounce
1 tablespoon	= ½ fluid ounce
1 tablespoon	= 3 teaspoons

Approximate Equivalents

1 average serving	= about 4 ounces
1 ounce fluid	= about 28 grams
1 cup fluid	
Cooking oil	= 200 grams
Water	= 220 grams
Milk, soups	= 240 grams
Syrup, honey	= 325 grams
1 cup dry	
Cereal flakes	= 50 grams
Flours	= 100 grams
Sugars	= 200 grams
1 tablespoon fluid	
Cooking oil	= 14 grams
Milk, water	= 15 grams
Syrup, honey	= 20 grams
1 tablespoon dry	= ⅙ ounce
Flours	= 8 grams
Sugars	= 12 grams
1 pat butter	= ½ tablespoon
1 teaspoon fluid	= about 5 grams
1 teaspoon dry	= about 4 grams
1 grain	= about 65 milligrams
1 minim	= about 1 drop water

Abbreviations and Symbols Used in the Tables

avg	average
cal	calorie
C	cup
ckd	cooked
diam	diameter
enr	enriched
g	gram
IU	International Unit
lb	pound
lge	large
mcg	microgram
mg	milligram
oz	ounce
reg	regular
sm	small
sq	square
svg	serving
t	trace
T	tablespoon
tsp	teaspoon
unsw	unsweetened
w	with
w/o	without
whl grd	whole ground
—	reliable data lacking
/	of; with; per
"	inches

Recommended Dietary Intake Chart

For more than 50 years, nutrition experts have produced a set of nutrient and energy standards known as the Recommended Dietary Allowances (RDA). A major revision is currently underway to replace the RDA. The revised recommendations are called Dietary Reference Intakes (DRI) and reflect the collaborative efforts of both the United States and Canada. Until 1997, the RDA were the only standards available and they will continue to serve health professionals until DRI can be established for all nutrients. For this reason, both the 1989 RDA and the 1997 DRI for selected nutrients are presented here.

Recommended Dietary Intakes

1989 Recommended Dietary Allowances (RDA)

Age, yr	Energy, kcal	Protein, g	Vitamin A, µg RE†	Vitamin E, mg α-TE†	Vitamin K, µg	Vitamin C, mg	Thiamin, mg	Riboflavin, mg	Niacin, mg NE	Vitamin B6, mg	Folate, µg	Vitamin B12, µg	Iron, mg	Zinc, mg	Iodine, µg	Selenium, µg
Infants																
0.0–0.5	650	13	375	3	5	30	0.3	0.4	5	0.3	25	0.3	6	5	40	10
0.5–1.0	850	14	375	4	10	35	0.4	0.5	6	0.6	35	0.5	10	5	50	15
Children																
1–3	1300	16	400	6	15	40	0.7	0.8	9	1.0	50	0.7	10	10	70	20
4–6	1800	24	500	7	20	45	0.9	1.1	12	1.1	75	1.0	10	10	90	20
7–10	2000	28	700	7	30	45	1.0	1.2	13	1.4	100	1.4	10	10	120	30
Males																
11–14	2500	45	1000	10	45	50	1.3	1.5	17	1.7	150	2.0	12	15	150	40
15–18	3000	59	1000	10	65	60	1.5	1.8	20	2.0	200	2.0	12	15	150	50
19–24	2900	58	1000	10	70	60	1.5	1.7	19	2.0	200	2.0	10	15	150	70
25–50	2900	63	1000	10	80	60	1.5	1.7	19	2.0	200	2.0	10	15	150	70
51+	2300	63	1000	10	80	60	1.2	1.4	15	2.0	200	2.0	10	15	150	70
Females																
11–14	2200	46	800	8	45	50	1.1	1.3	15	1.4	150	2.0	15	12	150	45
15–18	2200	44	800	8	55	60	1.1	1.3	15	1.5	180	2.0	15	12	150	50
19–24	2200	46	800	8	60	60	1.1	1.3	15	1.6	180	2.0	15	12	150	55
25–50	2200	50	800	8	65	60	1.1	1.3	15	1.6	180	2.0	15	12	150	55
51+	1900	50	800	8	65	60	1.0	1.2	13	1.6	180	2.0	10	12	150	55
Pregnant	+300	60	800	10	65	70	1.5	1.6	17	2.2	400	2.2	30	15	175	65
Lactating																
1st 6 mo	+500	65	1300	12	65	95	1.6	1.8	20	2.1	280	2.6	15	19	200	75
2nd 6 mo	+500	62	1200	11	65	90	1.6	1.7	20	2.1	260	2.6	15	16	200	75

1997 Dietary Reference Intakes (DRI)

Age, yr	Vitamin D, µg	Calcium, mg	Phosphorus, mg	Magnesium, mg	Fluoride, mg
Infants					
0.0–0.5	5	210	100	30	0.01
0.5–1.0	5	270	275	75	0.5
Children					
1–3	5	500	460	80	0.7
4–8	5	800	500	130	1.1
Males					
9–13	5	1300	1250	240	2.0
14–18	5	1300	1250	410	3.2
19–30	5	1000	700	400	3.8
31–50	5	1000	700	420	3.8
51–70	10	1200	700	420	3.8
71+	10	1200	700	420	3.8
Females					
9–13	5	1300	1250	240	2.0
14–18	5	1300	1250	360	2.9
19–30	5	1000	700	310	3.1
31–50	5	1000	700	320	3.1
51–70	10	1200	700	320	3.1
71+	10	1200	700	320	3.1
Pregnant	*	*	*	+40	*
Lactating	*	*	*	*	*

*Values are the same as for other women of comparable age.

†1 µg (1 mcg) is 1 microgram. To convert 1-µg RE (microgram of retinol equivalent) to IUs (International Units), multiply 1-µg RE by 3.33. To convert 1-mg α-TE (alpha tocopherol equivalent) to IUs, multiply 1-mg α-TE by 1.49.

Source: RDA reprinted with permission from Recommended Dietary Allowances, 10th edition © 1959 by the National Academy of Sciences. Courtesy of the National Academy Press, Washington, D.C.; Committee on Dietary Reference Intakes, Dietary Reference Intakes for Calcium, Phosphorus, Magnesium, Vitamin D, and Fluoride (Washington, D.C.: National Academy Press, 1997).

Dietary Reference Intakes: Recommended Intakes for Individuals

Life stage group	Calcium, mg/d	Phosphorus, mg/d	Magnesium, mg/d	Vitamin D, μg/d[a,b]	Fluoride, mg/d	Thiamin, mg/d	Riboflavin, mg/d	Niacin, mg/d[c]
Infants								
0–6 mo	210*	100*	30*	5*	0.01*	0.2*	0.3*	2*
7–12 mo	270*	275*	75*	5*	0.5*	0.3*	0.4*	4*
Children								
1–3 y	500*	**460**	**80**	5*	0.7*	**0.5**	0.5	6
4–8 y	800*	**500**	**130**	5*	1*	**0.6**	0.6	8
Males								
9–13 y	1300*	**1250**	**240**	5*	2*	**0.9**	0.9	12
14–18 y	1300*	**1250**	**410**	5*	3*	**1.2**	1.3	16
19–30 y	1000*	**700**	**400**	5*	4*	**1.2**	1.3	16
31–50 y	1000*	**780**	**420**	5*	4*	**1.2**	1.3	16
51–70 y	1200*	**700**	**420**	10*	4*	**1.2**	1.3	16
>70 y	1200*	**700**	**420**	15*	4*	**1.2**	1.3	16
Females								
9–13 y	1300*	**1250**	**240**	5*	2*	**0.9**	0.9	12
14–18 y	1300*	**1250**	**360**	5*	3*	**1.0**	1.0	14
19–30 y	1000*	**700**	**310**	5*	3*	**1.1**	1.1	14
31–50 y	1000*	**700**	**320**	5*	3*	**1.1**	1.1	14
51–70 y	1200*	**700**	**320**	10*	3*	**1.1**	1.1	14
>70 y	1200*	**700**	**320**	15*	3*	**1.1**	1.1	14
Pregnancy								
≤18 y	1300*	**1250**	**400**	5*	3*	**1.4**	1.4	18
19–30 y	1000*	**700**	**350**	5*	3*	**1.4**	1.4	18
31–50 y	1000*	**700**	**360**	5*	3*	**1.4**	1.4	18
Lactation								
≤18 y	1300*	**1250**	**360**	5*	3*	**1.4**	1.6	17
19–30 y	1000*	**700**	**310**	5*	3*	**1.4**	1.6	17
31–50 y	1000*	**700**	**320**	5*	3*	**1.4**	1.6	17

Note: This table presents Recommended Dietary Allowances (RDAs) in **bold type** and Adequate Intakes (AIs) in ordinary type followed by an asterisk (*). RDAs and AIs may both be used as goals for individual intake. RDAs are set to meet the needs of almost all (97 to 98%) individuals in a group. For healthy breastfed infants, the AI is the mean intake. The AI for other life-stage and gender groups is believed to cover needs of all individuals in the group, but lack of data or uncertainty in the data prevent being able to specify with confidence the percentage of individuals covered by this intake.

[a]As cholecalciferol. 1-mg cholecalciferol = 40-IU vitamin D.

[b]In the absence of adequate exposure to sunlight.

[c]As niacin equivalents (NE). 1 mg of niacin = 60 mg of tryptophan; 0–6 months = preformed niacin (not NE).

Dietary Reference Intakes: Recommended Intakes for Individuals (*Continued*)

Vitamin B₆, mg/d	Folate, μg/d[d]	Vitamin B₁₂, μg/d	Pantothenic acid, mg/d	Biotin μg/d	Choline[e], mg/d	Vitamin C, mg/d	Vitamin E[f], mg/d	Selenium, μg/d	Life stage group
									Infants
0.1*	65*	0.4*	1.7*	5*	125*	40*	4*	15*	0–6 mo
0.3*	80*	0.5*	1.8*	6*	150*	50*	5*	20*	7–12 mo
									Children
0.5	150	0.9	2*	8*	200*	15	6	20	1–3 y
0.6	200	1.2	3*	12*	250*	25	7	30	4–8 y
									Males
1.0	300	1.8	4*	20*	375*	45	11	40	9–13 y
1.3	400	2.4	3*	25*	550*	75	15	55	14–18 y
1.3	400	2.4	5*	30*	550*	90	15	55	19–30 y
1.3	400	2.4	5*	30*	550*	90	15	55	31–50 y
1.7	400	2.4[g]	5*	30*	550*	90	15	55	51–70 y
1.7	400	2.4[g]	5*	30*	550*	90	15	55	>70 y
									Females
1.0	300	1.8	4*	20*	375*	45	11	40	9–13 y
1.2	400[h]	2.4	5*	25*	400*	65	15	55	14–18 y
1.3	400[h]	2.4	5*	30*	425*	75	15	55	19–30 y
1.3	400[h]	2.4	5*	30*	425*	75	15	55	31–50 y
1.5	400	2.4[g]	5*	30*	425*	75	15	55	51–70 y
1.5	400	2.4[g]	5*	30*	425*	75	15	55	>70 y
									Pregnancy
1.9	600[i]	2.6	6*	30*	450*	80	15	60	≤18 y
1.9	600[i]	2.6	6*	30*	450*	85	15	60	19–30 y
1.9	600[i]	2.6	6*	30*	450*	85	15	60	31–60 y
									Lactation
2.0	500	2.8	7*	35*	550*	115	19	70	≤18 y
2.0	500	2.8	7*	35*	550*	120	19	70	19–30 y
2.0	500	2.8	7*	35*	550*	120	19	70	31–50 y

[d]As dietary folate equivalents (DFE). 1 DFE = 1 μg (mcg) food folate = 0.6 μg of folic acid from fortified food or as a supplement consumed with food = 0.5 μg of a supplement taken on an empty stomach.

[e]Although AIs have been set for choline, there are few data to assess whether a dietary supply of choline is needed at all stages of the life cycle, and it may be that the choline requirement can be met by endogenous synthesis at some of these stages.

[f]As α-tocopherol. α-Tocopherol includes RRR-α-tocopherol, the only form of α-tocopherol that occurs naturally in foods, and the 2R-steroisomeric forms of α-tocopheral (*RRR*-, *RSR*-, *RRS*-, and *RSS*-α-tocopherol) that occur in fortified foods and supplements. It does not include the 2S-steroisomeric forms of α-tocopherol (*SRR*-, *SSR*-, *SRS*-, *SSS*-α-tocopherol) also found in fortified foods and supplements.

[g]Because 10 to 30% of older people may malabsorb food-bound B₁₂, it is advisable for those older than 50 years to meet their RDA mainly by consuming foods fortified with B₁₂ or a supplement containing B₁₂.

[h]In view of evidence linking folate intake with neural tube defects in the fetus, it is recommended that all women capable of becoming pregnant consume 400 pg (mcg) from supplements or fortified foods in addition to intake of food folate from a varied diet.

[i]It is assumed that women will continue consuming 400 μg from supplements or fortified food until their pregnancy is confirmed and they enter prenatal care, which ordinarily occurs after the end of the periconceptional period—the critical time for formation of the neural tube.

Source: Food and Nutrition Board, Institute of Medicine—National Academy of Sciences.

Table of Food Composition

The foods in the following table have been divided according to food groups and run alphabetically. All figures are averages of different food samples. The dash (—) indicates that meaningful analysis of the food for that nutrient is lacking. The zero confirms the absence of a nutrient. The content of trace minerals depends on the soil in which the foods are grown and where they are grown and will vary significantly in foods from area to area. Updated values are from the U.S. Department of Agriculture *Nutrient Database for Standard Reference,* Release 13, November 1999.

Food Groups

Beverages

Dairy and Eggs

Fats and Oils

Fruits and Fruit
  Juices

Grains

Legumes

Meats

Nuts and Seeds

Poultry

Seafood and Seaweed

Vegetables and
  Vegetable Juices

Beverages

	Beer, reg.	Coffee, reg.	Coffee substitute, cereal grain	Cola	Tea, brewed
Measure	12 oz	6 oz	6 oz	12 oz	6 oz
Weight, g	356	178	180	370	178
Calories	146	6	9	152	1.8
Protein, g	1.1	0.18	0.18	0	0
Carbohydrate, g	13	0.71	1.8	39	0.53
Fiber, g	0.7	0	0	0	0
Vitamin A, IU	0	0	0	0	0
Vitamin B$_1$, mg	0.02	0	0.01	0	0
Vitamin B$_2$, mg	0.09	0	t	0	0.03
Vitamin B$_6$, mg	0.18	0	0.02	0	0
Vitamin B$_{12}$, mcg	0.07	0	0	0	0
Niacin, mg	1.6	0.4	0.4	0	0
Pantothenic acid, mg	0.21	T	0.02	0	0.02
Folic acid, mcg	21	0.18	0.54	0	9.3
Vitamin C, mg	0	0	0	0	0
Vitamin E, IU	0	0	0	0	0
Calcium, mg	18	3.6	5	11	0
Copper, mg	0.03	0.01	0.02	0.04	0.02
Iron, mg	0.11	0.09	0.01	0.11	0.04
Magnesium, mg	21	9	7	4	0.3
Manganese, mg	0.04	0.05	0.03	0.13	0.4
Phosphorus, mg	43	1.8	13	44	1.8
Potassium, mg	89	96	43	4	66
Selenium, mcg	4.3	0.18	0.36	0.37	0
Sodium, mg	18	3.6	7	15	5
Zinc, mg	0.1	0.04	0.05	0.04	0.04
Total lipid, g	0	0	0	0	0
Total saturated, g	0	t	0.01	0	t
Total unsaturated, g	0	0	0.04	0	t
Total monounsaturated, g	0	t	t	0	t
Cholesterol, mg	0	0	0	0	0
Tryptophan, g	0.01	—	t	—	0
Threonine, g	0.02	—	t	—	0
Isoleucine, g	0.02	—	t	—	0
Leucine, g	0.02	—	t	—	0
Lycine, g	0.03	—	t	—	0
Methionine, g	t	—	t	—	0
Cystine, g	0.01	—	t	—	0
Phenylalanine, g	0.02	—	t	—	0
Tyrosine, g	0.05	—	t	—	0
Valine, g	0.03	—	t	—	0
Arginine, g	0.03	—	t	—	0
Histidine, g	0.02	—	t	—	0
Alanine, g	0.04	—	t	—	0
Aspartic acid, g	0.04	—	t	—	0
Glutamic acid, g	0.11	—	0.03	—	0
Glycine, g	0.03	—	t	—	0
Proline, g	0.11	—	0.01	—	0
Serine, g	0.02	—	t	—	0

Beverages

Beverages

	Tea, herb, brewed	Wine, table, red	Wine, table, white
Measure	6 oz	3.5 oz	3.5 oz
Weight, g	178	103	103
Calories	1.8	74	70
Protein, g	0	0.21	0.1
Carbohydrate, g	0.36	1.8	0.8
Fiber, g	0	0	0
Vitamin A, IU	0	0	0
Vitamin B_1, mg	0.02	0.01	t
Vitamin B_2, mg	t	0.03	0.01
Vitamin B_6, mg	0	0.04	0.01
Vitamin B_{12}, mcg	0	0.01	0
Niacin, mg	0	0.08	0.07
Pantothenic acid, mg	0.02	0.04	0.02
Folic acid, mcg	1	2	0.2
Vitamin C, mg	0	0	0
Vitamin E, IU	0	—	—
Calcium, mg	3.6	8	9
Copper, mg	0.03	0.02	0.02
Iron, mg	0.14	0.44	0.33
Magnesium, mg	1.8	13	10
Manganese, mg	0.08	0.62	0.47
Phosphorus, mg	0	14	14
Potassium, mg	16	115	82
Selenium, mcg	0	0.21	0.21
Sodium, mg	1.8	5	5
Zinc, mg	0.07	0.09	0.07
Total lipid, g	0	0	0
Total saturated, g	t	0	0
Total unsaturated, g	t	0	0
Total monounsaturated, g	t	0	0
Cholesterol, mg	0	0	0
Tryptophan, g	—	—	—
Threonine, g	—	—	—
Isoleucine, g	—	—	—
Leucine, g	—	—	—
Lycine, g	—	—	—
Methionine, g	—	—	—
Cystine, g	—	—	—
Phenylalanine, g	—	—	—
Tyrosine, g	—	—	—
Valine, g	—	—	—
Arginine, g	—	—	—
Histidine, g	—	—	—
Alanine, g	—	—	—
Aspartic acid, g	—	—	—
Glutamic acid, g	—	—	—
Glycine, g	—	—	—
Proline, g	—	—	—
Serine, g	—	—	—

Beverages

Cheese

	Blue	Brick	Brie	Camembert	Cheddar
Measure	1 oz	1 oz	1 oz	1 oz	1 oz
Weight, g	28	28	28	28	28
Calories	100	105	95	85	114
Protein, g	6.07	6.59	5.88	5.61	7.06
Carbohydrate, g	0.66	0.79	0.13	0.13	0.36
Fiber, g	0	0	0	0	0
Vitamin A, IU	204	307	189	262	300
Vitamin B_1, mg	0.008	0.004	0.02	0.008	0.008
Vitamin B_2, mg	0.108	0.1	0.147	0.138	0.106
Vitamin B_6, mg	0.047	0.018	0.067	0.064	0.021
Vitamin B_{12}, mcg	0.345	0.356	0.468	0.367	0.234
Niacin, mg	0.288	0.033	0.108	0.179	0.023
Pantothenic acid, mg	0.49	0.082	0.196	0.387	0.117
Folic acid, mcg	10	6	18	18	5
Vitamin C, mg	0	0	0	0	0
Vitamin E, IU	0.27	0.21	0.28	0.28	0.15
Calcium, mg	150	191	52	110	204
Copper, mg	0.011	0.007	t	0.022	0.031
Iron, mg	0.09	0.12	0.14	0.09	0.19
Magnesium, mg	7	7	5.7	6	8
Manganese, mg	0.003	0.003	0.01	0.011	0.003
Phosphorus, mg	110	128	53	98	145
Potassium, mg	73	38	43	53	28
Selenium, mcg	4	4	4	4	3.9
Sodium, mg	396	159	178	239	176
Zinc, mg	0.75	0.74	0.68	0.68	0.88
Total lipid, gm	8.15	8.41	7.85	6.88	9.4
Total saturated, gm	5.3	5.32	5	4.33	5.98
Total unsaturated, gm	0.23	0.22	0.23	0.21	0.27
Total monounsaturated, gm	2.2	2.4	2.3	2	2.66
Cholesterol, mg	21	27	28	20	30
Tryptophan, g	0.089	0.092	0.091	0.087	0.091
Threonine, g	0.223	0.25	0.213	0.203	0.251
Isoleucine, g	0.319	0.322	0.288	0.275	0.438
Leucine, g	0.545	0.636	0.547	0.522	0.676
Lycine, g	0.526	0.602	0.525	0.501	0.588
Methionine, g	0.166	0.16	0.168	0.16	0.185
Cystine, g	0.03	0.037	0.032	0.031	0.035
Phenylalanine, g	0.309	0.349	0.328	0.313	0.372
Tyrosine, g	0.368	0.316	0.34	0.325	0.341
Valine, g	0.442	0.417	0.38	0.362	0.471
Arginine, g	0.202	0.248	0.208	0.199	0.267
Histidine, g	0.215	0.233	0.203	0.194	0.248
Alanine, g	0.183	0.19	0.243	0.232	0.199
Aspartic acid, g	0.408	0.45	0.383	0.365	0.454
Glutamic acid, g	1.47	1.56	1.24	1.18	1.72
Glycine, g	0.115	0.124	0.112	0.107	0.122
Proline, g	0.596	0.73	0.697	0.665	0.796
Serine, g	0.318	0.366	0.331	0.316	0.413

Dairy and Eggs

Cheese

	Cheshire	Colby	Cottage, creamed, sm curd	Cottage, low-fat, 1%	Cream
Measure	1 oz	1 oz	1 C	1 C	1 oz
Weight, g	28	28	225	226	28
Calories	110	112	232	164	99
Protein, g	6.62	6.74	28	28	2.14
Carbohydrate, g	1.36	0.73	5.6	6	0.75
Fiber, g	0	0	0	0	0
Vitamin A, IU	279	293	367	83	405
Vitamin B$_1$, mg	0.013	0.004	0.05	0.05	0.005
Vitamin B$_2$, mg	0.083	0.106	0.37	0.37	0.056
Vitamin B$_6$, mg	0.02	0.022	0.15	0.15	0.013
Vitamin B$_{12}$, mcg	0.23	0.234	1.4	1.4	0.12
Niacin, mg	0.02	0.026	0.28	0.29	0.029
Pantothenic acid, mg	0.12	0.06	0.48	0.49	0.077
Folic acid, mcg	5.2	5.2	27	28	4
Vitamin C, mg	0	0	0	0	0
Vitamin E, IU	—	0.15	0.4	0.37	0.4
Calcium, mg	182	194	135	137	23
Copper, mg	0.01	0.012	0.06	0.06	0.011
Iron, mg	0.06	0.22	0.32	0.32	0.34
Magnesium, mg	6	7	12	12	2
Manganese, mg	t	0.003	t	t	0.001
Phosphorus, mg	131	129	297	302	30
Potassium, mg	27	36	190	193	34
Selenium, mcg	4	4	20	20	0.68
Sodium, mg	198	171	910	917	84
Zinc, mg	0.8	0.87	0.83	0.86	0.15
Total lipid, g	8.68	9.1	10	2.3	9.89
Total saturated, g	5.5	5.73	6.4	1.5	6.23
Total unsaturated, g	0.25	0.27	0.3	0.07	0.36
Total monounsaturated, g	2.5	2.6	2.9	0.66	2.8
Cholesterol, mg	29	27	34	10	31
Tryptophan, g	0.085	0.087	0.313	0.312	0.019
Threonine, g	0.236	0.24	1.25	1.24	0.091
Isoleucine, g	0.411	0.418	1.65	1.65	0.113
Leucine, g	0.635	0.645	2.9	2.88	0.207
Lycine, g	0.551	0.561	2.3	2.27	0.192
Methionine, g	0.173	0.176	0.846	0.843	0.051
Cystine, g	0.033	0.034	0.26	0.26	0.019
Phenylalanine, g	0.349	0.355	1.5	1.5	0.119
Tyrosine, g	0.32	0.325	1.5	1.5	0.102
Valine, g	0.442	0.45	1.7	1.7	0.125
Arginine, g	0.25	0.254	1.3	1.28	0.081
Histidine, g	0.233	0.236	0.93	0.93	0.077
Alanine, g	0.187	0.19	1.46	1.45	0.065
Aspartic acid, g	0.426	0.433	1.9	1.9	0.151
Glutamic acid, g	1.62	1.64	6	6.1	0.486
Glycine, g	0.114	0.116	0.6	0.6	0.042
Proline, g	0.747	0.759	3.3	3.2	0.195
Serine, g	0.387	0.394	1.6	1.6	0.113

Dairy and Eggs

Cheese

	Edam	Feta	Fontina	Gjetost	Gouda
Measure	1 oz	1 oz	1 oz	1 oz	1 oz
Weight, g	28	28	28	28	28
Calories	101	75	110	132	101
Protein, g	7.08	4	7.26	2.74	7.07
Carbohydrate, g	0.4	1.16	0.44	12	0.63
Fiber, g	0	0	0	0	0
Vitamin A, IU	260	127	333	316	183
Vitamin B$_1$, mg	0.01	0.04	0.006	0.09	0.009
Vitamin B$_2$, mg	0.11	0.24	0.058	0.4	0.095
Vitamin B$_6$, mg	0.022	0.12	0.024	0.07	0.023
Vitamin B$_{12}$, mcg	0.435	0.48	0.48	0.69	0.44
Niacin, mg	0.023	0.28	0.043	0.23	0.018
Pantothenic acid, mg	0.08	0.27	0.122	0.95	0.096
Folic acid, mcg	5	9	1.7	1	6
Vitamin C, mg	0	0	0.	0	0
Vitamin E, IU	0.31	t	0.15	—	0.15
Calcium, mg	207	140	156	113	198
Copper, mg	0.008	—	t	0.023	0.01
Iron, mg	0.12	0.18	0.06	0.15	0.07
Magnesium, mg	8	5	4	20	8
Manganese, mg	0.003	t	t	0.01	t
Phosphorus, mg	152	96	98	126	155
Potassium, mg	53	18	18	400	34
Selenium, mcg	4	4.3	4	4	4
Sodium, mg	274	316	227	170	232
Zinc, mg	1.06	0.82	0.99	0.32	1.11
Total lipid, g	7.88	6	8.83	8.37	7.78
Total saturated, g	4.98	4.24	5.44	5.43	4.99
Total unsaturated, g	0.19	0.17	0.47	0.27	0.19
Total monounsaturated, g	2.3	1.3	2.5	2.2	2.2
Cholesterol, mg	25	25	33	27	32
Tryptophan, g	0.1	0.06	0.1	0.038	0.1
Threonine, g	0.264	0.18	0.27	0.111	0.264
Isoleucine, g	0.371	0.23	0.4	0.147	0.370
Leucine, g	0.720	0.4	0.76	0.281	0.727
Lycine, g	0.754	0.35	0.66	0.231	0.752
Methionine, g	0.204	0.1	0.2	0.09	0.204
Cystine, g	0.07	0.024	0.074	0.016	0.07
Phenylalanine, g	0.406	0.2	0.424	0.153	0.406
Tyrosine, g	0.413	0.19	0.43	0.154	0.412
Valine, g	0.513	0.3	0.55	0.217	0.512
Arginine, g	0.273	0.133	0.24	0.093	0.273
Histidine, g	0.293	0.113	0.27	0.083	0.293
Alanine, g	0.217	0.18	0.23	0.092	0.216
Aspartic acid, g	0.495	0.22	0.4	0.201	0.494
Glutamic acid, g	1.74	0.69	1.46	0.563	1.74
Glycine, g	0.138	0.03	0.13	0.054	0.137
Proline, g	0.922	0.4	0.94	0.334	0.92
Serine, g	0.439	0.33	0.42	0.133	0.438

Dairy and Eggs

Cheese

	Gruyere	Limburger	Monterey Jack	Mozzarella	Mozzarella part skim
Measure	1 oz	1 oz	1 oz	1 oz	1 oz
Weight, g	28	28	28	28	28
Calories	117	93	106	80	72
Protein, g	8.45	5.68	6.94	5.5	6.88
Carbohydrate, g	0.1	0.14	0.19	0.63	0.78
Fiber, g	0	0	0	0	0
Vitamin A, IU	346	363	269	225	166
Vitamin B_1, mg	0.017	0.023	t	0.004	0.005
Vitamin B_2, mg	0.079	0.143	0.111	0.069	0.086
Vitamin B_6, mg	0.023	0.024	0.02	0.016	0.02
Vitamin B_{12}, mcg	0.454	0.295	0.23	0.185	0.232
Niacin, mg	0.03	0.045	0.03	0.024	0.03
Pantothenic acid, mg	0.159	0.334	0.06	0.018	0.022
Folic acid, mcg	3	16	5	2	2
Vitamin C, mg	0	0	0	0	0
Vitamin E, IU	0.15	0.27	0.15	0.15	0.18
Calcium, mg	287	141	212	147	183
Copper, mg	t	t	0.009	t	0.008
Iron, mg	0.05	0.04	0.2	0.05	0.06
Magnesium, mg	10	6	8	5	7
Manganese, mg	t	0.01	0.003	t	0.003
Phosphorus, mg	172	111	126	105	131
Potassium, mg	23	36	23	19	24
Selenium, mcg	4	4	4	4	4.1
Sodium, mg	95	227	152	106	132
Zinc, mg	1	0.6	0.85	0.63	0.78
Total lipid, g	9.17	7.72	8.58	6.12	4.51
Total saturated, g	5.36	4.75	5.4	3.73	2.87
Total unsaturated, g	0.5	0.14	0.26	0.22	0.13
Total monounsaturated, g	2.85	2.44	2.5	1.86	1.3
Cholesterol, mg	31	26	25	22	16
Tryptophan, g	0.119	0.082	0.089	0.08	0.1
Threonine, g	0.309	0.209	0.247	0.21	0.262
Isoleucine, g	0.457	0.346	0.431	0.264	0.33
Leucine, g	0.88	0.593	0.665	0.537	0.671
Lycine, g	0.768	0.475	0.578	0.559	0.699
Methionine, g	0.233	0.176	0.182	0.154	0.192
Cystine, g	0.086	0.03	0.035	0.033	0.041
Phenylalanine, g	0.494	0.316	0.365	0.287	0.359
Tyrosine, g	0.503	0.339	0.335	0.318	0.398
Valine, g	0.636	0.408	0.463	0.344	0.430
Arginine, g	0.276	0.198	0.262	0.236	0.295
Histidine, g	0.317	0.164	0.244	0.207	0.259
Alanine, g	0.272	0.189	0.196	0.168	0.21
Aspartic acid, g	0.466	0.419	0.446	0.399	0.498
Glutamic acid, g	1.69	1.27	1.69	1.28	1.6
Glycine, g	0.151	0.116	0.12	0.105	0.132
Proline, g	1.09	0.691	0.782	0.567	0.708
Serine, g	0.487	0.324	0.406	0.321	0.401

Cheese

	Muenster	Neufchatel	Parmesan, hard	Parmesan, grated	Port du salut
Measure	1 oz	1 oz	1 oz	1 T	1 oz
Weight, g	28	28	28	5	28
Calories	104	74	111	23	100
Protein, g	6.64	2.82	10	2	6.74
Carbohydrate, g	0.32	0.83	0.91	0.19	0.16
Fiber, g	0	0	0	0	0
Vitamin A, IU	318	321	171	35	378
Vitamin B_1, mg	0.004	0.004	0.011	0.002	t
Vitamin B_2, mg	0.091	0.055	0.094	0.019	0.068
Vitamin B_6, mg	0.016	0.012	0.026	0.005	0.015
Vitamin B_{12}, mcg	0.418	0.075	0.34	0.07	0.425
Niacin, mg	0.029	0.036	0.077	0.016	0.017
Pantothenic acid, mg	0.054	0.16	0.128	0.026	0.06
Folic acid, mcg	3	3	2	t	5
Vitamin C, mg	0	0	0	0	0
Vitamin E, IU	0.19	—	0.34	0.06	0.21
Calcium, mg	203	21	336	69	184
Copper, mg	0.009	t	0.101	0.018	t
Iron, mg	0.12	0.08	0.23	0.05	0.12
Magnesium, mg	8	2	12	3	6.9
Manganese, mg	0.002	t	0.006	t	t
Phosphorus, mg	133	39	197	40	102
Potassium, mg	38	32	26	5	39
Selenium, mcg	4	0.85	6.4	1.3	4
Sodium, mg	178	113	454	93	151
Zinc, mg	0.8	0.15	0.78	0.16	0.74
Total lipid, g	8.52	6.64	7.32	1.5	8
Total saturated, g	5.42	4.2	4.65	0.95	4.73
Total unsaturated, g	0.19	0.18	0.16	0.03	0.21
Total monounsaturated, g	2.5	1.9	2	0.44	2.7
Cholesterol, mg	27	22	19	4	35
Tryptophan, g	0.093	0.025	0.137	0.028	0.097
Threonine, g	0.252	0.12	0.373	0.077	0.248
Isoleucine, g	0.325	0.149	0.537	0.11	0.41
Leucine, g	0.641	0.274	0.979	0.201	0.704
Lycine, g	0.606	0.253	0.937	0.192	0.563
Methionine, g	0.161	0.068	0.272	0.056	0.208
Cystine, g	0.037	0.025	0.067	0.014	0.04
Phenylalanine, g	0.352	0.157	0.545	0.112	0.375
Tyrosine, g	0.318	0.135	0.566	0.116	0.403
Valine, g	0.42	0.166	0.696	0.143	0.484
Arginine, g	0.25	0.107	0.373	0.077	0.235
Histidine, g	0.235	0.101	0.392	0.08	0.194
Alanine, g	0.191	0.086	0.297	0.061	0.224
Aspartic acid, g	0.454	0.199	0.634	0.13	0.497
Glutamic acid, g	1.57	0.641	2.32	0.477	1.51
Glycine, g	0.125	0.056	0.176	0.036	0.137
Proline, g	0.735	0.258	1.18	0.243	0.82
Serine, g	0.368	0.149	0.586	0.12	0.385

Dairy and Eggs

Cheese

	Provolone	Ricotta	Ricotta, part skim	Romano	Roquefort
Measure	1 oz	1 C	1 C	1 oz	1 oz
Weight, g	28	246	246	28	28
Calories	100	428	340	110	105
Protein, g	7.25	27.7	28	9	6.11
Carbohydrate, g	0.61	7.48	12.6	1	0.57
Fiber, g	0	0	0	0	0
Vitamin A, IU	231	1205	1063	162	297
Vitamin B_1, mg	0.005	0.032	0.052	0.01	0.011
Vitamin B_2, mg	0.091	0.48	0.455	0.105	0.166
Vitamin B_6, mg	0.021	0.106	0.049	0.024	0.035
Vitamin B_{12}, mcg	0.415	0.831	0.716	0.32	0.182
Niacin, mg	0.044	0.256	0.192	0.022	0.208
Pantothenic acid, mg	0.135	0.52	0.6	0.12	0.491
Folic acid, mcg	3	30	32	2	14
Vitamin C, mg	0	0	0	0	0
Vitamin E, IU	0.15	1.34	0.79	0.3	—
Calcium, mg	214	509	669	302	188
Copper, mg	0.007	0.085	0.08	t	0.01
Iron, mg	0.15	0.94	1.08	0.22	0.16
Magnesium, mg	8	28	36	12	8
Manganese, mg	0.003	0.024	0.03	t	0.009
Phosphorus, mg	141	389	449	215	111
Potassium, mg	39	257	308	25	26
Selenium, mcg	4	36	41	4	4
Sodium, mg	248	207	307	340	513
Zinc, mg	0.92	2.85	3.3	0.73	0.59
Total lipid, g	7.55	31.9	19.4	7.64	8.69
Total saturated, g	4.84	20.4	12.1	4.8	5.46
Total unsaturated, g	0.22	1	0.63	0.17	0.37
Total monounsaturated, g	2.1	8.9	5.7	2.2	2.4
Cholesterol, mg	20	124	76	29	26
Tryptophan, g	0.1	0.31	0.31	0.12	0.086
Threonine, g	0.278	1.27	1.28	0.33	0.274
Isoleucine, g	0.309	1.45	1.46	0.48	0.345
Leucine, g	0.651	3	3.03	0.87	0.6
Lycine, g	0.75	3.29	3.32	0.834	0.524
Methionine, g	0.194	0.69	0.698	0.24	0.16
Cystine, g	0.033	0.243	0.246	0.06	0.036
Phenylalanine, g	0.365	1.36	1.38	0.49	0.3
Tyrosine, g	0.431	1.45	1.46	0.5	0.29
Valine, g	0.465	1.7	1.72	0.62	0.46
Arginine, g	0.29	1.55	1.57	0.33	0.2
Histidine, g	0.316	1.12	1.14	0.35	0.17
Alanine, g	0.2	1.22	1.24	0.26	0.275
Aspartic acid, g	0.494	2.44	2.47	0.56	0.335
Glutamic acid, g	1.76	6	6.08	2.1	1
Glycine, g	0.123	0.725	0.733	0.16	0.04
Proline, g	0.784	2.62	2.65	1.1	0.6
Serine, g	0.417	1.41	1.43	0.52	0.5

Cheese

	Swiss	Tilsit	Processed, American	Processed, Swiss	Cheese spread, American
Measure	1 oz	1 oz	1 oz	1 oz	1 oz
Weight, g	28	28	28	28	28
Calories	107	96	106	95	82
Protein, g	8.06	6.92	6.28	7	4.65
Carbohydrate, g	0.96	0.53	0.45	0.6	2.48
Fiber, g	0	0	0	0	0
Vitamin A, IU	240	296	343	229	223
Vitamin B_1, mg	0.006	0.017	0.008	0.004	0.014
Vitamin B_2, mg	0.103	0.102	0.1	0.078	0.122
Vitamin B_6, mg	0.024	0.02	0.02	0.01	0.033
Vitamin B_{12}, mcg	0.475	0.595	0.197	0.348	0.113
Niacin, mg	0.026	0.058	0.02	0.011	0.037
Pantothenic acid, mg	0.122	0.098	0.137	0.074	0.194
Folic acid, mcg	2	5.67	2	1.7	2
Vitamin C, mg	0	0	0	0	0
Vitamin E, IU	0.21	0.3	0.19	0.28	—
Calcium, mg	272	198	174	219	159
Copper, mg	0.036	t	0.017	t	t
Iron, mg	0.05	0.06	0.11	0.17	0.09
Magnesium, mg	10	4	6	8	8
Manganese, mg	0.005	t	t	t	t
Phosphorus, mg	171	142	211	216	202
Potassium, mg	31	18	46	61	69
Selenium, mcg	3.6	4	4.1	4.5	3.2
Sodium, mg	74	213	406	388	381
Zinc, mg	1.11	0.99	0.85	1.02	0.73
Total lipid, g	7.78	7.36	8.86	7.09	6.02
Total saturated, g	5.04	4.76	5.58	4.55	3.78
Total unsaturated, g	0.276	0.2	0.28	2.18	0.18
Total monounsaturated, g	2.1	2	2.54	—	1.76
Cholesterol, mg	26	29	27	24	16
Tryptophan, g	0.114	0.1	0.092	0.102	0.07
Threonine, g	0.294	0.255	0.204	0.227	0.178
Isoleucine, g	0.436	0.421	0.29	0.324	0.236
Leucine, g	0.839	0.722	0.555	0.62	0.505
Lycine, g	0.733	0.578	0.623	0.696	0.427
Methionine, g	0.222	0.214	0.162	0.181	0.152
Cystine, g	0.082	0.04	0.04	0.045	0.03
Phenylalanine, g	0.471	0.385	0.319	0.356	0.264
Tyrosine, g	0.48	0.413	0.344	0.384	0.252
Valine, g	0.606	0.497	0.376	0.42	0.387
Arginine, g	0.263	0.241	0.263	0.293	0.155
Histidine, g	0.302	0.2	0.256	0.286	0.144
Alanine, g	0.259	0.23	0.157	0.176	0.171
Aspartic acid, g	0.445	0.51	0.386	0.431	0.313
Glutamic acid, g	1.61	1.55	1.3	1.45	0.985
Glycine, g	0.144	0.141	0.103	0.115	0.088
Proline, g	1.04	0.842	0.639	0.713	0.658
Serine, g	0.465	0.395	0.303	0.338	0.294

Dairy and Eggs

Cream

	Half and half	Coffee	Whipping, light	Whipping, heavy	Whipped, pressurized
Measure	1 C	1 T	1 C	1 C	1 C
Weight, g	242	15	239	238	60
Calories	315	29	699	821	154
Protein, g	7.16	0.4	5.19	4.88	1.92
Carbohydrate, g	10.4	0.55	7.07	6.64	7.49
Fiber, g	0	0	0	0	0
Vitamin A, IU	1050	108	2694	3499	548
Vitamin B$_1$, mg	0.085	0.005	0.057	0.052	0.022
Vitamin B$_2$, mg	0.361	0.022	0.299	0.262	0.039
Vitamin B$_6$, mg	0.094	0.005	0.067	0.062	0.025
Vitamin B$_{12}$, mcg	0.796	0.033	0.466	0.428	0.175
Niacin, mg	0.189	0.009	0.1	0.093	0.042
Pantothenic acid, mg	0.699	0.041	0.619	0.607	0.183
Folic acid, mcg	6	t	9	9	1.56
Vitamin C, mg	2.08	0.11	1.46	1.38	0
Vitamin E, IU	0.4	0.03	2.1	2.2	0.54
Calcium, mg	254	14	166	154	61
Copper, mg	0.024	0.033	0.02	0.014	t
Iron, mg	0.17	0.01	0.07	0.07	0.03
Magnesium, mg	25	1	17	17	6
Manganese, mg	t	0	t	t	t
Phosphorus, mg	230	12	146	149	54
Potassium, mg	314	18	231	179	88
Selenium, mcg	4.4	0.09	1.2	1.2	0.84
Sodium, mg	98	6	82	89	78
Zinc, mg	1.23	0.04	0.6	0.55	0.22
Total lipid, g	27.8	2.9	73.8	88	13
Total saturated, g	17.3	1.8	46.2	54.8	8.3
Total unsaturated, g	1	0.11	2	3.3	0.5
Total monounsaturated, g	8	0.84	22	25	3.9
Cholesterol, mg	89	10	265	326	45.6
Tryptophan, g	0.101	0.006	0.073	0.069	0.027
Threonine, g	0.323	0.018	0.234	0.22	0.087
Isoleucine, g	0.433	0.025	0.314	0.295	0.116
Leucine, g	0.702	0.04	0.508	0.478	0.188
Lysine, g	0.568	0.032	0.411	0.387	0.152
Methionine, g	0.18	0.01	0.130	0.122	0.048
Cystine, g	0.066	0.004	0.048	0.045	0.018
Phenylalanine, g	0.346	0.02	0.25	0.236	0.093
Tyrosine, g	0.346	0.02	0.25	0.236	0.093
Valine, g	0.479	0.027	0.347	0.327	0.129
Arginine, g	0.259	0.015	0.188	0.177	0.07
Histidine, g	0.194	0.011	0.141	0.132	0.052
Alanine, g	0.247	0.014	0.179	0.168	0.066
Aspartic acid, g	0.543	0.031	0.393	0.37	0.146
Glutamic acid, g	1.5	0.085	1.08	1.02	0.402
Glycine, g	0.152	0.009	0.110	0.103	0.041
Proline, g	0.694	0.039	0.502	0.473	0.186
Serine, g	0.39	0.022	0.282	0.265	0.104

Dairy and Eggs

	Cream	Frozen Desserts		Milk	
	Sour cream	Ice cream, vanilla	Sherbet, orange	Whole, 3.25% milkfat	Low-fat, 2% added vitamin A
Measure	1 C	½ C	½ C	1 C	1 C
Weight, g	230	66	74	244	244
Calories	493	133	102	150	121
Protein, g	7.27	2.3	0.8	8.03	8.12
Carbohydrate, g	9.82	15.6	23	11.37	11.7
Fiber, g	0	0	0	0	0
Vitamin A, IU	1817	543	56	307	500
Vitamin B$_1$, mg	0.081	0.03	0.02	0.093	0.095
Vitamin B$_2$, mg	0.343	0.16	0.06	0.395	0.403
Vitamin B$_6$, mg	0.037	0.03	0.02	0.102	0.105
Vitamin B$_{12}$, mcg	0.69	0.26	0.14	0.871	0.888
Niacin, mg	0.154	0.08	0.044	0.205	0.21
Pantothenic acid, mg	0.828	0.38	0.133	0.766	0.781
Folic acid, mcg	25	3.3	3.7	12	12
Vitamin C, mg	1.98	0.4	2.3	2.29	2.32
Vitamin E, IU	1.9	0	0.09	0.36	0.25
Calcium, mg	268	85	40	291	297
Copper, mg	0.04	0.02	0.02	0.02	0.02
Iron, mg	0.14	0.06	0.1	0.12	0.12
Magnesium, mg	26	9.2	5.9	33	33
Manganese, mg	t	t	t	0.01	t
Phosphorus, mg	195	69	30	228	232
Potassium, mg	331	131	71	370	377
Selenium, mcg	5.1	1.7	0.96	4.9	5.4
Sodium, mg	123	53	34	120	122
Zinc, mg	0.62	0.46	0.36	0.93	0.95
Total lipid, g	48.2	7.3	1.48	8.15	4.68
Total saturated, g	30	4.48	0.86	5.07	2.92
Total unsaturated, g	1.8	0.27	0.06	0.3	0.17
Total monounsaturated, g	14	2.1	0.4	2.35	1.35
Cholesterol, mg	102	29	4.4	33	18
Tryptophan, g	0.1	0.03	0.01	0.113	0.115
Threonine, g	0.33	0.1	0.03	0.362	0.367
Isoleucine, g	0.44	0.13	0.04	0.486	0.492
Leucine, g	0.71	0.21	0.07	0.786	0.796
Lycine, g	0.58	0.17	0.06	0.637	0.644
Methionine, g	0.184	0.05	0.02	0.201	0.204
Cystine, g	0.067	0.02	0.007	0.074	0.075
Phenylalanine, g	0.35	0.1	0.036	0.388	0.392
Tyrosine, g	0.35	0.1	0.035	0.388	0.392
Valine, g	0.485	0.14	0.05	0.537	0.544
Arginine, g	0.26	0.08	0.03	0.291	0.294
Histidine, g	0.2	0.06	0.02	0.218	0.22
Alanine, g	0.25	0.08	0.03	0.277	0.28
Aspartic acid, g	0.55	0.17	0.06	0.609	0.616
Glutamic acid, g	1.5	0.45	0.15	1.68	1.7
Glycine, g	0.154	0.06	0.016	0.17	0.172
Proline, g	0.7	0.22	0.074	0.778	0.787
Serine, g	0.4	0.117	0.04	0.437	0.442

Milk

	Low-fat, 1%, added vitamin A	Nonfat, added vitamin A	Buttermilk, low-fat	Whole, dry	Nonfat, dry
Measure	1 C	1 C	1 C	1 C	1 C
Weight, g	244	245	245	128	120
Calories	102	86	99	635	435
Protein, g	8	8.35	8.11	33.6	43.4
Carbohydrate, g	11.8	11.8	11.7	49	62.3
Fiber, g	0	0	0	0	0
Vitamin A, IU	500	500	81	1180	43
Vitamin B_1, mg	0.095	0.088	0.083	0.362	0.498
Vitamin B_2, mg	0.41	0.343	0.377	1.54	1.86
Vitamin B_6, mg	0.11	0.098	0.083	0.387	0.433
Vitamin B_{12}, mcg	0.9	0.926	0.537	4.16	4.84
Niacin, mg	0.212	0.216	0.142	0.827	1.14
Pantothenic acid, mg	0.79	0.806	0.674	2.9	4.28
Folic acid, mcg	12.4	13	12.3	47	60
Vitamin C, mg	2.4	2.4	2.4	11	8.11
Vitamin E, IU	0.15	0.15	0.22	2	0.04
Calcium, mg	300	302	285	1168	1508
Copper, mg	0.024	0.027	0.027	0.1	0.05
Iron, mg	0.1	0.1	0.12	0.6	0.38
Magnesium, mg	34	28	27	108	132
Manganese, mg	t	t	t	0.05	0.024
Phosphorus, mg	235	247	219	993	1162
Potassium, mg	381	406	371	1702	2153
Selenium, mcg	2.2	5	4.9	21	32.7
Sodium, mg	123	126	257	475	642
Zinc, mg	0.95	0.98	1.03	4.28	4.9
Total lipid, g	2.59	0.44	2.16	34.2	0.92
Total saturated, g	1.6	0.287	1.34	21.4	0.6
Total unsaturated, g	0.095	0.017	0.08	0.95	0.036
Total monounsaturated, g	0.75	0.115	0.62	10	0.24
Cholesterol, mg	9.8	4	9	124	24
Tryptophan, g	0.112	0.118	0.088	0.475	0.612
Threonine, g	0.364	0.377	0.386	1.52	1.96
Isoleucine, g	0.486	0.505	0.5	2.03	2.62
Leucine, g	0.786	0.818	0.807	3.3	4.25
Lycine, g	0.637	0.663	0.679	2.67	3.44
Methionine, g	0.2	0.21	0.198	0.845	1.08
Cystine, g	0.07	0.077	0.076	0.312	0.401
Phenylalanine, g	0.39	0.403	0.427	1.62	2.1
Tyrosine, g	0.39	0.403	0.339	1.62	2.1
Valine, g	0.54	0.559	0.596	2.25	2.9
Arginine, g	0.29	0.302	0.309	1.22	1.57
Histidine, g	0.22	0.227	0.233	0.914	1.17
Alanine, g	0.276	0.288	0.292	1.16	1.49
Aspartic acid, g	0.61	0.634	0.647	2.55	3.29
Glutamic acid, g	1.68	1.74	1.57	7.05	9.08
Glycine, g	0.17	0.177	0.178	0.713	0.918
Proline, g	0.78	0.809	0.819	3.26	4.2
Serine, g	0.44	0.454	0.422	1.83	2.36

Dairy and Eggs

Milk

	Nonfat, dry, instant	Condensed, sweetened	Evaporated	Evaporated, nonfat	Chocolate
Measure	1 C	1 C	½ C	½ C	1 C
Weight, g	68	306	126	128	250
Calories	244	982	169	99	208
Protein, g	23.8	24.2	8.58	9.63	7.92
Carbohydrate, g	35.5	166	12.6	14.4	25.8
Fiber, g	0	0	0	0	0.15
Vitamin A, IU	18.3	1004	306	500	302
Vitamin B_1, mg	0.281	0.275	0.059	0.057	0.092
Vitamin B_2, mg	1.18	1.27	0.398	0.394	0.405
Vitamin B_6, mg	0.235	0.156	0.063	0.07	0.1
Vitamin B_{12}, mcg	2.71	1.36	0.205	0.305	0.835
Niacin, mg	0.606	0.643	0.244	0.222	0.313
Pantothenic acid, mg	2.2	2.29	0.804	0.941	0.738
Folic acid, mcg	34	34	10	11	12
Vitamin C, mg	3.79	7.96	2.37	1.58	2.28
Vitamin E, IU	0.02	0.98	0.34	0.009	0.34
Calcium, mg	837	868	329	369	280
Copper, mg	0.03	0.046	0.02	0.02	0.16
Iron, mg	0.21	0.58	0.24	0.37	0.6
Magnesium, mg	80	78	30	34	33
Manganese, mg	0.014	0.018	t	t	0.19
Phosphorus, mg	670	775	255	248	251
Potassium, mg	1160	1136	382	423	417
Selenium, mcg	18.6	45.3	2.89	3.2	4.75
Sodium, mg	373	389	133	147	149
Zinc, mg	3	2.88	0.97	1.15	1.02
Total lipid, g	0.49	26.6	9.53	0.26	8.48
Total saturated, g	0.32	16.8	5.78	0.155	5.26
Total unsaturated, g	0.02	1.03	0.31	0.008	0.31
Total monounsaturated, g	0.127	7.4	2.94	0.079	2.48
Cholesterol, mg	12	104	37	5	30
Tryptophan, g	0.337	0.341	0.121	0.136	0.112
Threonine, g	1.07	1.09	0.387	0.435	0.358
Isoleucine, g	1.44	1.46	0.519	0.582	0.479
Leucine, g	2.33	2.37	0.841	0.943	0.776
Lycine, g	1.89	1.92	0.681	0.763	0.629
Methionine, g	0.599	0.607	0.215	0.241	0.199
Cystine, g	0.221	0.224	0.079	0.089	0.073
Phenylalanine, g	1.15	1.16	0.414	0.465	0.383
Tyrosine, g	1.15	1.16	0.414	0.465	0.383
Valine, g	1.59	1.62	0.574	0.644	0.53
Arginine, g	0.864	0.876	0.311	0.349	0.287
Histidine, g	0.647	0.656	0.233	0.261	0.215
Alanine, g	0.823	0.835	0.296	0.332	0.273
Aspartic acid, g	1.81	1.83	0.651	0.73	0.601
Glutamic acid, g	4.99	5.07	1.79	2.01	1.66
Glycine, g	0.505	0.512	0.182	0.204	0.168
Proline, g	2.31	2.34	0.831	0.932	0.768
Serine, g	1.29	1.31	0.467	0.524	0.431

Dairy and Eggs

Dairy and Eggs

	Milk			Yogurt	
	Eggnog	Goat	Human, mature	Plain, whole milk	Plain, low-fat
Measure	1 C	1 C	1 C	1 C	1 C
Weight, g	254	244	246	227	227
Calories	342	168	171	139	144
Protein, g	9.68	8.69	2.53	7.88	11.9
Carbohydrate, g	34.4	10.9	17	10.5	16
Fiber, g	0	0	0	0	0
Vitamin A, IU	894	451	593	279	150
Vitamin B$_1$, mg	0.086	0.117	0.034	0.066	0.1
Vitamin B$_2$, mg	0.483	0.337	0.089	0.322	0.486
Vitamin B$_6$, mg	0.127	0.112	0.027	0.073	0.111
Vitamin B$_{12}$, mcg	1.14	0.159	0.111	0.844	1.27
Niacin, mg	0.267	0.676	0.435	0.17	0.259
Pantothenic acid, mg	1.06	0.756	0.549	0.883	1.34
Folic acid, mcg	2	1	13	17	25
Vitamin C, mg	3.81	3.15	12.3	1.2	1.82
Vitamin E, IU	0.86	0.33	3.3	0.32	0.15
Calcium, mg	330	326	79	274	415
Copper, mg	0.033	0.112	0.12	0.022	0.03
Iron, mg	0.51	0.12	0.07	0.11	0.18
Magnesium, mg	47	34	8	26	40
Manganese, mg	0.013	0.044	0.064	0.01	0.01
Phosphorus, mg	278	270	34	215	326
Potassium, mg	420	499	126	351	531
Selenium, mcg	10.7	3.4	4.43	5.4	8.1
Sodium, mg	138	122	42	105	159
Zinc, mg	1.17	0.73	0.42	1.34	2.02
Total lipid, g	19	10	10.7	7.38	3.52
Total saturated, g	11.3	6.51	4.94	4.76	2.27
Total unsaturated, g	0.86	0.36	1.22	0.225	0.108
Total monounsaturated, g	5.67	2.7	4.08	2.18	1.04
Cholesterol, mg	149	28	31	29	14
Tryptophan, g	0.137	0.106	0.041	0.044	0.067
Threonine, g	0.444	0.398	0.112	0.323	0.489
Isoleucine, g	0.583	0.505	0.137	0.43	0.65
Leucine, g	0.937	0.765	0.233	0.794	1.2
Lycine, g	0.758	0.708	0.160	0.706	1.06
Methionine, g	0.222	0.196	0.052	0.232	0.351
Cystine, g	0.097	0.113	0.047	0.078	0.118
Phenylalanine, g	0.463	0.377	0.113	0.43	0.65
Tyrosine, g	0.462	0.437	0.129	0.398	0.601
Valine, g	0.643	0.585	0.156	0.652	0.986
Arginine, g	0.378	0.291	0.105	0.237	0.359
Histidine, g	0.24	0.218	0.057	0.195	0.295
Alanine, g	0.346	0.287	0.089	0.337	0.51
Aspartic acid, g	0.74	0.512	0.201	0.625	0.945
Glutamic acid, g	1.95	1.52	0.414	1.54	2.33
Glycine, g	0.213	0.123	0.064	0.19	0.288
Proline, g	0.89	0.899	0.203	0.933	1.41
Serine, g	0.55	0.441	0.107	0.488	0.738

Yogurt   Eggs

	Plain, nonfat	Fruit, low-fat	Whole, raw	White, raw	Yolk, raw	Whole, dried
Measure	1 C	1 C	1 lge	1 lge	1 lge	1 T
Weight, g	227	227	50	33	17	5
Calories	127	225	79	16	63	30
Protein, g	13	9.04	6.07	3.35	2.79	2.29
Carbohydrate, g	17.4	42.3	0.6	0.41	0.04	0.24
Fiber, g	0	0.27	0	0	0	0
Vitamin A, IU	16	111	260	0	313	98
Vitamin B$_1$, mg	0.109	0.077	0.044	0.002	0.043	0.015
Vitamin B$_2$, mg	0.531	0.368	0.15	0.094	0.074	0.059
Vitamin B$_6$, mg	0.120	0.084	0.06	0.001	0.053	0.02
Vitamin B$_{12}$, mcg	1.39	0.967	0.773	0.021	0.647	0.5
Niacin, mg	0.281	0.195	0.031	0.029	0.012	0.012
Pantothenic acid, mg	1.45	1.01	0.864	0.08	0.753	0.319
Folic acid, mcg	28	19	32	5	26	9
Vitamin C, mg	1.98	1.36	0	0	0	0
Vitamin E, IU	0.018	0.11	0.78	0	0.78	0.33
Calcium, mg	452	314	28	4	26	11
Copper, mg	0.037	0.194	0.007	0.102	0.004	0.009
Iron, mg	0.2	0.14	1.04	0.01	0.95	0.39
Magnesium, mg	43	30	6	3	3	2
Manganese, mg	0.012	0.157	0.012	0.001	0.015	0.006
Phosphorus, mg	355	247	90	4	86	34
Potassium, mg	579	402	65	45	15	24
Selenium, mcg	8.8	6.86	15.4	5.8	7.5	5.98
Sodium, mg	174	121	69	50	8	26
Zinc, mg	2.2	1.52	0.72	0.01	0.58	0.27
Total lipid, g	0.41	2.61	5.58	0	5.6	2.09
Total saturated, g	0.264	1.68	1.67	0	1.68	0.63
Total unsaturated, g	0.012	0.081	0.68	0	0.698	0.29
Total monounsaturated, g	0.12	0.774	1.9	0	1.9	0.767
Cholesterol, mg	4	10	212	0	212	86
Tryptophan, g	0.073	0.051	0.097	0.051	0.041	0.037
Threonine, g	0.534	0.371	0.298	0.149	0.151	0.113
Isoleucine, g	0.709	0.493	0.380	0.204	0.16	0.143
Leucine, g	1.31	0.911	0.533	0.291	0.237	0.201
Lycine, g	1.16	0.81	0.41	0.206	0.189	0.155
Methionine, g	0.383	0.266	0.196	0.13	0.071	0.074
Cystine, g	0.127	0.08	0.145	0.083	0.05	0.055
Phenylalanine, g	0.709	0.493	0.343	0.21	0.121	0.129
Tyrosine, g	0.656	0.456	0.253	0.134	0.12	0.095
Valine, g	1.07	0.748	0.437	0.251	0.17	0.165
Arginine, g	0.391	0.272	0.388	0.195	0.193	0.147
Histidine, g	0.322	0.224	0.147	0.076	0.067	0.055
Alanine, g	0.557	0.387	0.354	0.216	0.14	0.134
Aspartic acid, g	1.03	0.717	0.602	0.296	0.233	0.227
Glutamic acid, g	2.54	1.77	0.773	0.467	0.341	0.292
Glycine, g	0.314	0.218	0.202	0.125	0.084	0.076
Proline, g	1.54	1.07	0.241	0.126	0.116	0.091
Serine, g	0.805	0.559	0.461	0.247	0.231	0.174

Dairy and Eggs

Fats and Oils

	Almond	Apricot kernel	Avocado	Beef tallow	Butter
Measure	1 T	1 T	1 T	1 T	1 T
Weight, g	13.6	13.6	14	12.8	14.1
Calories	120	120	124	115	101
Protein, g	0	0	0	0	0.12
Carbohydrate, g	0	0	0	0	0.008
Fiber, g	0	0	0	0	0
Vitamin A, IU	0	0	0	0	433
Vitamin B_1, mg	0	0	0	0	t
Vitamin B_2, mg	0	0	0	0	0.004
Vitamin B_6, mg	0	0	0	0	t
Vitamin B_{12}, mcg	0	0	0	0	0.018
Niacin, mg	0	0	0	0	0.006
Pantothenic acid, mg	0	0	0	0	0.016
Folic acid, mcg	0	0	0	0	0.375
Vitamin C, mg	0	0	0	0	0
Vitamin E, IU	7.96	1.76	—	0.52	0.33
Calcium, mg	0	0	0	0	3.37
Copper, mg	0	0	0	0	0.004
Iron, mg	0	0	0	0	0.022
Magnesium, mg	0	0	0	0	0.25
Manganese, mg	0	0	0	0	0.006
Phosphorus, mg	0	0	0	0	3.25
Potassium, mg	0	0	0	t	3.62
Selenium, mcg	0	0	0	0.03	0.142
Sodium, mg	0	0	0	t	117
Zinc, mg	0	0	0	0	0.007
Total lipid, g	13.6	13.6	14	12.8	11.5
Total saturated, g	1.1	0.857	1.62	6.4	7.15
Total unsaturated, g	2.37	3.99	9.5	0.512	0.43
Total monounsaturated, g	9.51	8.16	1.88	5.35	3.33
Cholesterol, mg	0	0	—	14	31
Tryptophan, g	0	0	—	0	0.002
Threonine, g	0	0	—	0	0.005
Isoleucine, g	0	0	—	0	0.007
Leucine, g	0	0	—	0	0.011
Lycine, g	0	0	—	0	0.009
Methionine, g	0	0	—	0	0.003
Cystine, g	0	0	—	0	0.001
Phenylalanine, g	0	0	—	0	0.005
Tyrosine, g	0	0	—	0	0.005
Valine, g	0	0	—	0	0.008
Arginine, g	0	0	—	0	0.004
Histidine, g	0	0	—	0	0.003
Alanine, g	0	0	—	0	0.004
Aspartic acid, g	0	0	—	0	0.009
Glutamic acid, g	0	0	—	0	0.025
Glycine, g	0	0	—	0	0.002
Proline, g	0	0	—	0	0.011
Serine, g	0	0	—	0	0.006

Fats and Oils

Fats and Oils

	Canola	Chicken fat	Coconut	Cod liver	Corn
Measure	1 T	1 T	1 T	1 T	1 T
Weight, g	14	12.8	13.6	13.6	13.6
Calories	124	115	117	123	120
Protein, g	0	0	0	0	0
Carbohydrate, g	0	0	0	0	0
Fiber, g	0	0	0	0	0
Vitamin A, IU	0	0	0	13,600	0
Vitamin B_1, mg	0	0	0	0	0
Vitamin B_2, mg	0	0	0	0	0
Vitamin B_6, mg	0	0	0	0	0
Vitamin B_{12}, mcg	0	0	0	0	0
Niacin, mg	0	0	0	0	0
Pantothenic acid, mg	0	0	0	0	0
Folic acid, mcg	0	0	0	0	0
Vitamin C, mg	0	0	0	0	0
Vitamin E, IU	4.37	0.52	0.057	—	4.28
Calcium, mg	0	0	0	0	0
Copper, mg	0	0	0	0	0
Iron, mg	0	0	t	0	0
Magnesium, mg	0	0	0	0	0
Manganese, mg	0	0	0	0	0
Phosphorus, mg	0	0	0	0	0
Potassium, mg	0	0	0	0	0
Selenium, mcg	0	0.026	0	0	0
Sodium, mg	0	0	0	0	0
Zinc, mg	0	0	0	0	0
Total lipid, g	14	12.8	13.6	13.6	13.6
Total saturated, g	0.994	3.8	11.8	3.08	1.7
Total unsaturated, g	4.14	2.68	0.245	3.07	7.98
Total monounsaturated, g	8.25	5.7	0.79	6.35	3.3
Cholesterol, mg	0	11	0	77.5	0
Tryptophan, g	—	0	0	—	0
Threonine, g	—	0	0	—	0
Isoleucine, g	—	0	0	—	0
Leucine, g	—	0	0	—	0
Lycine, g	—	0	0	—	0
Methionine, g	—	0	0	—	0
Cystine, g	—	0	0	—	0
Phenylalanine, g	—	0	0	—	0
Tyrosine, g	—	0	0	—	0
Valine, g	—	0	0	—	0
Arginine, g	—	0	0	—	0
Histidine, g	—	0	0	—	0
Alanine, g	—	0	0	—	0
Aspartic acid, g	—	0	0	—	0
Glutamic acid, g	—	0	0	—	0
Glycine, g	—	0	0	—	0
Proline, g	—	0	0	—	0
Serine, g	—	0	0	—	0

Fats and Oils

Fats and Oils

	Cottonseed	Grapeseed	Hazelnut	Margarine	Olive
Measure	1 T	1 T	1 T	1 T	1 T
Weight, g	13.6	13.6	13.6	14.1	13.5
Calories	120	120	120	101	119
Protein, g	0	0	0	0	0
Carbohydrate, g	0	0	0	0	0
Fiber, g	0	0	0	0	0
Vitamin A, IU	0	0	0	465	0
Vitamin B_1, mg	0	0	0	0	0
Vitamin B_2, mg	0	0	0	0.006	0
Vitamin B_6, mg	0	0	0	0	0
Vitamin B_{12}, mcg	0	0	0	0.012	0
Niacin, mg	0	0	0	0.003	0
Pantothenic acid, mg	0	0	0	0.012	0
Folic acid, mcg	0	0	0	0.24	0
Vitamin C, mg	0	0	0	0.024	0
Vitamin E, IU	7.75	—	—	2.68	2.49
Calcium, mg	0	0	0	4.23	0.02
Copper, mg	0	0	0	0	0
Iron, mg	0	0	0	t	0.05
Magnesium, mg	0	0	0	0.36	t
Manganese, mg	0	0	0	—	—
Phosphorus, mg	0	0	0	3.24	0.16
Potassium, mg	0	0	0	5.97	—
Selenium, mcg	0	0	0	0	0
Sodium, mg	0	0	0	133	t
Zinc, mg	0	0	0	0	0.01
Total lipid, g	13.6	13.6	13.6	11.4	13.5
Total saturated, g	3.5	1.31	1	2.2	1.8
Total unsaturated, g	7.1	9.51	1.39	3.57	1.13
Total monounsaturated, g	2.4	2.2	10.6	5.04	9.95
Cholesterol, mg	0	0	0	0	0
Tryptophan, g	0	0	0	0.003	0
Threonine, g	0	0	0	0.006	0
Isoleucine, g	0	0	0	0.006	0
Leucine, g	0	0	0	0.012	0
Lycine, g	0	0	0	0.009	0
Methionine, g	0	0	0	0.003	0
Cystine, g	0	0	0	0	0
Phenylalanine, g	0	0	0	0.006	0
Tyrosine, g	0	0	0	0.006	0
Valine, g	0	0	0	0.009	0
Arginine, g	0	0	0	0.003	0
Histidine, g	0	0	0	0.003	0
Alanine, g	0	0	0	0.003	0
Aspartic acid, g	0	0	0	0.009	0
Glutamic acid, g	0	0	0	0.024	0
Glycine, g	0	0	0	0.003	0
Proline, g	0	0	0	0.012	0
Serine, g	0	0	0	0.006	0

Fats and Oils

Fats and Oils

	Palm	Palm kernel	Peanut	Safflower	Sesame
Measure	1 T	1 T	1 T	1 T	1 T
Weight, g	13.6	13.6	13.5	13.6	13.6
Calories	120	117	119	120	120
Protein, g	0	0	0	0	0
Carbohydrate, g	0	0	0	0	0
Fiber, g	0	0	0	0	0
Vitamin A, IU	0	0	0	0	0
Vitamin B$_1$, mg	0	0	0	0	0
Vitamin B$_2$, mg	0	0	0	0	0
Vitamin B$_6$, mg	0	0	0	0	0
Vitamin B$_{12}$, mcg	0	0	0	0	0
Niacin, mg	0	0	0	0	0
Pantothenic acid, mg	0	0	0	0	0
Folic acid, mcg	0	0	0	0	0
Vitamin C, mg	0	0	0	0	0
Vitamin E, IU	4.4	0.77	2.59	6.97	0.83
Calcium, mg	0	0	0.01	0	0
Copper, mg	0	0	0.001	0	0
Iron, mg	T	0	0	0	0
Magnesium, mg	0	0	0.01	0	0
Manganese, mg	0	0	—	0	0
Phosphorus, mg	0.02	0	0	0	0
Potassium, mg	0	0	0	0	0
Selenium, mcg	0	0	0	0	0
Sodium, mg	0	0	0.01	0	0
Zinc, mg	0	0	t	0	0
Total lipid, g	13.6	13.6	13.5	13.6	13.6
Total saturated, g	6.7	11	2.3	0.84	1.9
Total unsaturated, g	1.27	0.22	4.3	1.95	5.67
Total monounsaturated, g	5	1.55	6.24	10	5.4
Cholesterol, mg	0	0	0	0	0
Tryptophan, g	0	0	0	0	0
Threonine, g	0	0	0	0	0
Isoleucine, g	0	0	0	0	0
Leucine, g	0	0	0	0	0
Lycine, g	0	0	0	0	0
Methionine, g	0	0	0	0	0
Cystine, g	0	0	0	0	0
Phenylalanine, g	0	0	0	0	0
Tyrosine, g	0	0	0	0	0
Valine, g	0	0	0	0	0
Arginine, g	0	0	0	0	0
Histidine, g	0	0	0	0	0
Alanine, g	0	0	0	0	0
Aspartic acid, g	0	0	0	0	0
Glutamic acid, g	0	0	0	0	0
Glycine, g	0	0	0	0	0
Proline, g	0	0	0	0	0
Serine, g	0	0	0	0	0

Fats and Oils

Fats and Oils

	Soybean	Sunflower	Vegetable shortening	Walnut	Wheat germ
Measure	1 T	1 T	1 T	1 T	1 T
Weight, g	13.6	13.6	12.8	13.6	13.6
Calories	120	120	115	120	120
Protein, g	0	0	0	0	0
Carbohydrate, g	0	0	0	0	0
Fiber, g	0	0	0	0	0
Vitamin A, IU	0	0	0	0	0
Vitamin B_1, mg	0	0	0	0	0
Vitamin B_2, mg	0	0	0	0	0
Vitamin B_6, mg	0	0	0	0	0
Vitamin B_{12}, mcg	0	0	0	0	0
Niacin, mg	0	0	0	0	0
Pantothenic acid, mg	0	0	0	0	0
Folic acid, mcg	0	0	0	0	0
Vitamin C, mg	0	0	0	0	0
Vitamin E, IU	3.68	1.3	0.23	0.65	39
Calcium, mg	0.01	0.03	0	0	0
Copper, mg	0	0	0	0	0
Iron, mg	t	t	0	0	0
Magnesium, mg	t	0.03	0	0	0
Manganese, mg	0	0	0	0	0
Phosphorus, mg	0.03	0	0	0	0
Potassium, mg	0	0	0	0	0
Selenium, mcg	0	0	0	0	0
Sodium, mg	0	0.01	0	0	0
Zinc, mg	0	0	0	0	0
Total lipid, g	13.6	13.6	12.8	13.6	13.6
Total saturated, g	2	1.4	5.2	1.24	2.6
Total unsaturated, g	7.9	5.45	1.4	8.6	8.4
Total monounsaturated, g	3.17	6.17	5.68	3.1	2.05
Cholesterol, mg	0	0	7.2	0	0
Tryptophan, g	0	0	0	0	0
Threonine, g	0	0	0	0	0
Isoleucine, g	0	0	0	0	0
Leucine, g	0	0	0	0	0
Lycine, g	0	0	0	0	0
Methionine, g	0	0	0	0	0
Cystine, g	0	0	0	0	0
Phenylalanine, g	0	0	0	0	0
Tyrosine, g	0	0	0	0	0
Valine, g	0	0	0	0	0
Arginine, g	0	0	0	0	0
Histidine, g	0	0	0	0	0
Alanine, g	0	0	0	0	0
Aspartic acid, g	0	0	0	0	0
Glutamic acid, g	0	0	0	0	0
Glycine, g	0	0	0	0	0
Proline, g	0	0	0	0	0
Serine, g	0	0	0	0	0

Fruits and Fruit Juices

	Apple, med	Apple, dried	Apple juice	Applesauce, unsw.	Apricot
Measure	1	10 rings	1 C	1 C	3
Weight, g	138	64	248	244	105
Calories	81	155	116	106	51
Protein, g	0.27	0.59	0.15	0.4	1.48
Carbohydrate, g	21	42	29	27.5	11.7
Fiber, g	3.7	5.57	0.52	2.9	2.5
Vitamin A, IU	74	0	2	70	2769
Vitamin B$_1$, mg	0.023	0	0.052	0.032	0.032
Vitamin B$_2$, mg	0.019	0.102	0.042	0.061	0.042
Vitamin B$_6$, mg	0.066	0.08	0.074	0.063	0.057
Vitamin B$_{12}$, mcg	0	0	0	0	0
Niacin, mg	0.106	0.593	0.248	0.459	0.636
Pantothenic acid, mg	0.084	0.16	0.156	0.232	0.254
Folic acid, mcg	3.9	0	0.2	1.4	9.1
Vitamin C, mg	7.8	2.5	2.3	2.9	10.6
Vitamin E, IU	0.66	0.52	0.04	0.036	1.39
Calcium, mg	10	9	16	7	15
Copper, mg	0.057	0.122	0.055	0.063	0.094
Iron, mg	0.25	0.9	0.92	0.29	0.58
Magnesium, mg	6	10	8	7	8
Manganese, mg	0.062	0.058	0.28	0.183	0.084
Phosphorus, mg	10	25	18	18	21
Potassium, mg	159	288	296	183	313
Selenium, mcg	0.7	0.83	0.25	0.488	0.42
Sodium, mg	1	56	7	5	1
Zinc, mg	0.05	0.13	0.07	0.06	0.28
Total lipid, g	0.49	0.2	0.28	0.12	0.41
Total saturated, g	0.08	0.033	0.047	0.02	0.029
Total unsaturated, g	0.145	0.06	0.082	0.034	0.027
Total monounsaturated, g	0.021	0.01	0.012	0.005	0.06
Cholesterol, mg	0	0	0	0	0
Tryptophan, g	0.003	0.006	—	0.005	0.016
Threonine, g	0.01	0.021	—	0.015	0.05
Isoleucine, g	0.011	0.024	—	0.015	0.043
Leucine, g	0.017	0.036	—	0.024	0.082
Lycine, g	0.017	0.037	—	0.024	0.103
Methionine, g	0.003	0.006	—	0.005	0.006
Cystine, g	0.004	0.008	—	0.005	0.003
Phenylalanine, g	0.007	0.017	—	0.012	0.055
Tyrosine, g	0.006	0.011	—	0.007	0.031
Valine, g	0.012	0.028	—	0.02	0.05
Arginine, g	0.008	0.019	—	0.012	0.048
Histidine, g	0.004	0.01	—	0.007	0.029
Alanine, g	0.01	0.021	—	0.015	0.072
Aspartic acid, g	0.047	0.104	—	0.068	0.333
Glutamic acid, g	0.028	0.062	—	0.041	0.166
Glycine, g	0.011	0.024	—	0.015	0.042
Proline, g	0.01	0.02	—	0.015	0.107
Serine, g	0.011	0.024	—	0.017	0.088

Fruits/Juices

Fruits and Fruit Juices

	Apricot, dried	Apricot nectar	Avocado	Banana, med.	Blackberries
Measure	10 halves	1 C	1	1	1 C
Weight, g	35	251	272	175	144
Calories	83	141	324	105	74
Protein, g	1.28	0.92	3.99	1.18	1.04
Carbohydrate, g	21.6	36	14.8	26.7	18.3
Fiber, g	3.15	1.5	10	2.8	7.6
Vitamin A, IU	2534	3304	1230	92	237
Vitamin B_1, mg	0.003	0.023	0.217	0.051	0.043
Vitamin B_2, mg	0.053	0.035	0.245	0.114	0.058
Vitamin B_6, mg	0.055	0.055	0.563	0.659	0.084
Vitamin B_{12}, mcg	0	0	0	0	0
Niacin, mg	1.05	0.653	3.86	0.616	0.576
Pantothenic acid, mg	0.264	0.24	1.95	0.296	0.346
Folic acid, mcg	3.6	3.3	124	21.8	49
Vitamin C, mg	0.8	1.4	15.9	10.3	30.2
Vitamin E, IU	0.775	0.3	0.4	0.55	1.52
Calcium, mg	16	17	22	7	46
Copper, mg	0.15	0.183	0.527	0.119	0.202
Iron, mg	1.65	0.96	2.05	0.35	0.83
Magnesium, mg	16	13	79	33	29
Manganese, mg	0.096	0.08	0.454	0.173	1.86
Phosphorus, mg	41	23	83	22	30
Potassium, mg	482	286	1204	451	282
Selenium, mcg	0.77	0.5	0.8	1.5	0.864
Sodium, mg	3	9	21	1	0
Zinc, mg	0.26	0.23	0.84	0.19	0.39
Total lipid, g	0.16	0.23	30.8	0.55	0.56
Total saturated, g	0.011	0.015	4.9	0.21	0.02
Total unsaturated, g	0.03	0.043	3.9	0.12	0.32
Total monounsaturated, g	0.07	0.095	19.3	0.056	0.055
Cholesterol, mg	0	0	0	0	0
Tryptophan, g	0.023	—	0.042	0.014	—
Threonine, g	0.046	—	0.133	0.039	—
Isoleucine, g	0.039	—	0.143	0.038	—
Leucine, g	0.075	—	0.247	0.081	—
Lysine, g	0.089	—	0.189	0.055	—
Methionine, g	0.006	—	0.074	0.013	—
Cystine, g	0.004	—	0.042	0.019	—
Phenylalanine, g	0.053	—	0.137	0.043	—
Tyrosine, g	0.03	—	0.098	0.027	—
Valine, g	0.047	—	0.195	0.054	—
Arginine, g	0.049	—	0.119	0.054	—
Histidine, g	0.021	—	0.058	0.092	—
Alanine, g	0.063	—	0.239	0.044	—
Aspartic acid, g	0.293	—	0.569	0.129	—
Glutamic acid, g	0.129	—	0.416	0.127	—
Glycine, g	0.04	—	0.167	0.042	—
Proline, g	0.076	—	0.155	0.046	—
Serine, g	0.074	—	0.163	0.054	—

Fruits/Juices

Fruits and Fruit Juices

	Blueberries	Boysenberries, frozen	Cherimoya w/o skin, seeds	Cherries, w/o pits	Cherry, sour
Measure	1 C	1 C	1	1 C	1 C
Weight, g	145	132	547	145	103
Calories	82	66	514	104	51
Protein, g	0.97	1.46	7	1.74	1
Carbohydrate, g	20.5	16	131	24	12.5
Fiber, g	3.9	3.56	13	3.3	1.65
Vitamin A, IU	145	89	55	310	1322
Vitamin B_1, mg	0.07	0.07	0.547	0.073	0.031
Vitamin B_2, mg	0.073	0.049	0.6	0.087	0.041
Vitamin B_6, mg	0.052	0.074	—	0.052	0.045
Vitamin B_{12}, mcg	0	0	0	0	0
Niacin, mg	0.521	1.01	7	0.58	0.412
Pantothenic acid, mg	0.135	0.330	—	0.184	0.147
Folic acid, mcg	9.3	83.6	—	6.1	7.73
Vitamin C, mg	18.9	4.1	49	10.2	10
Vitamin E, IU	2.16	0.885	—	0.28	0.134
Calcium, mg	9	36	126	21	16.5
Copper, mg	0.088	0.106	—	0.138	0.11
Iron, mg	0.24	1.12	2.7	0.56	0.33
Magnesium, mg	7	21	—	16	9.27
Manganese, mg	0.409	0.722	—	0.133	0.115
Phosphorus, mg	15	36	219	28	15.5
Potassium, mg	129	183	—	325	178
Selenium, mcg	0.87	0.79	—	0.87	0.412
Sodium, mg	9	2	—	1	3.1
Zinc, mg	0.16	0.29	—	0.09	0.103
Total lipid, g	0.55	0.35	2.2	1.39	0.309
Total saturated, g	0.046	0.012	—	0.313	0.07
Total unsaturated, g	0.24	0.195	—	0.419	0.093
Total monounsaturated, g	0.078	0.033	—	0.38	0.084
Cholesterol, mg	0	0	0	0	0
Tryptophan, g	0.004	—	—	—	—
Threonine, g	0.026	—	—	—	—
Isoleucine, g	0.03	—	—	—	—
Leucine, g	0.058	—	—	—	—
Lycine, g	0.017	—	—	—	—
Methionine, g	0.016	—	—	—	—
Cystine, g	0.01	—	—	—	—
Phenylalanine, g	0.035	—	—	—	—
Tyrosine, g	0.012	—	—	—	—
Valine, g	0.041	—	—	—	—
Arginine, g	0.049	—	—	—	—
Histidine, g	0.015	—	—	—	—
Alanine, g	0.041	—	—	—	—
Aspartic acid, g	0.075	—	—	—	—
Glutamic acid, g	0.12	—	—	—	—
Glycine, g	0.041	—	—	—	—
Proline, g	0.036	—	—	—	—
Serine, g	0.029	—	—	—	—

Fruits/Juices

Fruits and Fruit Juices

	Crabapple, slices	Cranberries	Currants, black	Dates	Elderberries
Measure	1 C	1 C	1 C	10	1 C
Weight, g	110	95	112	83	145
Calories	0.83	46	71	228	105
Protein, g	0.44	0.37	1.57	1.63	0.95
Carbohydrate, g	21.9	12	17.2	61	26.6
Fiber, g	—	4	—	6.2	10
Vitamin A, IU	44	44	258	42	870
Vitamin B$_1$, mg	0.033	0.029	0.056	0.075	0.102
Vitamin B$_2$, mg	0.022	0.019	0.056	0.083	0.087
Vitamin B$_6$, mg	—	0.062	0.074	0.159	0.334
Vitamin B$_{12}$, mcg	0	0	0	0	0
Niacin, mg	0.11	0.095	0.336	1.82	0.725
Pantothenic acid, mg	—	0.208	0.446	0.647	0.203
Folic acid, mcg	—	1.6	—	10.4	8.7
Vitamin C, mg	8.8	12.8	202	0	52.2
Vitamin E, IU	—	0.14	0.167	0.012	2.16
Calcium, mg	20	7	61	27	55
Copper, mg	0.074	0.055	0.096	0.239	0.088
Iron, mg	0.39	0.19	1.72	0.96	2.32
Magnesium, mg	7	5	27	29	7.25
Manganese, mg	0.127	0.149	0.287	0.247	—
Phosphorus, mg	17	8	66	33	57
Potassium, mg	213	67	361	541	406
Selenium, mcg	—	0.57	—	0.158	0.87
Sodium, mg	1	1	2	2	8.7
Zinc, mg	—	0.12	0.3	0.24	0.16
Total lipid, g	0.33	0.19	0.45	0.37	0.73
Total saturated, g	0.053	0.016	0.038	0.016	0.033
Total unsaturated, g	0.097	0.084	0.2	0.003	0.358
Total monounsaturated, g	0.013	0.027	0.065	0.012	0.116
Cholesterol, mg	0	0	0	0	0
Tryptophan, g	0.004	—	—	0.042	0.019
Threonine, g	0.015	—	—	0.043	0.039
Isoleucine, g	0.018	—	—	0.039	0.039
Leucine, g	0.028	—	—	0.073	0.087
Lysine, g	0.028	—	—	0.05	0.038
Methionine, g	0.004	—	—	0.018	0.02
Cystine, g	0.006	—	—	0.037	0.022
Phenylalanine, g	0.012	—	—	0.046	0.058
Tyrosine, g	0.009	—	—	0.025	0.074
Valine, g	0.021	—	—	0.055	0.048
Arginine, g	0.014	—	—	0.055	0.068
Histidine, g	0.007	—	—	0.025	0.022
Alanine, g	0.015	—	—	0.083	0.044
Aspartic acid, g	0.077	—	—	0.105	0.084
Glutamic acid, g	0.046	—	—	0.177	0.139
Glycine, g	0.018	—	—	0.079	0.052
Proline, g	0.015	—	—	0.088	0.036
Serine, g	0.018	—	—	0.055	0.046

Fruits and Fruit Juices

	Fig	Fig, dried	Gooseberries	Grapefruit, med.	Grapefruit juice
Measure	1	10	1 C	½	1 C
Weight, g	64	190	150	128	247
Calories	47	480	67	38	96
Protein, g	0.48	5.7	1.32	0.75	1.24
Carbohydrate, g	12.2	122	15.2	9.7	22.7
Fiber, g	2.1	23	6.5	1.4	0.247
Vitamin A, IU	91	248	435	149	17.3
Vitamin B_1, mg	0.038	0.133	0.06	0.043	0.099
Vitamin B_2, mg	0.032	0.165	0.045	0.024	0.049
Vitamin B_6, mg	0.072	0.419	0.12	0.05	0.049
Vitamin B_{12}, mcg	0	0	0	0	0
Niacin, mg	0.256	1.3	0.45	0.3	0.494
Pantothenic acid, mg	0.192	0.813	0.429	0.34	0.321
Folic acid, mcg	3.84	14.1	9	12.2	25.7
Vitamin C, mg	1.3	1.6	41.6	41.3	93.9
Vitamin E, IU	0.85	—	0.826	0.26	0.185
Calcium, mg	22	269	38	14	22
Copper, mg	0.045	0.585	0.105	0.056	0.082
Iron, mg	0.23	4.18	0.47	0.1	0.49
Magnesium, mg	11	111	15	10	30
Manganese, mg	0.082	0.726	0.216	0.014	0.049
Phosphorus, mg	9	128	40	10	37
Potassium, mg	148	1332	297	167	400
Selenium, mcg	0.384	2.47	0.9	1.79	0.247
Sodium, mg	1	20	1	0	2
Zinc, mg	0.09	0.94	0.18	0.09	0.13
Total lipid, g	0.19	2.18	0.87	0.12	0.25
Total saturated, g	0.038	0.438	0.057	0.017	0.035
Total unsaturated, g	0.092	1.06	0.475	0.031	0.057
Total monounsaturated, g	0.042	0.49	0.076	0.017	0.032
Cholesterol, mg	0	0	0	0	0
Tryptophan, g	0.004	0.049	—	0.002	—
Threonine, g	0.015	0.187	—	—	—
Isoleucine, g	0.015	0.174	—	—	—
Leucine, g	0.021	0.249	—	—	—
Lycine, g	0.019	0.228	—	0.019	—
Methionine, g	0.004	0.047	—	0.002	—
Cystine, g	0.008	0.094	—	—	—
Phenylalanine, g	0.012	0.138	—	—	—
Tyrosine, g	0.02	0.247	—	—	—
Valine, g	0.018	0.215	—	—	—
Arginine, g	0.011	0.131	—	—	—
Histidine, g	0.007	0.08	—	—	—
Alanine, g	0.029	0.344	—	—	—
Aspartic acid, g	0.113	1.34	—	—	—
Glutamic acid, g	0.046	0.552	—	—	—
Glycine, g	0.016	0.193	—	—	—
Proline, g	0.031	0.376	—	—	—
Serine, g	0.024	0.282	—	—	—

Fruits/Juices

Fruits and Fruit Juices

	Grapes, slipskin	Grapes, seedless	Grape juice	Guava	Kiwi, med.
Measure	1 C	1 C	1 C	1	1
Weight, g	92	160	253	90	76
Calories	62	114	155	45	46
Protein, g	0.58	1.06	1.41	0.74	0.75
Carbohydrate, g	15.7	28.4	37.8	10.7	11.3
Fiber, g	0.92	1.6	0.25	5.04	2.6
Vitamin A, IU	92	117	20	713	133
Vitamin B_1, mg	0.085	0.147	0.066	0.045	0.015
Vitamin B_2, mg	0.052	0.091	0.094	0.045	0.038
Vitamin B_6, mg	0.1	0.176	0.164	0.129	0.068
Vitamin B_{12}, mcg	0	0	0	0	0
Niacin, mg	0.276	0.48	0.663	1.08	0.38
Pantothenic acid, mg	0.022	0.038	0.104	0.135	—
Folic acid, mcg	3.6	6.3	6.5	12.6	29
Vitamin C, mg	3.7	17.3	0.2	165	74.5
Vitamin E, IU	0.466	1.67	—	1.5	1.27
Calcium, mg	13	17	22	18	20
Copper, mg	0.037	0.144	0.071	0.093	0.119
Iron, mg	0.27	0.41	0.6	0.28	0.31
Magnesium, mg	5	10	24	9	23
Manganese, mg	0.661	0.093	0.911	0.13	—
Phosphorus, mg	9	21	27	23	31
Potassium, mg	176	296	334	256	252
Selenium, mcg	0.184	0.32	0.25	0.54	0.456
Sodium, mg	2	3	7	2	4
Zinc, mg	0.04	0.09	0.13	0.21	0.129
Total lipid, g	0.32	0.92	0.19	0.54	0.34
Total saturated, g	0.105	0.302	0.063	0.155	0.022
Total unsaturated, g	0.094	0.27	0.056	0.228	0.183
Total monounsaturated, g	0.013	0.037	0.008	0.05	0.03
Cholesterol, mg	0	0	0	0	0
Tryptophan, g	0.003	0.005	—	0.006	—
Threonine, g	0.016	0.029	0.04	0.028	—
Isoleucine, g	0.005	0.008	0.018	0.027	—
Leucine, g	0.012	0.022	0.03	0.05	—
Lycine, g	0.013	0.024	0.025	0.021	—
Methionine, g	0.019	0.035	0.003	0.005	—
Cystine, g	0.009	0.018	—	—	—
Phenylalanine, g	0.012	0.022	0.03	0.002	—
Tyrosine, g	0.01	0.019	0.008	0.009	—
Valine, g	0.016	0.029	0.025	0.025	—
Arginine, g	0.042	0.078	0.119	0.019	—
Histidine, g	0.021	0.038	0.018	0.006	—
Alanine, g	0.024	0.045	0.218	0.037	—
Aspartic acid, g	0.071	0.13	0.056	0.047	—
Glutamic acid, g	0.121	0.221	0.278	0.096	—
Glycine, g	0.017	0.032	0.03	0.037	—
Proline, g	0.019	0.035	0.04	0.023	—
Serine, g	0.028	0.051	0.033	0.022	—

Fruits/Juices

Fruits and Fruit Juices

	Kumquat	Lemon juice	Lime juice	Loganberries, frozen	Loquat
Measure	1	1 T	1 T	1 C	1
Weight, g	19	15.2	15.4	147	13.6
Calories	12	3	4	80	6.4
Protein, g	0.17	0.06	0.07	2.23	0.06
Carbohydrate, g	3.12	0.99	1.39	19	1.65
Fiber, g	1.25	0.06	0.06	7.2	0.23
Vitamin A, IU	57	2	2	52	208
Vitamin B$_1$, mg	0.015	0.006	0.003	0.074	0.003
Vitamin B$_2$, mg	0.019	0.001	0.002	0.05	0.003
Vitamin B$_6$, mg	0.01	0.007	0.007	0.096	0.014
Vitamin B$_{12}$, mcg	0	0	0	0	0
Niacin, mg	0.095	0.03	0.015	1.23	0.024
Pantothenic acid, mg	—	0.014	0.021	0.359	—
Folic acid, mcg	3	1.5	—	37.8	1.9
Vitamin C, mg	7.1	3.8	4.5	22.5	0.136
Vitamin E, IU	0.07	0.02	0.02	4.8	0.18
Calcium, mg	8	2	1	38	2
Copper, mg	0.02	0.006	0.005	0.172	0.004
Iron, mg	0.07	0.02	0	0.94	0.03
Magnesium, mg	2	1	1	32	1
Manganese, mg	0.016	0.003	0.001	1.83	0.015
Phosphorus, mg	4	1	1	38	3
Potassium, mg	37	15	17	213	36
Selenium, mcg	0.114	0.016	0.015	0.88	0.08
Sodium, mg	1	3	0	1	0.136
Zinc, mg	0.02	0.01	0.01	0.5	t
Total lipid, g	0.02	0	0.02	0.46	0.02
Total saturated, g	0.003	0	0.002	0.016	0.004
Total unsaturated, g	0.005	0	0.008	0.259	0.01
Total monounsaturated, g	0.002	0	0.003	0.044	0.001
Cholesterol, mg	0	0	0	0	0
Tryptophan, g	—	—	—	—	0.001
Threonine, g	—	—	—	—	0.002
Isoleucine, g	—	—	—	—	0.002
Leucine, g	—	—	—	—	0.004
Lycine, g	—	—	—	—	0.003
Methionine, g	—	—	—	—	0.001
Cystine, g	—	—	—	—	0.001
Phenylalanine, g	—	—	—	—	0.002
Tyrosine, g	—	—	—	—	0.002
Valine, g	—	—	—	—	0.003
Arginine, g	—	—	—	—	0.002
Histidine, g	—	—	—	—	0.001
Alanine, g	—	—	—	—	0.003
Aspartic acid, g	—	—	—	—	0.008
Glutamic acid, g	—	—	—	—	0.008
Glycine, g	—	—	—	—	0.003
Proline, g	—	—	—	—	0.004
Serine, g	—	—	—	—	0.003

Fruits/Juices

Fruits and Fruit Juices

	Lychee	Mango	Melon, cantaloupe, sm.	Melon, casaba	Melon, honeydew
Measure	1	1	1	$\frac{1}{10}$	$\frac{1}{10}$
Weight, g	16	207	441	164	125
Calories	6	135	154	43	46
Protein, g	0.08	1.06	3.9	1.48	0.59
Carbohydrate, g	1.59	35	37	10	11.8
Fiber, g	—	3.7	3.5	1.3	0.77
Vitamin A, IU	—	8060	14217	49	52
Vitamin B_1, mg	0.001	0.12	0.159	0.098	0.099
Vitamin B_2, mg	0.006	0.118	0.09	0.033	0.023
Vitamin B_6, mg	—	0.277	0.5	0.197	0.076
Vitamin B_{12}, mcg	0	0	0	0	0
Niacin, mg	0.058	1.21	2.5	0.656	0.774
Pantothenic acid, mg	—	0.331	0.56	—	0.267
Folic acid, mcg	—	29	75	28	7.5
Vitamin C, mg	6.9	57.3	186	26.2	32
Vitamin E, IU	—	3.46	0.66	0.367	0.28
Calcium, mg	0	21	49	8	8
Copper, mg	0.014	0.228	0.19	0.066	0.053
Iron, mg	0.03	0.26	0.93	0.66	0.09
Magnesium, mg	1	18	49	13	9
Manganese, mg	0.005	0.056	0.2	—	0.023
Phosphorus, mg	3	22	75	11	13
Potassium, mg	16	322	1363	344	350
Selenium, mcg	—	1.24	1.76	0.49	0.5
Sodium, mg	0	4	40	20	13
Zinc, mg	0.01	0.07	0.71	0.26	—
Total lipid, g	—	0.57	1.23	0.16	0.13
Total saturated, g	—	0.137	0.313	0.041	0.031
Total unsaturated, g	—	0.106	0.485	0.064	0.049
Total monounsaturated, g	—	0.209	0.031	0.003	0.003
Cholesterol, mg	0	0	0	0	0
Tryptophan, g	0.001	0.017	—	—	—
Threonine, g	—	0.039	—	—	—
Isoleucine, g	—	0.037	—	—	—
Leucine, g	—	0.064	—	—	—
Lycine, g	0.004	0.085	—	—	—
Methionine, g	0.001	0.01	—	—	—
Cystine, g	—	—	—	—	—
Phenylalanine, g	—	0.035	—	—	—
Tyrosine, g	—	0.021	—	—	—
Valine, g	—	0.054	—	—	—
Arginine, g	—	0.039	—	—	—
Histidine, g	—	0.025	—	—	—
Alanine, g	—	0.106	—	—	—
Aspartic acid, g	—	0.087	—	—	—
Glutamic acid, g	—	0.124	—	—	—
Glycine, g	—	0.043	—	—	—
Proline, g	—	0.037	—	—	—
Serine, g	—	0.046	—	—	—

Fruits and Fruit Juices

	Mulberries	Nectarine	Orange	Orange juice	Papaya
Measure	1 C	1	1	1 C	1
Weight, g	140	136	131	248	304
Calories	61	67	62	111	117
Protein, g	2.02	1.28	1.23	1.74	1.86
Carbohydrate, g	13.7	16	15.4	25.8	30
Fiber, g	2.4	2.2	3.1	0.49	5.5
Vitamin A, IU	35	1001	269	496	6122
Vitamin B$_1$, mg	0.041	0.023	0.114	0.223	0.082
Vitamin B$_2$, mg	0.141	0.056	0.052	0.074	0.097
Vitamin B$_6$, mg	0.07	0.034	0.079	0.099	0.058
Vitamin B$_{12}$, mcg	0	0	0	0	0
Niacin, mg	0.868	1.34	0.369	0.992	1.02
Pantothenic acid, mg	—	0.215	0.328	0.471	0.663
Folic acid, mcg	8.4	5.1	39.7	75	116
Vitamin C, mg	51	7.3	69.7	124	187
Vitamin E, IU	0.94	1.8	0.468	0.33	5
Calcium, mg	55	6	52	27	72
Copper, mg	0.08	0.099	0.059	0.109	0.049
Iron, mg	2.59	0.21	0.13	0.5	0.3
Magnesium, mg	25	11	13	27	31
Manganese, mg	—	0.06	0.033	0.035	0.033
Phosphorus, mg	53	22	18	42	16
Potassium, mg	271	288	237	496	780
Selenium, mcg	0.84	0.54	0.655	0.248	1.8
Sodium, mg	14	0	0	2	8
Zinc, mg	0.168	0.12	0.09	0.13	0.22
Total lipid, g	0.55	0.62	0.16	0.5	0.43
Total saturated, g	0.038	0.069	0.02	0.06	0.131
Total unsaturated, g	0.29	0.313	0.033	0.099	0.094
Total monounsaturated, g	0.057	0.237	0.03	0.089	0.116
Cholesterol, mg	0	0	0	0	0
Tryptophan, g	—	—	0.012	0.005	0.024
Threonine, g	—	—	0.02	0.02	0.033
Isoleucine, g	—	—	0.033	0.02	0.024
Leucine, g	—	—	0.03	0.032	0.049
Lycine, g	—	—	0.062	0.022	0.076
Methionine, g	—	—	0.026	0.007	0.006
Cystine, g	—	—	0.013	0.012	—
Phenylalanine, g	—	—	0.041	0.022	0.027
Tyrosine, g	—	—	0.021	0.01	0.015
Valine, g	—	—	0.052	0.027	0.03
Arginine, g	—	—	0.085	0.117	0.03
Histidine, g	—	—	0.024	0.007	0.015
Alanine, g	—	—	0.066	0.037	0.043
Aspartic acid, g	—	—	0.149	0.186	0.149
Glutamic acid, g	—	—	0.123	0.082	0.1
Glycine, g	—	—	0.123	0.022	0.055
Proline, g	—	—	0.06	0.109	0.03
Serine, g	—	—	0.042	0.032	0.046

Fruits/Juices

Fruits and Fruit Juices

	Passion fruit	Peach	Peach, dried	Peach nectar	Pear
Measure	1	1	10 halves	1 C	1
Weight, g	18	98	130	249	166
Calories	18	42	311	134	98
Protein, g	0.4	0.69	4.69	0.67	0.65
Carbohydrate, g	4.21	9.65	79.7	34.6	25
Fiber, g	1.97	2	10	1.5	4
Vitamin A, IU	126	524	2812	643	33
Vitamin B$_1$, mg	0	0.015	0.003	0.007	0.033
Vitamin B$_2$, mg	0.023	0.036	0.276	0.035	0.066
Vitamin B$_6$, mg	0.018	0.016	0.087	0.017	0.03
Vitamin B$_{12}$, mcg	0	0	0	0	0
Niacin, mg	0.27	0.861	5.68	0.717	0.166
Pantothenic acid, mg	—	0.148	0.73	0.169	0.116
Folic acid, mcg	2.5	3	0.39	3.5	12.1
Vitamin C, mg	5.4	6.5	6.3	13.1	6.6
Vitamin E, IU	0.3	1.17	—	0.037	1.24
Calcium, mg	2	5	37	13	19
Copper, mg	0.015	0.059	0.473	0.172	0.188
Iron, mg	0.29	0.1	5.28	0.47	0.41
Magnesium, mg	5	6	54	11	9
Manganese, mg	—	0.041	0.397	0.047	0.126
Phosphorus, mg	12	11	155	16	18
Potassium, mg	63	193	1295	101	208
Selenium, mcg	0.11	0.46	2.86	0.5	1.2
Sodium, mg	5	0	9	17	1
Zinc, mg	0.018	0.12	0.75	0.2	0.2
Total lipid, g	0.13	0.08	0.99	0.05	0.66
Total saturated, g	0.011	0.009	0.107	0.005	0.037
Total unsaturated, g	0.074	0.044	0.48	0.027	0.156
Total monounsaturated, g	0.015	0.033	0.36	0.02	0.139
Cholesterol, mg	0	0	0	0	0
Tryptophan, g	—	0.002	0.013	—	—
Threonine, g	—	0.023	0.183	—	0.017
Isoleucine, g	—	0.017	0.135	—	0.018
Leucine, g	—	0.035	0.265	—	0.033
Lycine, g	—	0.02	0.151	—	0.023
Methionine, g	—	0.015	0.113	—	0.008
Cystine, g	—	0.005	0.038	—	0.007
Phenylalanine, g	—	0.019	0.148	—	0.017
Tyrosine, g	—	0.016	0.122	—	0.005
Valine, g	—	0.033	0.256	—	0.023
Arginine, g	—	0.016	0.12	—	0.012
Histidine, g	—	0.011	0.087	—	0.007
Alanine, g	—	0.037	0.28	—	0.022
Aspartic acid, g	—	0.102	0.783	—	0.128
Glutamic acid, g	—	0.092	0.712	—	0.046
Glycine, g	—	0.021	0.164	—	0.018
Proline, g	—	0.025	0.198	—	0.018
Serine, g	—	0.028	0.217	—	0.023

Fruits and Fruit Juices

	Pear, Asian	Pear, dried	Pear nectar	Persimmon	Pineapple
Measure	1	10 halves	1 C	1	1 C
Weight, g	275	175	250	168	155
Calories	116	459	149	118	77
Protein, g	1.4	3.28	0.27	0.98	0.6
Carbohydrate, g	29	122	39.4	31.2	19.2
Fiber, g	10	13	1.5	6	1.9
Vitamin A, IU	0	6	1	3640	35
Vitamin B$_1$, mg	0.025	0.014	0.005	0.05	0.143
Vitamin B$_2$, mg	0.028	0.254	0.033	0.034	0.056
Vitamin B$_6$, mg	0.06	0.126	0.035	0.168	0.135
Vitamin B$_{12}$, mcg	0	0	0	0	0
Niacin, mg	0.6	2.4	0.32	0.168	0.651
Pantothenic acid, mg	0.19	0.268	0.055	—	0.248
Folic acid, mcg	22	—	3	12.6	16.4
Vitamin C, mg	10.5	12.3	2.7	12.6	23.9
Vitamin E, IU	1.38	—	0.253	1.48	0.23
Calcium, mg	11	59	11	13	11
Copper, mg	0.14	0.649	0.168	0.19	0.171
Iron, mg	0	3.68	0.65	0.26	0.57
Magnesium, mg	22	58	6	15	21
Manganese, mg	0.17	0.572	0.075	0.596	2.55
Phosphorus, mg	30	103	7	28	11
Potassium, mg	333	932	33	270	175
Selenium, mcg	1.65	7.9	1.25	1	0.93
Sodium, mg	0	10	9	3	1
Zinc, mg	0.06	0.68	0.16	0.18	0.12
Total lipid, g	0.63	1.1	0.03	0.31	0.66
Total saturated, g	0.03	0.061	0.003	0.034	0.05
Total unsaturated, g	0.15	0.259	0.007	0.072	0.226
Total monounsaturated, g	0.135	0.231	0.007	0.062	0.074
Cholesterol, mg	0	0	0	0	9
Tryptophan, g	0.014	—	—	0.017	0.008
Threonine, g	0.036	0.086	—	0.05	0.019
Isoleucine, g	0.038	0.095	—	0.042	0.02
Leucine, g	0.069	0.165	—	0.071	0.029
Lycine, g	0.047	0.116	—	0.055	0.039
Methionine, g	0.017	0.039	—	0.008	0.017
Cystine, g	0.014	0.032	—	0.022	0.003
Phenylalanine, g	0.036	0.086	—	0.044	0.019
Tyrosine, g	0.011	0.028	—	0.027	0.019
Valine, g	0.049	0.116	—	0.05	0.025
Arginine, g	0.025	0.056	—	0.042	0.028
Histidine, g	0.014	0.035	—	0.02	0.014
Alanine, g	0.047	0.109	—	0.049	0.026
Aspartic acid, g	0.27	0.644	—	0.096	0.088
Glutamic acid, g	0.1	0.236	—	0.128	0.07
Glycine, g	0.04	0.095	—	0.042	0.026
Proline, g	0.044	0.089	—	0.037	0.02
Serine, g	0.05	0.117	—	0.037	0.039

Fruits and Fruit Juices

	Pineapple juice	Plantain	Plum	Plum, sapotes	Pomegranate
Measure	1 C	1 C	1	1	1
Weight, g	250	148	70	225	154
Calories	139	181	36	302	104
Protein, g	0.8	1.92	0.52	1.8	1.47
Carbohydrate, g	34.4	47.2	8.59	76	26.4
Fiber, g	0.5	3.4	0.99	5.9	0.92
Vitamin A, IU	12	1668	213	923	0
Vitamin B_1, mg	0.138	0.077	0.028	0.022	0.046
Vitamin B_2, mg	0.055	0.08	0.063	0.045	0.046
Vitamin B_6, mg	0.24	0.443	0.053	—	0.162
Vitamin B_{12}, mcg	0	0	0	0	0
Niacin, mg	0.643	1.01	0.330	4.1	0.462
Pantothenic acid, mg	0.25	0.385	0.120	—	0.918
Folic acid, mcg	57.7	32.6	1.4	—	9.24
Vitamin C, mg	26.7	27.2	6.3	45	9.4
Vitamin E, IU	0.075	0.6	0.59	—	1.26
Calcium, mg	42	4	2	88	5
Copper, mg	0.225	0.12	0.028	—	0.108
Iron, mg	0.65	0.89	0.07	2.25	0.46
Magnesium, mg	34	55	4	68	4.6
Manganese, mg	2.47	—	0.032	—	—
Phosphorus, mg	20	50	7	63	12
Potassium, mg	334	739	113	774	399
Selenium, mcg	0.25	2.22	0.33	—	0.92
Sodium, mg	2	6	0	23	5
Zinc, mg	0.29	0.21	0.06	—	0.185
Total lipid, g	0.2	0.55	0.41	1.35	0.46
Total saturated, g	0.013	0.212	0.032	—	0.059
Total unsaturated, g	0.07	0.102	0.088	—	0.097
Total monounsaturated, g	0.022	0.047	0.268	—	0.071
Cholesterol, mg	0	0	0	0	0
Tryptophan, g	—	0.022	—	0.052	—
Threonine, g	—	0.05	0.011	0.131	—
Isoleucine, g	—	0.053	0.011	0.103	—
Leucine, g	—	0.087	0.014	0.189	—
Lysine, g	—	0.080	0.011	0.216	—
Methionine, g	—	0.025	0.004	0.036	—
Cystine, g	—	0.03	0.003	—	—
Phenylalanine, g	—	0.065	0.011	0.119	—
Tyrosine, g	—	0.047	0.004	0.124	—
Valine, g	—	0.068	0.013	0.173	—
Arginine, g	—	0.16	0.009	0.124	—
Histidine, g	—	0.095	0.009	0.095	—
Alanine, g	—	0.075	0.019	0.259	—
Aspartic acid, g	—	0.16	0.164	1.2	—
Glutamic acid, g	—	0.172	0.024	0.486	—
Glycine, g	—	0.067	0.008	0.128	—
Proline, g	—	0.074	0.022	0.128	—
Serine, g	—	0.061	0.013	0.511	—

Fruits/Juices

Fruits and Fruit Juices

	Prickly pear	Prune	Prune juice	Quince	Raisins packed
Measure	1	10	1 C	1	1 C
Weight, g	103	84	256	92	165
Calories	42	201	181	53	488
Protein, g	0.75	2.19	1.55	0.37	4.16
Carbohydrate, g	9.86	52.7	44.6	14	12.9
Fiber, g	3.7	6	2.5	1.56	6.6
Vitamin A, IU	53	1669	9	37	0
Vitamin B$_1$, mg	0.014	0.068	0.041	0.018	0.185
Vitamin B$_2$, mg	0.062	0.136	0.179	0.028	0.3
Vitamin B$_6$, mg	0.062	0.222	0.558	0.037	0.31
Vitamin B$_{12}$, mcg	0	0	0	0	0
Niacin, mg	0.474	1.64	2.01	0.184	1.83
Pantothenic acid, mg	—	0.386	0.274	0.075	—
Folic acid, mcg	6.2	3.1	1	2.76	5.5
Vitamin C, mg	14.4	2.8	10.6	13.8	9
Vitamin E, IU	0.015	3.28	0.04	0.75	1.7
Calcium, mg	58	43	30	10	46
Copper, mg	0.08	0.361	0.174	0.12	0.498
Iron, mg	0.31	2.08	3.03	0.64	4.27
Magnesium, mg	88	38	36	7	49
Manganese, mg	—	0.185	0.387	—	0.441
Phosphorus, mg	25	66	64	16	124
Potassium, mg	226	626	706	181	1362
Selenium, mcg	0.62	1.93	1.54	0.55	1.15
Sodium, mg	6	3	11	4	47
Zinc, mg	0.124	0.45	0.52	0.037	0.3
Total lipid, g	0.53	0.43	0.08	0.09	0.9
Total saturated, g	0.069	0.034	0.008	0.009	0.294
Total unsaturated, g	0.219	0.009	0.018	0.046	0.223
Total monounsaturated, g	0.077	0.029	0.054	0.033	0.03
Cholesterol, mg	0	0	0	0	0
Tryptophan, g	—	—	—	—	—
Threonine, g	—	—	—	—	—
Isoleucine, g	—	—	—	—	—
Leucine, g	—	—	—	—	—
Lycine, g	—	—	—	—	—
Methionine, g	—	—	—	—	—
Cystine, g	—	—	—	—	—
Phenylalanine, g	—	—	—	—	—
Tyrosine, g	—	—	—	—	—
Valine, g	—	—	—	—	—
Arginine, g	—	—	—	—	—
Histidine, g	—	—	—	—	—
Alanine, g	—	—	—	—	—
Aspartic acid, g	—	—	—	—	—
Glutamic acid, g	—	—	—	—	—
Glycine, g	—	—	—	—	—
Proline, g	—	—	—	—	—
Serine, g	—	—	—	—	—

Fruits and Fruit Juices

	Raspberries	Rhubarb	Straw-berries	Tangerine (mandarin)	Tangerine juice	Water-melon
Measure	1 C	1 C	1 C halves	1	1 C	1 C
Weight, g	123	122	152	84	247	160
Calories	61	26	45	37	106	50
Protein, g	1.11	1.09	0.91	0.53	1.24	0.99
Carbohydrate, g	14.2	5.53	10.4	9.4	25	11.5
Fiber, g	8.4	2.2	3.5	1.9	0.5	0.77
Vitamin A, IU	160	122	41	773	1037	585
Vitamin B_1, mg	0.037	0.024	0.03	0.088	0.148	0.128
Vitamin B_2, mg	0.111	0.037	0.098	0.018	0.049	0.032
Vitamin B_6, mg	0.07	0.029	0.088	0.056	0.104	0.23
Vitamin B_{12}, mcg	0	0	0	0	0	0
Niacin, mg	1.1	0.366	0.343	0.134	0.247	0.32
Pantothenic acid, mg	0.295	0.104	0.507	0.168	0.31	0.339
Folic acid, mcg	32	8.7	26.4	17.1	11.4	3.4
Vitamin C, mg	30.8	9.8	84.5	26	76.6	15.4
Vitamin E, IU	0.82	0.364	0.32	0.3	0.22	0.34
Calcium, mg	27	105	21	12	44	13
Copper, mg	0.091	0.026	0.073	0.024	0.062	0.051
Iron, mg	0.7	0.27	0.57	0.09	0.49	0.28
Magnesium, mg	22	14	16	10	20	17
Manganese, mg	1.24	0.239	0.432	0.027	0.091	0.059
Phosphorus, mg	15	17	28	8	35	14
Potassium, mg	187	351	247	132	440	186
Selenium, mcg	0.74	1.34	1.06	0.42	0.247	0.154
Sodium, mg	0	5	2	1	2	3
Zinc, mg	0.57	0.13	0.19	0.202	0.06	0.11
Total lipid, g	0.68	0.24	0.55	0.16	0.49	0.68
Total saturated, g	0.023	0.065	0.03	0.018	0.059	0.074
Total unsaturated, g	0.385	0.121	0.28	0.031	0.099	0.225
Total monounsaturated, g	0.065	0.048	0.079	0.029	0.089	0.165
Cholesterol, mg	0	0	0	0	0	0
Tryptophan, g	—	—	0.01	0.005	0.002	0.011
Threonine, g	—	—	0.028	0.008	0.015	0.043
Isoleucine, g	—	—	0.021	0.014	0.012	0.03
Leucine, g	—	—	0.046	0.013	0.025	0.029
Lycine, g	—	—	0.037	0.027	0.017	0.099
Methionine, g	—	—	0.001	0.011	0.005	0.01
Cystine, g	—	—	0.007	0.006	0.01	0.003
Phenylalanine, g	—	—	0.027	0.018	0.015	0.024
Tyrosine, g	—	—	0.031	0.009	0.007	0.019
Valine, g	—	—	0.027	0.023	0.02	0.026
Arginine, g	—	—	0.039	0.037	0.084	0.094
Histidine, g	—	—	0.018	0.01	0.005	0.01
Alanine, g	—	—	0.046	0.029	0.027	0.027
Aspartic acid, g	—	—	0.206	0.065	0.131	0.062
Glutamic acid, g	—	—	0.134	0.054	0.059	0.101
Glycine, g	—	—	0.036	0.054	0.017	0.016
Proline, g	—	—	0.028	0.026	0.077	0.038
Serine, g	—	—	0.034	0.018	0.022	0.026

Fruits/Juices

Grains

	Amaranth	Barley, pot or scotch	Barley, pearled	Buckwheat groats	Bulgur
Measure	1 C	1 C	1 C	1 C	1 C
Weight, g	195	184	200	164	140
Calories	729	651	704	567	478
Protein, g	28	23	20	19	19
Carbohydrate, g	129	135	155	123	106
Fiber, g	30	32	31	17	25
Vitamin A, IU	0	41	44	0	0
Vitamin B$_1$, mg	0.16	1.19	0.38	0.37	0.32
Vitamin B$_2$, mg	0.41	0.5	0.23	0.44	0.16
Vitamin B$_6$, mg	0.44	0.59	0.52	0.58	0.48
Vitamin B$_{12}$, mcg	0	0	0	0	0
Niacin, mg	2.5	7.4	9	8.4	7.8
Pantothenic acid, mg	2	0.52	0.56	2	1.5
Folic acid, mcg	96	40	46	69	38
Vitamin C, mg	8.2	0	0	0	0
Vitamin E, IU	2.98	1.64	0.39	2.5	0.33
Calcium, mg	298	68	58	28	49
Copper, mg	1.5	0.92	0.84	1	0.47
Iron, mg	15	5.4	5	4	3.4
Magnesium, mg	519	245	158	362	230
Manganese, mg	4.4	3.6	2.6	2.7	4.3
Phosphorus, mg	887	485	442	523	420
Potassium, mg	714	832	560	525	574
Selenium, mcg	—	—	75	14	3.2
Sodium, mg	41	22	18	18	24
Zinc, mg	6.2	5	4.3	4	2.7
Total lipid, g	12.7	4	2.3	4.4	2.5
Total saturated, g	3.2	0.88	0.49	0.97	0.34
Total unsaturated, g	5.64	2.1	1.12	1.36	0.76
Total monounsaturated, g	2.8	0.54	0.3	1.36	0.24
Cholesterol, mg	0	0	0	0	—
Tryptophan, g	0.35	0.38	0.33	0.28	0.266
Threonine, g	1.1	0.78	0.67	0.74	0.5
Isoleucine, g	1.14	0.84	0.72	0.723	0.64
Leucine, g	1.7	1.56	1.35	1.2	1.2
Lycine, g	1.46	0.86	0.74	0.976	0.475
Methionine, g	0.44	0.44	0.38	0.25	0.266
Cystine, g	0.37	0.51	0.44	0.33	0.4
Phenylalanine, g	1.1	1.3	1.1	0.756	0.8
Tyrosine, g	0.64	0.66	0.57	0.35	0.5
Valine, g	1.3	1.13	0.97	0.98	0.776
Arginine, g	2.1	1.2	0.99	1.4	0.81
Histidine, g	0.76	0.52	0.45	0.45	0.4
Alanine, g	1.56	0.9	0.77	1.1	0.6
Aspartic acid, g	2.5	1.4	1.24	1.65	0.88
Glutamic acid, g	4.4	6	5.2	2.97	5.43
Glycine, g	3.2	0.8	0.72	1.5	0.7
Proline, g	1.36	2.7	2.4	0.74	1.78
Serine, g	2.24	0.97	0.84	0.99	0.8

Grains

Grains

	Cornmeal, degermed, enr.	Cornmeal, whl. grain	Millet	Oats	Pasta, corn
Measure	1 C	1 C	1 C	1 C	1 C
Weight, g	138	122	200	156	105
Calories	505	441	756	607	375
Protein, g	11	10.6	22.6	26	7.8
Carbohydrate, g	107	93	146	103	83
Fiber, g	10	9	17	17	12
Vitamin A, IU	0	0	0	0	179
Vitamin B_1, mg	0.987	0.47	0.84	1.2	0.24
Vitamin B_2, mg	0.56	0.25	0.58	0.22	0.09
Vitamin B_6, mg	0.355	0.37	0.77	0.19	0.216
Vitamin B_{12}, mcg	0	0	0	0	0
Niacin, mg	6.95	4.4	9.4	1.5	2.55
Pantothenic acid, mg	—	0.52	1.7	2	0.51
Folic acid, mcg	258	31	170	87	26
Vitamin C, mg	0	0	0	0	0
Vitamin E, IU	0.68	0.6	0.54	1.64	1.58
Calcium, mg	6.9	7.3	16	84	4.2
Copper, mg	0.11	0.24	1.5	0.98	0.212
Iron, mg	5.7	4	6	7.4	0.98
Magnesium, mg	55	155	228	276	125
Manganese, mg	0.145	0.61	3.3	7.7	0.51
Phosphorus, mg	116	294	570	816	266
Potassium, mg	223	350	390	670	309
Selenium, mcg	11	19	5.4	—	8.3
Sodium, mg	4	43	10	3	3.2
Zinc, mg	0.99	2.1	3.4	6.2	1.9
Total lipid, g	2.3	4	8.5	11	2.18
Total saturated, g	0.31	0.46	1.4	1.9	0.3
Total unsaturated, g	0.98	2	4.3	3.95	0.97
Total monounsaturated, g	0.57	1.2	1.55	3.4	0.57
Cholesterol, mg	0	0	0	0	0
Tryptophan, g	—	0.07	0.24	0.365	0.056
Threonine, g	—	0.37	0.7	0.9	0.3
Isoleucine, g	—	0.36	0.9	1.1	0.28
Leucine, g	—	1.2	2.8	2	0.96
Lycine, g	—	0.28	0.4	1.1	0.22
Methionine, g	—	0.21	0.44	0.49	0.164
Cystine, g	—	0.178	0.4	0.64	0.14
Phenylalanine, g	—	0.49	1.16	1.4	0.384
Tyrosine, g	—	0.4	0.68	0.9	0.32
Valine, g	—	0.5	1.16	1.5	0.4
Arginine, g	—	0.5	0.76	1.9	0.4
Histidine, g	—	0.3	0.47	0.63	0.24
Alanine, g	—	0.7	1.97	1.4	0.6
Aspartic acid, g	—	0.69	1.45	2.26	0.545
Glutamic acid, g	—	1.86	4.8	5.8	1.5
Glycine, g	—	0.41	0.57	1.3	0.32
Proline, g	—	0.87	1.75	1.46	0.684
Serine, g	—	0.47	1.3	1.2	0.37

Grains

Grains

	Pasta, couscous	Pasta, macaroni, enr.	Pasta, macaroni, whole wheat, spiral	Pasta, spaghetti, enr.	Pasta, spaghetti, whole wheat
Measure	1 C	1 C	1 C	2 oz	2 oz
Weight, g	173	105	105	57	57
Calories	650	390	365	211	198
Protein, g	22	13	15	7.3	8.4
Carbohydrate, g	134	78	78	43	43
Fiber, g	8.7	2.5	8.7	1.4	—
Vitamin A, IU	0	0	0	0	0
Vitamin B_1, mg	0.28	1.1	0.5	0.59	0.278
Vitamin B_2, mg	0.135	0.67	0.15	0.25	0.08
Vitamin B_6, mg	0.19	0.1	0.23	0.06	0.13
Vitamin B_{12}, mcg	0	0	0	0	0
Niacin, mg	6.04	7.9	5.4	4.3	2.9
Pantothenic acid, mg	2.2	0.45	1.03	0.25	0.56
Folic acid, mcg	35	243	60	132	33
Vitamin C, mg	0	0	0	0	0
Vitamin E, IU	—	0.2	—	0.13	—
Calcium, mg	42	19	42	10	23
Copper, mg	0.43	0.27	0.48	0.145	0.26
Iron, mg	1.9	4.1	3.8	2.2	2
Magnesium, mg	76	50	150	27	82
Manganese, mg	1.35	0.73	3.2	0.4	1.7
Phosphorus, mg	294	158	271	86	147
Potassium, mg	287	170	226	92	123
Selenium, mcg	—	65	—	3.5	42
Sodium, mg	17	7.4	8.4	4	4.6
Zinc, mg	1.44	1.3	2.5	0.7	1.4
Total lipid, g	1.11	1.66	1.47	0.9	0.8
Total saturated, g	0.2	0.24	0.27	0.13	0.147
Total unsaturated, g	0.44	0.68	0.58	0.37	0.317
Total monounsaturated, g	0.15	0.2	0.21	0.11	0.111
Cholesterol, mg	0	0	0	0	0
Tryptophan, g	0.28	0.17	0.197	0.09	0.11
Threonine, g	0.58	0.355	0.4	0.19	0.22
Isoleucine, g	0.85	0.52	0.6	0.28	0.325
Leucine, g	1.5	0.92	1.05	0.5	0.57
Lycine, g	0.42	0.26	0.34	0.14	0.185
Methionine, g	0.34	0.21	0.25	0.11	0.135
Cystine, g	0.62	0.38	0.32	0.21	0.174
Phenylalanine, g	1.1	0.65	0.76	0.354	0.415
Tyrosine, g	0.58	0.35	0.4	0.19	0.22
Valine, g	0.94	0.57	0.667	0.31	0.36
Arginine, g	0.8	0.495	0.54	0.27	0.295
Histidine, g	0.45	0.27	0.36	0.15	0.196
Alanine, g	0.65	0.39	0.48	0.2	0.26
Aspartic acid, g	0.9	0.55	0.69	0.3	0.376
Glutamic acid, g	7.96	4.84	5.33	2.63	2.9
Glycine, g	0.7	0.4	0.56	0.23	0.3
Proline, g	2.43	1.48	1.64	0.8	0.9
Serine, g	0.75	0.63	0.75	0.34	0.41

Grains

	Popcorn, oil popped	Rice, brown	Rice cake, brown, plain	Rice, flour, brown	Rice, white, enr.
Measure	1 C	1 C	1	1 C	1 C
Weight, g	11	196	9	158	195
Calories	54	704	35	574	708
Protein, g	0.99	14.8	0.74	11	13.1
Carbohydrate, g	6.3	152	7	121	157
Fiber, g	1.1	6.5	0.38	7.3	2.7
Vitamin A, IU	17	0	4	0	0
Vitamin B_1, mg	0.015	0.68	t	0.7	1.1
Vitamin B_2, mg	0.02	0.08	0.015	0.13	0.09
Vitamin B_6, mg	0.03	1	0.013	1.2	0.3
Vitamin B_{12}, mcg	0	0	0	0	0
Niacin, mg	0.17	9.2	0.7	10	9.9
Pantothenic acid, mg	0.034	2.1	0.09	2.5	2.6
Folic acid, mcg	1.9	32	1.9	25	450
Vitamin C, mg	0	0	0	0	0
Vitamin E, IU	0.02	1.86	0.1	1.7	0.38
Calcium, mg	1	64	1	17	17
Copper, mg	0.04	0.4	0.04	0.36	0.2
Iron, mg	0.4	3.2	0.13	3	8.5
Magnesium, mg	12	272	12	177	68
Manganese, mg	0.1	7.1	0.34	6.3	2.1
Phosphorus, mg	28	502	32	532	211
Potassium, mg	25	509	26	457	168
Selenium, mcg	0.8	43	2.2	—	29
Sodium, mg	97	7.6	29	13	1.95
Zinc, mg	0.3	3.6	0.27	3.9	2.5
Total lipid, g	3.09	5.1	0.25	4.4	1.5
Total saturated, g	0.538	1	0.05	0.88	0.31
Total unsaturated, g	1.5	1.8	0.089	1.57	0.3
Total monounsaturated, g	0.9	1.85	0.09	1.59	0.35
Cholesterol, mg	0	0	0	0	0
Tryptophan, g	0.007	0.18	0.009	0.15	0.15
Threonine, g	0.037	0.52	0.027	0.42	0.46
Isoleucine, g	0.036	0.6	0.03	0.48	0.56
Leucine, g	0.12	1.18	0.06	0.95	1.1
Lycine, g	0.03	0.54	0.03	0.44	0.47
Methionine, g	0.02	0.3	0.02	0.26	0.3
Cystine, g	0.02	0.17	0.01	0.14	0.26
Phenylalanine, g	0.05	0.74	0.038	0.59	0.69
Tyrosine, g	0.04	0.5	0.03	0.43	0.4
Valine, g	0.05	0.84	0.04	0.67	0.79
Arginine, g	0.05	1.1	0.056	0.87	1.1
Histidine, g	0.03	0.36	0.02	0.3	0.3
Alanine, g	0.07	0.83	0.04	0.67	0.75
Aspartic acid, g	0.07	1.33	0.07	1.1	1.2
Glutamic acid, g	0.19	2.9	0.15	2.3	2.5
Glycine, g	0.04	0.7	0.04	0.56	0.59
Proline, g	0.086	0.67	0.034	0.54	0.61
Serine, g	0.05	0.73	0.04	0.6	0.67

Grains

Grains   Breads

	Rice, wild	Quinoa	Bagels, enr.	Cracked wheat, enr.
Measure	1 C	1 C	1 (4 in dia.)	1 slice
Weight, g	160	170	89	23
Calories	565	636	245	60
Protein, g	22.6	22	9	2
Carbohydrate, g	121	117	48	12
Fiber, g	9.9	10	2	1.4
Vitamin A, IU	30	0	0	0
Vitamin B$_1$, mg	0.18	0.337	0.48	0.09
Vitamin B$_2$, mg	0.42	0.67	0.28	0.06
Vitamin B$_6$, mg	0.63	0.38	0.045	0.076
Vitamin B$_{12}$, mcg	0	0	0	0
Niacin, mg	9.9	4.98	4	0.9
Pantothenic acid, mg	1.63	1.78	0.3	0.14
Folic acid, mcg	152	83	78	15
Vitamin C, mg	0	0	0	0
Vitamin E, IU	1.7	—	0.05	0.22
Calcium, mg	30	102	66	11
Copper, mg	0.84	1.4	0.145	0.056
Iron, mg	3	16	3.2	0.7
Magnesium, mg	283	357	26	13
Manganese, mg	2	3.8	0.48	0.34
Phosphorus, mg	692	697	85	38
Potassium, mg	683	1258	90	44
Selenium, mcg	4.5	—	28.5	6
Sodium, mg	11	36	475	135
Zinc, mg	9.5	5.6	0.78	0.3
Total lipid, g	1.7	9.9	1.4	0.98
Total saturated, g	0.25	1	0.24	0.23
Total unsaturated, g	1.1	2.6	0.11	0.17
Total monounsaturated, g	0.25	4	0.144	0.48
Cholesterol, mg	0	0	0	0
Tryptophan, g	0.286	—	0.136	0.03
Threonine, g	0.75	0.78	0.33	0.065
Isoleucine, g	0.99	0.8	0.44	0.085
Leucine, g	1.6	1.34	0.8	0.15
Lycine, g	1	1.25	0.276	0.06
Methionine, g	0.7	0.445	0.21	0.037
Cystine, g	0.28	—	0.25	0.05
Phenylalanine, g	1.2	0.9	0.57	0.1
Tyrosine, g	0.995	0.6	0.33	0.06
Valine, g	1.4	1	0.5	0.1
Arginine, g	1.8	1.56	0.4	0.087
Histidine, g	0.6	0.5	0.25	0.05
Alanine, g	1.3	1.1	0.38	0.076
Aspartic acid, g	2.3	1.6	0.53	0.11
Glutamic acid, g	4	2.65	0.854	0.7
Glycine, g	1.1	1.16	0.41	0.08
Proline, g	0.83	0.7	1.3	0.23
Serine, g	1.25	0.8	0.56	0.1

Grains

Breads

	English muffin, enr.	English muffin, whole-wheat	French, enr.	Mixed grain, 7 grain
Measure	1	1	1 slice	1 slice
Weight, g	57	66	20	26
Calories	130	134	58	65
Protein, g	4.4	5.8	1.8	2.6
Carbohydrate, g	26	27	11.1	12
Fiber, g	1.5	4.4	0.75	1.7
Vitamin A, IU	0	0	0	0
Vitamin B_1, mg	0.23	0.2	0.13	0.11
Vitamin B_2, mg	0.136	0.09	0.08	0.09
Vitamin B_6, mg	0.025	0.11	0.01	0.087
Vitamin B_{12}, mcg	0.023	0	0	0
Niacin, mg	2	2.25	1.2	1.14
Pantothenic acid, mg	0.25	0.46	0.08	0.133
Folic acid, mcg	46	32	24	21
Vitamin C, mg	0	0	0	0.078
Vitamin E, IU	0.14	0.69	0.1	0.25
Calcium, mg	99	175	19	24
Copper, mg	0.1	0.14	0.05	0.07
Iron, mg	1.08	1.62	0.6	0.9
Magnesium, mg	12	47	6.8	14
Manganese, mg	0.2	1.2	0.127	0.39
Phosphorus, mg	76	186	26	46
Potassium, mg	75	139	28	53
Selenium, mcg	1.2	27	7.9	7.7
Sodium, mg	265	420	152	127
Zinc, mg	0.4	1.06	0.22	0.33
Total lipid, g	1	1.39	0.64	0.088
Total saturated, g	0.48	0.22	0.14	0.2
Total unsaturated, g	0.51	0.55	0.17	0.24
Total monounsaturated, g	0.17	0.34	0.3	0.4
Cholesterol, mg	0	0	0	0
Tryptophan, g	0.5	0.085	0.025	0.034
Threonine, g	0.14	0.2	0.06	0.08
Isoleucine, g	0.18	0.23	0.085	0.1
Leucine, g	0.32	0.4	0.154	0.18
Lycine, g	0.14	0.2	0.05	0.08
Methionine, g	0.08	0.1	0.04	0.04
Cystine, g	0.09	0.125	0.05	0.056
Phenylalanine, g	0.22	0.275	0.1	0.13
Tyrosine, g	0.13	0.18	0.06	0.074
Valine, g	0.2	0.27	0.1	0.12
Arginine, g	0.17	0.275	0.08	0.115
Histidine, g	0.1	0.135	0.048	0.06
Alanine, g	0.16	0.23	0.07	0.1
Aspartic acid, g	0.23	0.337	0.1	0.15
Glutamic acid, g	1.4	1.7	0.75	0.78
Glycine, g	0.16	0.24	0.078	0.1
Proline, g	0.46	0.55	0.25	0.26
Serine, g	0.2	0.27	0.11	0.13

Grains

Breads

	Pita, enr.	Pita, whole wheat	Pumpernickel	Rolls, dinner, enr.
Measure	1 sm.	1 sm.	1 slice	1
Weight, g	28	28	32	28
Calories	77	75	79	85
Protein, g	2.55	2.7	2.9	2.4
Carbohydrate, g	15.6	15	17	14
Fiber, g	0.6	2.1	2.1	0.85
Vitamin A, IU	0	0	0	0
Vitamin B_1, mg	0.17	0.095	0.07	0.14
Vitamin B_2, mg	0.09	0.022	0.04	0.09
Vitamin B_6, mg	0.01	0.07	0.05	0.015
Vitamin B_{12}, mcg	0	0	0	0
Niacin, mg	1.3	0.795	0.99	1.14
Pantothenic acid, mg	0.1	0.23	0.16	0.14
Folic acid, mcg	27	9.8	26	27
Vitamin C, mg	0	0	0	0.03
Vitamin E, IU	0.02	0.38	0.21	0.37
Calcium, mg	24	4.2	27	34
Copper, mg	0.05	0.08	0.09	0.04
Iron, mg	0.7	0.857	0.8	0.9
Magnesium, mg	7.3	19	23	6.5
Manganese, mg	0.14	0.487	0.42	0.13
Phosphorus, mg	27	50	57	33
Potassium, mg	34	48	67	38
Selenium, mcg	7.6	13	7.8	7.7
Sodium, mg	150	149	215	148
Zinc, mg	0.235	0.43	0.365	0.22
Total lipid, g	0.336	0.728	0.9	2.1
Total saturated, g	0.046	0.115	0.14	0.497
Total unsaturated, g	0.15	0.295	0.396	0.34
Total monounsaturated, g	0.029	0.088	0.3	1.05
Cholesterol, mg	0	0	0	0.284
Tryptophan, g	0.029	0.042	0.03	0.028
Threonine, g	0.07	0.08	0.085	0.07
Isoleucine, g	0.1	0.1	0.1	0.1
Leucine, g	0.18	0.19	0.2	0.17
Lycine, g	0.06	0.074	0.08	0.067
Methionine, g	0.045	0.043	0.05	0.043
Cystine, g	0.055	0.064	0.06	0.05
Phenylalanine, g	0.125	0.13	0.135	0.12
Tyrosine, g	0.07	0.08	0.076	0.07
Valine, g	0.11	0.123	0.13	0.1
Arginine, g	0.09	0.127	0.115	0.1
Histidine, g	0.05	0.06	0.06	0.05
Alanine, g	0.085	0.1	0.1	0.08
Aspartic acid, g	0.114	0.14	0.15	0.114
Glutamic acid, g	0.85	0.88	0.87	0.8
Glycine, g	0.09	0.1	0.1	0.08
Proline, g	0.28	0.3	0.304	0.26
Serine, g	0.123	0.13	0.13	0.117

Grains

Breads

	Rolls dinner, whole wheat	Rolls, hamburger/ hotdog, enr.	Rye	Wheat incl. wheatberry
Measure	1	1	1 slice	1 slice
Weight, g	35	40	32	25
Calories	90	119	83	65
Protein, g	3.5	3.3	2.1	2.3
Carbohydrate, g	18.3	21.2	12	12
Fiber, g	2.7	1.16	1.9	1
Vitamin A, IU	t	0	2.24	0
Vitamin B_1, mg	0.12	0.21	0.14	0.1
Vitamin B_2, mg	0.05	0.13	0.11	0.07
Vitamin B_6, mg	0.07	0.02	0.02	0.024
Vitamin B_{12}, mcg	0	0	0	0
Niacin, mg	1.1	1.7	1.22	1
Pantothenic acid, mg	1.76	0.23	0.1	0.11
Folic acid, mcg	11	41	26	19
Vitamin C, mg	0	0.04	0.13	0
Vitamin E, IU	0.73	0.99	0.17	0.2
Calcium, mg	37	60	23	26
Copper, mg	0.086	0.05	0.06	0.05
Iron, mg	0.8	1.4	0.9	0.83
Magnesium, mg	40	8.6	10	12
Manganese, mg	0.8	0.14	0.3	0.26
Phosphorus, mg	98	34	40	38
Potassium, mg	102	61	53	50
Selenium, mcg	18	11	9.9	17
Sodium, mg	197	241	211	133
Zinc, mg	0.7	0.21	0.4	0.26
Total lipid, g	1.69	2.2	1.06	1.1
Total saturated, g	0.3	0.5	0.2	0.224
Total unsaturated, g	0.778	1.08	0.256	0.227
Total monounsaturated, g	0.4	0.36	0.42	0.43
Cholesterol, mg	0	0	0	0
Tryptophan, g	0.048	0.043	0.03	0.03
Threonine, g	0.09	0.1	0.08	0.07
Isoleucine, g	0.12	0.14	0.1	0.09
Leucine, g	0.216	0.26	0.185	0.16
Lycine, g	0.1	0.1	0.075	0.065
Methionine, g	0.05	0.065	0.044	0.04
Cystine, g	0.07	0.078	0.055	0.05
Phenylalanine, g	0.15	0.18	0.132	0.11
Tyrosine, g	0.09	0.1	0.07	0.067
Valine, g	0.145	0.16	0.12	0.1
Arginine, g	0.147	0.133	0.1	0.1
Histidine, g	0.07	0.08	0.06	0.05
Alanine, g	0.113	0.12	0.1	0.08
Aspartic acid, g	0.167	0.168	0.14	0.12
Glutamic acid, g	0.97	1.21	0.8	0.73
Glycine, g	0.125	0.13	0.1	0.086
Proline, g	0.32	0.41	0.3	0.24
Serine, g	0.15	0.177	0.13	0.1

Grains

Breads

	White, enr.	Whole wheat	Crackers, graham	Crackers, soda
Measure	1 slice	1 slice	1	1
Weight, g	23	28	14.2	2.8
Calories	62	69	55	12.5
Protein, g	2	2.4	1.1	0.26
Carbohydrate, g	11.6	11	10.4	2
Fiber, g	0.58	1.9	0.22	0.09
Vitamin A, IU	0	0	0	0
Vitamin B$_1$, mg	0.12	0.098	0.01	0.017
Vitamin B$_2$, mg	0.085	0.057	0.03	0.014
Vitamin B$_6$, mg	0.009	0.05	t	t
Vitamin B$_{12}$, mcg	t	0	0	0
Niacin, mg	0.99	1.1	0.2	0.03
Pantothenic acid, mg	0.1	0.174	0.075	0.014
Folic acid, mcg	24	13	8.4	3.7
Vitamin C, mg	0	0	0	0
Vitamin E, IU	0.14	0.3	0.43	0.07
Calcium, mg	20	23	3.4	3.6
Copper, mg	0.05	0.06	0.03	0.006
Iron, mg	0.6	0.9	0.2	0.16
Magnesium, mg	5	25	5.68	0.81
Manganese, mg	0.07	0.65	0.113	0.02
Phosphorus, mg	22	64	21	2.5
Potassium, mg	24	70	55	3.4
Selenium, mcg	6.44	10	1.4	0.59
Sodium, mg	117	148	95	31
Zinc, mg	0.155	0.5	0.113	0.023
Total lipid, g	0.79	1.17	1.3	0.37
Total saturated, g	0.16	0.257	0.3	0.075
Total unsaturated, g	0.475	0.28	0.53	0.05
Total monounsaturated, g	0.18	0.47	0.57	0.19
Cholesterol, mg	0.25	0	0	0
Tryptophan, g	0.024	0.04	0.013	0.004
Threonine, g	0.06	0.08	0.03	0.01
Isoleucine, g	0.08	0.1	0.034	0.01
Leucine, g	0.145	0.19	0.066	0.02
Lycine, g	0.056	0.085	0.023	0.01
Methionine, g	0.036	0.043	0.017	0.005
Cystine, g	0.04	0.06	0.02	0.006
Phenylalanine, g	0.1	0.13	0.05	0.014
Tyrosine, g	0.06	0.08	0.03	0.01
Valine, g	0.1	0.124	0.04	0.01
Arginine, g	0.08	0.126	0.04	0.01
Histidine, g	0.045	0.06	0.02	0.006
Alanine, g	0.07	0.1	0.03	0.01
Aspartic acid, g	0.1	0.15	0.04	0.01
Glutamic acid, g	0.66	0.83	0.32	0.09
Glycine, g	0.07	0.11	0.036	0.01
Proline, g	0.22	0.27	0.1	0.03
Serine, g	0.1	0.13	0.05	0.014

Grains

	Bread	Flours		
	Crackers, whole wheat	Buckwheat, whole groat	Corn, degermed	Corn, whole grain
Measure	1	1 C	1 C	1 C
Weight, g	4	120	126	117
Calories	17	402	472	431
Protein, g	0.35	15	7	8
Carbohydrate, g	2.7	85	104	89.9
Fiber, g	0.42	12	2.4	16
Vitamin A, IU	0	0	64	548
Vitamin B$_1$, mg	0.01	0.58	0.09	0.23
Vitamin B$_2$, mg	t	0.23	0.07	0.07
Vitamin B$_6$, mg	t	0.578	0.12	0.43
Vitamin B$_{12}$, mcg	0	0	0	0
Niacin, mg	0.18	7.4	3.35	1.6
Pantothenic acid, mg	0.03	0.53	0.07	0.77
Folic acid, mcg	1.1	65	61	29
Vitamin C, mg	0	0	0	0
Vitamin E, IU	0.06	1.85	0.62	0.43
Calcium, mg	2	49	2.5	7
Copper, mg	0.02	0.7	0.18	0.27
Iron, mg	0.12	5	1.15	2.1
Magnesium, mg	4	301	23	109
Manganese, mg	0.09	2.09	0.07	0.54
Phosphorus, mg	12	404	76	318
Potassium, mg	12	682	113	369
Selenium, mcg	0.59	6.8	11	18
Sodium, mg	27	13	1.3	6
Zinc, mg	0.086	3.7	0.47	2
Total lipid, g	0.69	3.7	1.75	4.5
Total saturated, g	0.136	0.8	0.215	0.635
Total unsaturated, g	0.264	1.14	0.876	2.1
Total monounsaturated, g	0.235	1.14	0.345	1.2
Cholesterol, mg	0	0	0	0
Tryptophan, g	0.005	0.22	—	0.057
Threonine, g	0.01	0.58	—	0.31
Isoleucine, g	0.013	0.57	—	0.29
Leucine, g	0.024	0.95	—	0.995
Lycine, g	0.01	0.77	—	0.23
Methionine, g	0.005	0.2	—	0.17
Cystine, g	0.01	0.26	—	0.146
Phenylalanine, g	0.017	0.6	—	0.4
Tyrosine, g	0.01	0.276	—	0.33
Valine, g	0.016	0.775	—	0.4
Arginine, g	0.017	1.12	—	0.4
Histidine, g	0.01	0.35	—	0.25
Alanine, g	0.013	0.85	—	0.6
Aspartic acid, g	0.02	1.3	—	0.56
Glutamic acid, g	0.112	2.34	—	1.5
Glycine, g	0.014	1.18	—	0.33
Proline, g	0.037	0.58	—	0.71
Serine, g	0.017	0.78	—	0.385

Grains

Flours

	Rye, dark	Rye, light	White, enr.	Whole wheat
Measure	1 C	1 C	1 C	1 C
Weight, g	128	102	110	120
Calories	419	374	455	400
Protein, g	20.9	8.6	11.6	16
Carbohydrate, g	87.2	81	95	85.2
Fiber, g	29	15	3	15
Vitamin A, IU	0	0	0	0
Vitamin B_1, mg	0.4	0.34	0.98	0.66
Vitamin B_2, mg	0.28	0.09	0.62	0.25
Vitamin B_6, mg	0.6	0.24	0.066	0.41
Vitamin B_{12}, mcg	0	0	0	0
Niacin, mg	5.5	0.82	7.4	5.2
Pantothenic acid, mg	1.7	0.68	0.51	1.32
Folic acid, mcg	77	22	193	65
Vitamin C, mg	0	0	0	0
Vitamin E, IU	4.9	0.85	0.11	2.19
Calcium, mg	69	18	18	49
Copper, mg	0.96	0.3	0.21	0.6
Iron, mg	8	1.8	5.8	4
Magnesium, mg	317	71	28	136
Manganese, mg	8.6	2	0.85	4.6
Phosphorus, mg	808	198	135	446
Potassium, mg	934	238	133	444
Selenium, mcg	45	36	42	77.4
Sodium, mg	1	2	2	4
Zinc, mg	7.2	1.8	0.87	2.88
Total lipid, g	3.3	1.4	1.1	2.4
Total saturated, g	0.42	0.15	0.19	0.386
Total unsaturated, g	0.5	0.576	0.52	0.98
Total monounsaturated, g	0.42	0.16	0.11	0.278
Cholesterol, mg	0	0	0	0
Tryptophan, g	0.2	0.097	0.16	0.254
Threonine, g	0.6	0.3	0.35	0.474
Isoleucine, g	0.7	0.3	0.45	0.6
Leucine, g	1.24	0.6	0.89	1.1
Lycine, g	0.6	0.3	0.285	0.45
Methionine, g	0.27	0.13	0.23	0.25
Cystine, g	0.355	0.17	0.27	0.38
Phenylalanine, g	0.91	0.43	0.65	0.775
Tyrosine, g	0.355	0.17	0.4	0.48
Valine, g	0.9	0.43	0.52	0.74
Arginine, g	0.8	0.4	0.5	0.77
Histidine, g	0.4	0.2	0.29	0.38
Alanine, g	0.74	0.35	0.42	0.58
Aspartic acid, g	1.24	0.59	0.54	0.84
Glutamic acid, g	5	2.4	4.35	5.2
Glycine, g	0.68	0.325	0.464	0.66
Proline, g	1.9	0.92	1.5	1.7
Serine, g	0.98	0.465	0.65	0.775

Grains

Legumes

	Adzuki beans, cooked	Black beans, cooked	Blackeyed peas, cooked	Carob, flour	Fava beans, cooked
Measure	1 C	1 C	1 C	1 C	1 C
Weight, g	230	172	165	103	170
Calories	294	227	178	229	187
Protein, g	17	15	13.4	4.8	13
Carbohydrate, g	57	41	29.9	92	33
Fiber, g	17	15	11	41	9
Vitamin A, IU	14	10	26	14	26
Vitamin B$_1$, mg	0.27	0.42	0.5	0.055	0.17
Vitamin B$_2$, mg	0.15	0.1	0.18	0.475	0.15
Vitamin B$_6$, mg	0.22	0.12	0.18	0.38	0.12
Vitamin B$_{12}$, mcg	0	0	0	0	0
Niacin, mg	1.6	0.87	0.85	1.95	1.2
Pantothenic acid, mg	0.99	0.42	0.66	0.05	0.27
Folic acid, mcg	279	256	357	30	177
Vitamin C, mg	0	0	0.68	0.2	0.5
Vitamin E, IU	—	—	0.72	0.967	0.224
Calcium, mg	64	46	40	358	61
Copper, mg	0.69	0.36	0.46	0.59	0.44
Iron, mg	4.6	3.6	3.5	3	2.5
Magnesium, mg	120	120	90.7	56	73
Manganese, mg	1.3	0.76	0.82	0.5	0.72
Phosphorus, mg	386	241	241	81	213
Potassium, mg	1224	611	428	851	456
Selenium, mcg	2.8	2	4.3	5.46	4.4
Sodium, mg	18	1.7	2	36	8.5
Zinc, mg	4	1.9	3	0.95	1.7
Total lipid, g	0.23	0.93	1.3	0.669	0.68
Total saturated, g	0.08	0.24	0.237	0.09	0.112
Total unsaturated, g	—	0.397	0.387	0.22	0.279
Total monounsaturated, g	—	0.08	0.076	0.2	0.134
Cholesterol, mg	0	0	0	0	0
Tryptophan, g	0.166	0.18	0.16	0.05	0.12
Threonine, g	0.59	0.64	0.51	0.28	0.46
Isoleucine, g	0.7	0.67	0.54	0.22	0.52
Leucine, g	1.45	1.2	1	0.455	0.97
Lycine, g	1.3	1.05	0.9	0.2	0.83
Methionine, g	0.18	0.23	0.19	0.08	0.105
Cystine, g	0.16	0.165	0.15	0.03	0.165
Phenylalanine, g	0.9	0.8	0.776	0.156	0.55
Tyrosine, g	0.52	0.4	0.43	0.124	0.4
Valine, g	0.9	0.8	0.63	0.46	0.58
Arginine, g	1.12	0.94	0.9	0.134	1.2
Histidine, g	0.455	0.43	0.4	0.13	0.33
Alanine, g	1	0.6	0.6	0.6	0.53
Aspartic acid, g	2.05	1.8	1.6	0.52	1.4
Glutamic acid, g	2.7	2.3	2.5	0.37	2.2
Glycine, g	0.66	0.6	0.55	0.275	0.54
Proline, g	0.76	0.65	0.6	0.365	0.54
Serine, g	0.85	0.83	0.67	0.3	0.6

Legumes

Legumes

	Garbanzos, cooked	Kidney beans, cooked	Lentils, cooked	Lentil sprouts, raw	Lima beans, cooked
Measure	1 C	1 C	1 C	1 C	1 C
Weight, g	164	177	200	77	188
Calories	269	225	212	81	208
Protein, g	15	14.4	15.6	6.9	14
Carbohydrate, g	45	39.6	38.6	17	40
Fiber, g	13	13	15	—	13
Vitamin A, IU	44	0	15	35	0
Vitamin B$_1$, mg	0.19	0.2	0.33	0.176	0.238
Vitamin B$_2$, mg	0.1	0.11	0.12	0.099	0.163
Vitamin B$_6$, mg	0.23	0.2	0.35	0.146	0.328
Vitamin B$_{12}$, mcg	0	0	0	0	0
Niacin, mg	0.86	1.3	2.1	0.869	0.8
Pantothenic acid, mg	0.47	0.4	1.26	0.445	0.8
Folic acid, mcg	282	230	358	76.9	156
Vitamin C, mg	2	2	3	12.7	0
Vitamin E, IU	0.85	0.21	0.325	—	0.5
Calcium, mg	80	50	38	19	32
Copper, mg	0.58	0.43	0.54	0.27	0.519
Iron, mg	4.7	5.2	6.6	2.47	4.2
Magnesium, mg	79	79	71	28	80
Manganese, mg	1.7	0.84	0.98	0.39	0.97
Phosphorus, mg	276	259	356	133	221
Potassium, mg	477	629	730	248	969
Selenium, mcg	6	2	5.5	0.46	8.5
Sodium, mg	11	3.5	4	8	4
Zinc, mg	2.5	1.9	2	1.16	1.34
Total lipid, g	4.3	0.9	0.75	0.43	0.7
Total saturated, g	0.4	0.13	0.1	0.044	0.167
Total unsaturated, g	1.9	0.487	0.35	0.17	0.32
Total monounsaturated, g	0.96	0.069	0.13	0.08	0.06
Cholesterol, mg	0	0	0	0	0
Tryptophan, g	0.14	0.18	0.16	—	0.17
Threonine, g	0.54	0.65	0.64	0.253	0.63
Isoleucine, g	0.6	0.68	0.77	0.251	0.745
Leucine, g	1	1.2	1.3	0.484	0.113
Lycine, g	0.97	1	1.25	0.548	0.98
Methionine, g	0.19	0.23	0.15	0.081	0.18
Cystine, g	0.195	0.17	0.23	0.257	0.16
Phenylalanine, g	0.78	0.8	0.88	0.34	0.84
Tyrosine, g	0.36	0.4	0.48	0.194	0.52
Valine, g	0.6	0.8	0.89	0.307	0.88
Arginine, g	1.4	0.95	1.4	0.47	0.9
Histidine, g	0.4	0.43	0.5	0.198	0.393
Alanine, g	0.6	0.64	0.75	0.274	0.75
Aspartic acid, g	1.7	1.86	1.98	1.1	1.9
Glutamic acid, g	2.5	2.3	2.77	0.969	2
Glycine, g	0.6	0.6	0.73	0.246	0.62
Proline, g	0.6	0.65	0.75	0.274	0.67
Serine, g	0.7	0.84	0.8	0.381	0.98

Legumes

	Miso	Mung sprouts, raw	Natto	Navy beans, cooked	Peanuts, raw
Measure	1 C	1 C	1 C	1 C	1 C
Weight, g	275	104	175	190	144
Calories	566	32	375	224	838
Protein, g	33	3	31	14.8	37.7
Carbohydrate, g	77	6	25	40.3	29.7
Fiber, g	15	1.8	9.45	12	12
Vitamin A, IU	240	22	0	3.6	0
Vitamin B_1, mg	0.267	0.088	0.28	0.27	0.46
Vitamin B_2, mg	0.688	0.128	0.33	0.13	0.19
Vitamin B_6, mg	0.59	0.092	0.23	0.3	0.576
Vitamin B_{12}, mcg	0	0	0	0	0
Niacin, mg	2.37	0.778	0	1.3	24.6
Pantothenic acid, mg	0.7	0.396	0.376	0.46	3
Folic acid, mcg	91	63	14	255	350
Vitamin C, mg	0	13.6	23	1.6	0
Vitamin E, IU	0.04	0.015	0.027	—	19
Calcium, mg	181	14	380	95	104
Copper, mg	1.2	0.17	1.17	0.54	0.62
Iron, mg	7.5	0.94	15	5.1	3.2
Magnesium, mg	116	22	201	107	252
Manganese, mg	2.36	0.19	2.67	1	2.17
Phosphorus, mg	421	56	305	281	586
Potassium, mg	451	154	1276	790	1009
Selenium, mcg	4.4	0.6	15	10	10
Sodium, mg	10.029	6	12	2	26
Zinc, mg	9	0.42	5.3	1.8	4.78
Total lipid, g	16.7	0.2	19	1.1	70.1
Total saturated, g	2.4	0.048	2.78	0.269	10
Total unsaturated, g	9.4	0.052	10.9	0.45	22
Total monounsaturated, g	3.7	0.023	4.25	0.1	36
Cholesterol, mg	0	0	0	0	0
Tryptophan, g	0.4	0.038	0.4	0.187	0.453
Threonine, g	1.76	0.08	1.4	0.67	1.09
Isoleucine, g	2.2	0.138	1.63	0.7	1.45
Leucine, g	3.1	0.182	2.6	1.3	2.8
Lycine, g	1.8	0.172	2	1.1	1.45
Methionine, g	0.4	0.036	0.36	0.24	0.384
Cystine, g	0.27	0.018	0.385	0.17	0.48
Phenylalanine, g	1.64	0.122	1.65	0.86	2.14
Tyrosine, g	0.995	0.054	0.97	0.45	1.8
Valine, g	2	0.136	1.78	0.8	1.7
Arginine, g	2	0.2	1.6	0.98	5.05
Histidine, g	0.91	0.072	0.9	0.44	1.09
Alanine, g	1.57	0.102	1.4	0.66	1.65
Aspartic acid, g	3.6	0.498	3.4	1.9	5.04
Glutamic acid, g	5.78	0.168	5.8	2.4	8.9
Glycine, g	1.5	0.066	1	0.62	2.59
Proline, g	2	—	2.5	0.67	1.82
Serine, g	2	0.034	1.96	0.86	2.09

Legumes

	Peanut butter, smooth	Peas, green	Peas, split, cooked	Pinto beans, cooked	Soybeans, cooked	Soybean, flour
Measure	1 T	1 C	1 C	1 C	1 C	1 C
Weight, g	15	146	200	171	172	84
Calories	86	118	230	234	298	366
Protein, g	3.9	7.9	16	14	29	29
Carbohydrate, g	3.2	21	41.6	44	17	29.5
Fiber, g	0.9	7.4	16	15	10	8
Vitamin A, IU	0	934	14	3.4	15	100
Vitamin B$_1$, mg	0.018	0.387	0.3	0.32	0.27	0.49
Vitamin B$_2$, mg	0.02	0.193	0.18	0.156	0.5	0.97
Vitamin B$_6$, mg	0.05	0.247	0.09	0.27	0.4	0.387
Vitamin B$_{12}$, mcg	0	0	0	0	0	0
Niacin, mg	2.4	3.05	1.8	0.68	0.69	3.6
Pantothenic acid, mg	0.147	0.152	1.2	0.49	0.31	1.34
Folic acid, mcg	7	95	127	294	93	290
Vitamin C, mg	0	58.4	0.78	3.6	3	0
Vitamin E, IU	2.4	0.84	1	2.38	5	1.64
Calcium, mg	6	36	22	82	175	173
Copper, mg	0.022	0.257	0.5	0.44	0.7	2.45
Iron, mg	0.3	2.14	3.4	4.5	8.8	5.35
Magnesium, mg	26	48	71	94	148	360
Manganese, mg	0.257	0.599	0.78	0.95	1.4	1.9
Phosphorus, mg	59	157	194	273	421	415
Potassium, mg	123	357	709	800	885	2112
Selenium, mcg	1.2	2.6	1.18	12	12	6.3
Sodium, mg	75	7	4	3	1.7	11
Zinc, mg	0.47	1.8	2	1.85	2	3.3
Total lipid, g	8.1	0.58	0.76	0.889	15	—
Total saturated, g	1.5	0.1	0.1	0.186	2.2	2.5
Total unsaturated, g	2.2	0.27	0.3	0.32	8.7	9.8
Total monounsaturated, g	3.9	0.05	0.16	0.18	3.4	3.8
Cholesterol, mg	0	0	0	0	0	0
Tryptophan, g	0.055	0.054	0.18	0.167	0.42	0.422
Threonine, g	0.132	0.296	0.58	0.6	1.24	1.26
Isoleucine, g	0.177	0.285	0.67	0.62	1.4	1.4
Leucine, g	0.342	0.472	1.2	1	2.3	3.37
Lycine, g	0.176	0.463	1.2	0.96	2	1.9
Methionine, g	0.047	0.12	0.17	0.2	0.385	0.4
Cystine, g	0.058	0.047	0.25	0.15	0.46	0.467
Phenylalanine, g	0.26	0.292	0.75	0.76	1.5	1.5
Tyrosine, g	0.219	0.165	0.47	0.4	1.1	1.1
Valine, g	0.206	0.343	0.77	0.74	1.4	1.45
Arginine, g	0.613	0.625	1.46	0.87	2	2.25
Histidine, g	0.133	0.156	0.4	0.4	0.77	0.78
Alanine, g	0.201	0.35	0.72	0.59	1.35	1.37
Aspartic acid, g	0.613	0.723	1.9	1.7	3.6	3.6
Glutamic acid, g	1.08	1.08	2.8	2	5.5	5.6
Glycine, g	0.315	0.269	0.7	0.55	1.3	1.34
Proline, g	0.221	0.253	0.67	0.6	1.7	1.7
Serine, g	0.255	0.264	0.72	0.76	1.66	1.68

Legumes

Legumes

	Soybean sprouts, raw	Soymilk	Tempeh	Tofu, firm
Measure	1 C	1 C		½ C
Weight, g	70	245	100	126
Calories	90	81	193	97
Protein, g	9	6.7	19	10
Carbohydrate, g	7.8	4.4	9.4	3.7
Fiber, g	0.77	3.2	—	0.5
Vitamin A, IU	8	78	0	10
Vitamin B_1, mg	0.238	0.4	0.078	0.12
Vitamin B_2, mg	0.082	0.17	0.358	0.13
Vitamin B_6, mg	0.124	0.1	0.215	0.08
Vitamin B_{12}, mcg	0	0	0.075	0
Niacin, mg	0.804	0.36	2.64	0.01
Pantothenic acid, mg	0.65	0.12	0.278	0.08
Folic acid, mcg	120	3.7	24	42
Vitamin C, mg	10.6	0	0	0.25
Vitamin E, IU	—	0.04	—	—
Calcium, mg	48	9.8	111	204
Copper, mg	0.3	0.3	0.56	0.3
Iron, mg	1.48	1.4	2.7	1.8
Magnesium, mg	50	47	81	58
Manganese, mg	0.492	0.42	1.3	0.9
Phosphorus, mg	114	120	266	185
Potassium, mg	338	346	412	222
Selenium, mcg	0.4	3.2	0.017	12
Sodium, mg	10	29	9	10
Zinc, mg	0.82	0.56	1.14	1.3
Total lipid, g	4.68	4.7	10.8	5.6
Total saturated, g	0.5	0.5	2.2	0.8
Total unsaturated, g	2	2.04	3.83	3.2
Total monounsaturated, g	1	0.8	3	1.24
Cholesterol, mg	0	0	0	0
Tryptophan, g	0.126	0.11	0.28	0.16
Threonine, g	0.32	0.28	0.796	0.4
Isoleucine, g	0.276	0.35	0.88	0.5
Leucine, g	0.464	0.6	1.43	0.77
Lycine, g	0.386	0.44	0.91	0.67
Methionine, g	0.062	0.1	0.174	0.13
Cystine, g	0.03	0.1	0.32	0.14
Phenylalanine, g	0.222	0.37	0.89	0.5
Tyrosine, g	0.182	0.27	0.664	0.34
Valine, g	0.3	0.345	0.9	0.5
Arginine, g	0.266	0.5	1.25	0.67
Histidine, g	0.148	0.17	0.466	0.3
Alanine, g	0.26	0.3	0.96	0.42
Aspartic acid, g	0.8	0.84	2	1
Glutamic acid, g	0.784	1.35	3.3	1.75
Glycine, g	0.214	0.3	0.75	0.4
Proline, g	0.47	0.4	1	0.55
Serine, g	0.414	0.35	1	0.48

Beef[1]

	Chuck roast	Corned, brisket	Dried	Flank steak	Ground beef, lean
Measure	1 lb	1 lb	1 oz	1 lb	4 oz
Weight, g	454	454	28	454	113
Calories	1164	896	47	888	298
Protein, g	83	66.58	8.25	87.4	20
Carbohydrate, g	0	0.63	0.44	0	0
Fiber, g	0	0	0	0	0
Vitamin A, IU	130	—	—	50	22.5
Vitamin B$_1$, mg	0.485	0.195	0.02	0.499	0.057
Vitamin B$_2$, mg	0.794	0.712	0.09	0.680	0.237
Vitamin B$_6$, mg	1.7	1.32	—	1.87	0.28
Vitamin B$_{12}$, mcg	13.7	8.07	0.52	13.4	2.64
Niacin, mg	14.6	16.6	1.06	20.6	5.1
Pantothenic acid, mg	1.4	2.59	—	1.46	0.418
Folic acid, mcg	32	—	—	32	9
Vitamin C, mg	0	0	—	0	0
Vitamin E, IU	—	—	—	—	—
Calcium, mg	32	30	2	22	9
Copper, mg	0.363	0.499	0.045	0.327	0.082
Iron, mg	9.44	7.66	1.28	8.9	1.99
Magnesium, mg	87	66	9	93	20
Manganese, mg	0.054	0.091	—	0.064	0.017
Phosphorus, mg	779	531	49	864	154
Potassium, mg	1374	1348	126	1585	295
Selenium, mcg	—	—	—	—	—
Sodium, mg	266	5519	984	321	78
Zinc, mg	18.06	12.9	1.49	15.7	4.36
Total lipid, g	90	67.6	1.11	57	23.4
Total saturated, g	38.4	21.44	0.45	25.6	9.39
Total unsaturated, g	—	—	—	—	—
Total monounsaturated, g	—	—	—	—	—
Cholesterol, mg	311	245	—	238	85
Tryptophan, g	0.93	0.608	0.067	0.98	0.246
Threonine, g	3.63	2.51	0.346	3.82	0.837
Isoleucine, g	3.74	2.88	0.338	3.9	0.857
Leucine, g	6.57	4.89	0.616	6.9	1.6
Lycine, g	6.9	5.1	0.673	7.27	1.67
Methionine, g	2.13	1.55	0.199	2.24	0.467
Cystine, g	0.93	0.853	0.098	0.98	0.192
Phenylalanine, g	3.24	2.4	0.309	3.4	0.758
Tyrosine, g	2.8	2.17	0.249	2.9	0.624
Valine, g	4.04	2.93	0.379	4.25	0.968
Arginine, g	5.25	4.1	0.557	5.5	1.35
Histidine, g	2.8	2.1	0.239	2.99	0.636
Alanine, g	5.01	4.8	0.545	5.27	1.3
Aspartic acid, g	7.6	6.5	0.733	7.98	1.8
Glutamic acid, g	12.5	10.8	1.19	13.1	3.14
Glycine, g	4.5	5.56	0.612	4.76	1.48
Proline, g	3.67	4.79	0.449	3.86	1.01
Serine, g	3.18	2.68	0.337	3.34	0.774

[1]Beef contains approx. .63 mg vitamin E/100 g; 13.6 mcg biotin/lb; 19 mg zinc/lb (lean, no fat).

Meats

Beef[1]

	Ground beef, regular	Liver	Pastrami	Porterhouse steak	Rib roast
Measure	4 oz	4 oz	1 oz	1 lb	1 lb
Weight, g	113	113	28	454	454
Calories	351	161	99	1289	1503
Protein, g	18.8	22.6	4.9	78.8	72.8
Carbohydrate, g	0	6.58	0.86	0	0
Fiber, g	0	0	0	0	0
Vitamin A, IU	40	39941	—	300	310
Vitamin B_1, mg	0.043	0.292	0.027	0.44	0.349
Vitamin B_2, mg	0.171	3.14	0.048	0.739	0.576
Vitamin B_6, mg	0.27	1.06	0.05	1.62	1.39
Vitamin B_{12}, mcg	2.99	78.2	0.5	11.85	12.45
Niacin, mg	5.06	14.4	1.44	15.3	12.4
Pantothenic acid, mg	0.39	8.6	—	1.32	1.35
Folic acid, mcg	8	281	—	27	22
Vitamin C, mg	0	25.3	0.9	0	0
Vitamin E, IU	—	1.59	—	—	—
Calcium, mg	10	6	2	29	39
Copper, mg	0.07	3.12	—	0.336	0.259
Iron, mg	1.96	7.71	0.54	7.83	7.63
Magnesium, mg	18	22	5	82	71
Manganese, mg	0.019	0.298	—	0.054	0.054
Phosphorus, mg	146	360	43	770	685
Potassium, mg	258	365	65	1305	1180
Selenium, mcg	23.5	51.5	—	—	—
Sodium, mg	77	82	348	222	241
Zinc, mg	4.01	4.43	1.21	13.64	16.2
Total lipid, g	30	4.34	8.27	105.6	132
Total saturated, g	12.18	1.69	2.95	45.15	57.4
Total unsaturated, g	—	—	—	—	—
Total monounsaturated, g	—	—	—	—	—
Cholesterol, mg	96	400	26	316	326
Tryptophan, g	0.232	0.325	0.045	0.885	0.816
Threonine, g	0.788	1.034	0.185	3.44	3.18
Isoleucine, g	0.806	1.034	0.211	3.54	3.27
Leucine, g	1.5	2.13	0.359	6.23	5.75
Lycine, g	1.56	1.57	0.375	6.56	6.05
Methionine, g	0.438	0.572	0.113	2.02	1.86
Cystine, g	0.181	0.347	0.063	0.885	0.816
Phenylalanine, g	0.712	1.2	0.176	3.08	2.84
Tyrosine, g	0.586	0.897	0.16	2.65	2.44
Valine, g	0.911	1.4	0.215	3.83	3.58
Arginine, g	1.26	1.42	0.302	4.98	4.6
Histidine, g	0.598	0.618	0.156	2.7	2.49
Alanine, g	1.23	1.4	0.352	4.75	4.39
Aspartic acid, g	1.7	2.17	0.479	7.2	6.65
Glutamic acid, g	2.95	3.06	0.796	11.8	10.9
Glycine, g	1.39	1.29	0.408	4.3	3.97
Proline, g	0.953	1.19	0.352	3.48	3.21
Serine, g	0.727	1.09	0.197	3.01	2.78

[1]Beef contains approx. .63 mg vitamin E/100 g; 13.6 mcg biotin/lb; 19 mg zinc/lb (lean, no fat).

Meats

Beef[1]

	Round steak	Short ribs	Sirloin steak	Smoked, chopped	T-bone steak	Tenderloin
Measure	1 lb	1 lb	1 lb	1 oz	1 lb	1 lb
Weight, g	454	454	454	28	454	454
Calories	1093	1761	1179	38	1394	1095
Protein, g	88	65.3	82.7	5.7	76	84.1
Carbohydrate, g	0	0	0	0.53	0	0
Fiber, g	0	0	0	0	0	0
Vitamin A, IU	110	—	220	—	300	—
Vitamin B_1, mg	0.435	0.322	0.503	0.024	0.422	0.54
Vitamin B_2, mg	0.748	0.535	0.88	0.05	0.712	0.97
Vitamin B_6, mg	2.02	1.34	1.71	0.1	1.58	1.74
Vitamin B_{12}, mcg	12.21	11.6	12.58	0.49	11.6	12
Niacin, mg	15.97	11.6	13.9	1.3	14.8	13.9
Pantothenic acid, mg	1.53	1.09	1.38	0.167	1.27	1.41
Folic acid, mcg	35	21	30	—	26	28
Vitamin C, mg	0	0	0	0	0	0
Vitamin E, IU	—	—	—	—	—	—
Calcium, mg	23	41	34	—	30	30
Copper, mg	0.322	0.24	0.37	—	0.322	0.435
Iron, mg	8.5	7.03	10.2	0.81	7.58	10.9
Magnesium, mg	92	62	89	6	79	93
Manganese, mg	0.059	0.05	0.054	—	0.054	0.059
Phosphorus, mg	846	624	798	51	703	842
Potassium, mg	1434	1053	1331	107	1248	1422
Selenium, mcg	165		—	—	—	—
Sodium, mg	232	224	234	357	217	223
Zinc, mg	13.7	14.3	15.5	1.11	13.1	14.2
Total lipid, g	79.5	164	91.5	1.25	118.5	81.6
Total saturated, g	33.73	71.5	39.15	0.51	50.9	34.7
Total unsaturated, g	—	—	—	—	—	—
Total monounsaturated, g	—	—	—	—	—	—
Cholesterol, mg	298	345	315	13	323	313
Tryptophan, g	0.984	0.73	0.925	0.047	0.853	0.943
Threonine, g	3.84	2.85	3.6	0.24	3.33	3.67
Isoleucine, g	3.95	2.93	3.7	0.234	3.42	3.78
Leucine, g	6.95	5.16	6.54	0.428	6.02	6.65
Lycine, g	7.32	5.43	6.88	0.467	6.33	6.99
Methionine, g	2.25	1.67	2.12	0.138	1.95	2.15
Cystine, g	0.984	0.73	0.925	0.068	0.853	0.943
Phenylalanine, g	3.43	2.55	3.23	0.214	2.97	3.28
Tyrosine, g	2.95	2.19	2.78	0.173	2.56	2.83
Valine, g	4.27	3.18	4.02	0.263	3.7	4.09
Arginine, g	5.55	4.13	5.23	0.386	4.81	5.32
Histidine, g	3.01	2.24	2.83	0.166	2.6	2.88
Alanine, g	5.3	3.94	4.99	0.378	4.59	5.07
Aspartic acid, g	8.03	5.96	7.56	0.508	6.95	7.68
Glutamic acid, g	13.2	9.8	12.4	0.825	11.4	12.6
Glycine, g	4.8	3.56	4.51	0.425	4.16	4.59
Proline, g	3.88	2.88	3.65	0.311	3.36	3.72
Serine, g	3.36	2.5	3.16	0.234	2.91	3.22

[1]Beef contains approx. .63 mg vitamin E/100 g; 13.6 mcg biotin/lb; 19 mg zinc/lb (lean, no fat).

Meats

Lamb[1]

	Leg	Chops	Liver	Shoulder
Measure	1 lb	1 lb	1 lb	1 lb
Weight, g	454	454	454	454
Calories	845	1146	617	1082
Protein, g	67.7	63.7	95.3	59
Carbohydrate, g	0	0	13.2	0
Fiber, g	0	0	0	0
Vitamin A, IU	0	0	229070	0
Vitamin B$_1$, mg	0.59	0.57	1.81	0.53
Vitamin B$_2$, mg	0.82	0.79	14.9	0.73
Vitamin B$_6$, mg	1.05	1.05	1.36	1.05
Vitamin B$_{12}$, mcg	8.2	8.2	472	8.2
Niacin, mg	19	18.5	76.5	17.1
Pantothenic acid, mg	2	2	32.7	2
Folic acid, mcg	18	18	990	18
Vitamin C, mg	0	0	152	0
Vitamin E, IU	1.4	1.4	—	1.48
Calcium, mg	0.39	35	45	35
Copper, mg	0.27	0.73	25	0.44
Iron, mg	5.1	4.7	49.4	3.9
Magnesium, mg	61	55	64	50
Manganese, mg	0.09	—	1.04	0.086
Phosphorus, mg	593	567	1583	516
Potassium, mg	1083	1019	916	942
Selenium, mcg	94	78	—	87
Sodium, mg	237	223	236	206
Zinc, mg	15	—	—	18
Total lipid, g	77	0.97	19.6	97
Total saturated, g	35	54.3	6.9	42
Total unsaturated, g	6	—	—	7
Total monounsaturated, g	31	—	—	40
Cholesterol, mg	265	270	1361	270
Tryptophan, g	0.95	—	—	0.88
Threonine, g	3.5	—	—	3.2
Isoleucine, g	3.9	—	—	3.6
Leucine, g	6.3	—	—	5.85
Lycine, g	7.2	—	—	6.6
Methionine, g	2.1	—	—	1.9
Cystine, g	0.97	—	—	0.9
Phenylalanine, g	3.3	—	—	3
Tyrosine, g	2.7	—	—	2.5
Valine, g	4.4	—	—	4
Arginine, g	4.8	—	—	4.5
Histidine, g	2.57	—	—	2.4
Alanine, g	4.9	—	—	4.5
Aspartic acid, g	7	—	—	6.6
Glutamic acid, g	11.8	—	—	11
Glycine, g	4	—	—	3.67
Proline, g	3.4	—	—	3.2
Serine, g	3	—	—	2.8

[1]Lamb contains approx. 13.6 mg zinc/lb (lean, no fat); 13.6 mcg biotin/lb.

Pork

	Bacon	Bacon, Canadian style	Feet	Ham	Leg
Measure	1 lb	1 lb	½	1 lb	1 lb
Weight, g	454	454	95	454	454
Calories	2523	714	251	827	1182
Protein, g	39	93.6	21	79.6	77.4
Carbohydrate, g	0.42	7.61	0	14.1	0
Fiber, g	0	0	0	0	0
Vitamin A, IU	0	0	0	0	31
Vitamin B₁, mg	1.67	3.4	0.04	3.9	3.24
Vitamin B₂, mg	0.472	0.78	0.1	1.14	0.889
Vitamin B₆, mg	0.64	1.77	—	1.52	1.81
Vitamin B₁₂, mcg	4.2	3.02	—	3.75	2.79
Niacin, mg	12.6	28.2	1.05	23.8	20.5
Pantothenic acid, mg	1.6	2.36	—	2.02	3.04
Folic acid, mcg	9	18	—	15	33
Vitamin C, mg	0	0	0	—	3.2
Vitamin E, IU	0.41	—	—	—	1.9
Calcium, mg	34	36	56	0.32	25
Copper, mg	0.29	0.204	—	0.449	0.295
Iron, mg	2.7	3.07	—	4.5	3.87
Magnesium, mg	39	79	7	85	91
Manganese, mg	0.032	0.104	—	0.141	0.014
Phosphorus, mg	646	1102	52	1122	867
Potassium, mg	631	1560	216	1508	1405
Selenium, mcg	—	—	—	—	133
Sodium, mg	3107	6391	49	5974	214
Zinc, mg	5.23	6.31	—	9.69	8.6
Total lipid, g	261	31.6	17.9	47.9	94.4
Total saturated, g	96.4	10	6.18	15.4	34
Total unsaturated, g	—	—	—	—	9
Total monounsaturated, g	—	—	—	—	38
Cholesterol, mg	306	228	101	259	335
Tryptophan, g	0.376	0.93	0.042	0.957	0.993
Threonine, g	1.5	3.76	0.545	3.54	3.57
Isoleucine, g	1.6	3.53	0.335	3.49	3.63
Leucine, g	2.73	6.6	0.881	6.32	6.23
Lycine, g	2.9	7.37	0.902	6.75	7.55
Methionine, g	0.866	2.54	0.21	2.1	1.86
Cystine, g	0.404	1.17	—	1.2	0.98
Phenylalanine, g	1.5	3.04	0.566	3.44	3.08
Tyrosine, g	1.14	2.83	0.314	2.6	2.67
Valine, g	1.89	3.73	0.483	3.45	4.12
Arginine, g	2.4	5.1	1.59	5.17	5.53
Histidine, g	1.13	3.4	0.252	2.85	3.74
Alanine, g	2.2	4.70	1.76	4.7	4.31
Aspartic acid, g	3.24	7.8	1.46	7.54	6.75
Glutamic acid, g	5.39	13	2.28	13	11.3
Glycine, g	2.8	4.03	3.48	4.14	3.32
Proline, g	2.09	3.5	2.3	3.4	2.75
Serine, g	1.47	3.55	0.839	3.26	2.99

Meats

Pork

Measure	Loin, chop	Shoulder	Spareribs
Measure	1 chop	1 lb	1 lb
Weight, g	151	454	454
Calories	345	1249	804
Protein, g	20	73	48
Carbohydrate, g	0	0	0
Fiber, g	0	0	0
Vitamin A, IU	9	30	30
Vitamin B$_1$, mg	0.948	3.08	1.74
Vitamin B$_2$, mg	0.294	1.19	0.768
Vitamin B$_6$, mg	0.45	1.26	1.18
Vitamin B$_{12}$, mcg	0.86	3.25	2.45
Niacin, mg	5.33	16.8	13.6
Pantothenic acid, mg	0.788	2.87	2.23
Folic acid, mcg	4	16	11
Vitamin C, mg	0.8	3	—
Vitamin E, IU	0.48	1.9	—
Calcium, mg	7	24	19
Copper, mg	0.076	0.376	0.239
Iron, mg	0.85	4.59	2.78
Magnesium, mg	21	77	62
Manganese, mg	0.013	0.05	0.028
Phosphorus, mg	224	803	671
Potassium, mg	346	1325	728
Selenium, mcg	28	115	—
Sodium, mg	63	286	212
Zinc, mg	2.09	11.3	7.58
Total lipid, g	28.7	103	66.3
Total saturated, g	10.3	37.3	26.3
Total unsaturated, g	2.8	9	—
Total monounsaturated, g	11.8	36	—
Cholesterol, mg	81	329	218
Tryptophan, g	0.256	0.934	0.647
Threonine, g	0.923	3.38	2.26
Isoleucine, g	0.939	3.43	2.32
Leucine, g	1.6	5.9	3.9
Lycine, g	1.95	7.14	4.73
Methionine, g	0.481	1.75	1.18
Cystine, g	0.253	0.925	0.624
Phenylalanine, g	0.797	2.91	1.92
Tyrosine, g	0.689	2.52	1.71
Valine, g	1.06	3.89	2.57
Arginine, g	1.43	5.24	3.34
Histidine, g	0.963	3.53	2.44
Alanine, g	1.1	4.06	2.84
Aspartic acid, g	1.73	6.36	4.46
Glutamic acid, g	2.9	10.6	7.47
Glycine, g	0.852	3.13	2.19
Proline, g	0.708	2.6	1.82
Serine, g	0.769	2.82	1.97

Meats

Veal[2]

	Breast	Chuck	Cutlet	Liver	Rib roast
Measure	1 lb	1 lb	1 lb	1 lb	1 lb
Weight, g	454	454	454	454	454
Calories	828	628	681	635	723
Protein, g	65.6	70.4	72.3	87.1	65.7
Carbohydrate, g	0	0	0	18.6	0
Fiber, g	0	0	0	0	0
Vitamin A, IU	0	0	0	102060	0
Vitamin B$_1$, mg	0.48	0.52	0.53	0.9	0.48
Vitamin B$_2$, mg	0.87	0.94	0.96	12.3	0.87
Vitamin B$_6$, mg	1.22	1.22	1.22	3.04	1.22
Vitamin B$_{12}$, mcg	5.7	5.7	5.7	272	5.7
Niacin, mg	22	23.6	24.2	51.8	22
Pantothenic acid, mg	3.23	3.23	3.23	36.3	3.23
Folic acid, mcg	37	23	23	—	23
Vitamin C, mg	0	0	0	161	0
Vitamin E, IU	—	—	—	—	1.55
Calcium, mg	39	40	41	36	38
Copper, mg	—	—	1.14	36	1.14
Iron, mg	9.7	10.5	10.9	39.9	9.8
Magnesium, mg	81	—	73	73	52
Manganese, mg	0.045	—	—	—	0.136
Phosphorus, mg	652	722	734	1510	664
Potassium, mg	1050	1126	1157	1275	1051
Selenium, mcg	30	—	—	—	37
Sodium, mg	230	246	253	331	230
Zinc, mg	11	—	—	17	15
Total lipid, g	66	36	41	21.3	49
Total saturated, g	29.3	17	19.7	—	23.5
Total unsaturated, g	4	—	—	—	2.8
Total monounsaturated, g	32	—	—	—	15
Cholesterol, mg	254	320	254	1361	254
Tryptophan, g	0.8	—	—	—	0.86
Threonine, g	3.5	—	—	—	3.74
Isoleucine, g	3.9	—	—	—	4
Leucine, g	6.3	—	—	—	6.8
Lycine, g	6.5	—	—	—	7
Methionine, g	1.8	—	—	—	2
Cystine, g	0.9	—	—	—	0.97
Phenylalanine, g	3	—	—	—	3.45
Tyrosine, g	2.5	—	—	—	2.7
Valine, g	4.4	—	—	—	4.7
Arginine, g	4.7	—	—	—	5
Histidine, g	2.9	—	—	—	3
Alanine, g	4.7	—	—	—	5
Aspartic acid, g	6.8	—	—	—	7.4
Glutamic acid, g	12.5	—	—	—	13.5
Glycine, g	4	—	—	—	4.4
Proline, g	3	—	—	—	3.57
Serine, g	2.9	—	—	—	3

[2]Veal contains approx. 12.7 mg zinc/lb (lean, no fat).

Meats

Veal

Wild Game

	Rump roast	Sweetbreads	Rabbit	Venison
Measure	1 lb	1 lb	1 lb	1 lb
Weight, g	454	454	454	454
Calories	573	426	581	572
Protein, g	68	80.7	75	95
Carbohydrate, g	0	0	0	0
Fiber, g	0	0	0	0
Vitamin A, IU	0	0	136	—
Vitamin B_1, mg	0.5	0.37	0.29	1.03
Vitamin B_2, mg	0.9	0.76	0.2	2.19
Vitamin B_6, mg	1.22	—	1.58	—
Vitamin B_{12}, mcg	5.7	63.6	—	—
Niacin, mg	22.8	11.7	45.9	28.6
Pantothenic acid, mg	3.23	—	2.8	—
Folic acid, mcg	23	—	—	—
Vitamin C, mg	0	0	—	0
Vitamin E, IU	—	—	4.5	—
Calcium, mg	38	41	72	45
Copper, mg	—	0.27	—	—
Iron, mg	10	4.54	4.7	22.7
Magnesium, mg	—	68	—	150
Manganese, mg	—	—	—	—
Phosphorus, mg	699	1521	1261	1129
Potassium, mg	1090	1130	1379	1525
Selenium, mcg	—	—	—	—
Sodium, mg	238	281	154	318
Zinc, mg	—	—	—	—
Total lipid, g	31	9.1	29	18
Total saturated, g	14.9	—	11	11
Total unsaturated, g	—	—	—	—
Total monounsaturated, g	—	—	—	—
Cholesterol, mg	254	1135	295	—
Tryptophan, g	—	—	—	—
Threonine, g	—	—	—	—
Isoleucine, g	—	—	—	—
Leucine, g	—	—	—	—
Lycine, g	—	—	—	—
Methionine, g	—	—	—	—
Cystine, g	—	—	—	—
Phenylalanine, g	—	—	—	—
Tyrosine, g	—	—	—	—
Valine, g	—	—	—	—
Arginine, g	—	—	—	—
Histidine, g	—	—	—	—
Alanine, g	—	—	—	—
Aspartic acid, g	—	—	—	—
Glutamic acid, g	—	—	—	—
Glycine, g	—	—	—	—
Proline, g	—	—	—	—
Serine, g	—	—	—	—

Meats

Luncheon and Sausage

	Bologna, beef	Bologna, beef and pork	Bologna, pork	Bratwurst, ckd	Braun-schweiger
Measure	1 oz	1 oz	1 oz	1 link	1 oz
Weight, g	28	28	28	85	28
Calories	89	89	70	256	102
Protein, g	3.31	3.31	4.34	12	3.83
Carbohydrate, g	0.55	0.79	0.21	1.76	0.89
Fiber, g	0	0	0	—	0
Vitamin A, IU	—	—	—	—	3984
Vitamin B$_1$, mg	0.016	0.049	0.148	0.429	0.071
Vitamin B$_2$, mg	0.036	0.039	0.045	0.156	0.432
Vitamin B$_6$, mg	0.05	0.05	0.08	0.18	0.09
Vitamin B$_{12}$, mcg	0.4	0.38	0.26	0.81	5.69
Niacin, mg	0.746	0.731	1.1	2.72	2.37
Pantothenic acid, mg	0.08	0.08	0.2	0.27	0.96
Folic acid, mcg	1	1	1	—	—
Vitamin C, mg	t	t	t	1	t
Vitamin E, IU	—	—	—	—	—
Calcium, mg	3	3	3	38	2
Copper, mg	0.01	0.02	0.02	0.08	0.07
Iron, mg	0.4	0.43	0.22	1.09	2.65
Magnesium, mg	3	3	4	12	3
Manganese, mg	0.008	0.011	0.01	0.039	0.044
Phosphorus, mg	23	26	39	126	48
Potassium, mg	44	51	80	180	57
Selenium, mcg	—	—	—	—	—
Sodium, mg	284	289	336	473	324
Zinc, mg	0.57	0.55	0.57	1.96	0.8
Total lipid, g	8.04	8.01	5.63	22	9.1
Total saturated, g	3.31	3.03	1.95	7.93	3.09
Total unsaturated, g	—	—	—	—	—
Total monounsaturated, g	—	—	—	—	—
Cholesterol, mg	16	16	17	51	44
Tryptophan, g	0.03	0.03	0.042	0.096	0.041
Threonine, g	0.125	0.145	0.182	0.473	0.151
Isoleucine, g	0.143	0.144	0.188	0.437	0.137
Leucine, g	0.244	0.255	0.331	0.802	0.293
Lycine, g	0.254	0.25	0.341	0.91	0.258
Methionine, g	0.077	0.079	0.117	0.291	0.088
Cystine, g	0.042	0.039	0.048	0.121	0.07
Phenylalanine, g	0.119	0.131	0.166	0.4	0.157
Tyrosine, g	0.108	0.102	0.137	0.345	0.122
Valine, g	0.146	0.176	0.209	0.481	0.175
Arginine, g	0.205	0.198	0.285	0.706	0.217
Histidine, g	0.105	0.09	0.137	0.345	0.091
Alanine, g	0.238	0.207	0.278	0.671	0.216
Aspartic acid, g	0.324	0.291	0.398	0.996	0.319
Glutamic acid, g	0.54	0.531	0.651	1.65	0.462
Glycine, g	0.277	0.245	0.305	0.726	0.251
Proline, g	0.238	0.212	0.219	0.558	0.217
Serine, g	0.134	0.144	0.18	0.463	0.167

Meats

Meats

Luncheon and Sausage

	Brotwurst	Frankfurter, beef	Frankfurter, beef and pork	Italian sausage, ckd	Kielbasa
Measure	1 oz	1	1	1 link	1 oz
Weight, g	28	45	45	67	28
Calories	92	145	144	216	88
Protein, g	4.04	5.08	5.08	13.4	3.76
Carbohydrate, g	0.84	1.08	1.15	1	0.61
Fiber, g	—	0	0	0	0
Vitamin A, IU	—	—	—	—	—
Vitamin B₁, mg	0.071	0.023	0.09	0.417	0.065
Vitamin B₂, mg	0.064	0.046	0.054	0.156	0.061
Vitamin B₆, mg	0.04	0.05	0.06	0.22	0.05
Vitamin B₁₂, mcg	0.58	0.74	0.58	0.87	0.46
Niacin, mg	0.936	1.13	1.18	2.79	0.816
Pantothenic acid, mg	0.02	0.13	0.16	0.3	0.23
Folic acid, mcg	—	2	2	—	—
Vitamin C, mg	t	t	t	1	t
Vitamin E, IU	—	—	—	—	—
Calcium, mg	14	6	5	16	12
Copper, mg	0.02	0.03	0.04	0.05	0.03
Iron, mg	0.29	0.6	0.52	1	0.41
Magnesium, mg	4	4	5	12	5
Manganese, mg	0.011	0.015	0.014	0.055	0.011
Phosphorus, mg	38	37	38	114	42
Potassium, mg	80	71	75	204	77
Selenium, mcg	—	—	—	—	—
Sodium, mg	315	461	504	618	305
Zinc, mg	0.6	0.95	0.83	1.6	0.57
Total lipid, g	7.88	13.2	13.1	17.2	7.7
Total saturated, g	2.81	5.38	4.84	6.08	2.81
Total unsaturated, g	—	—	—	—	—
Total monounsaturated, g	—	—	—	—	—
Cholesterol, mg	18	22	22	52	19
Tryptophan, g	0.037	0.046	0.037	0.108	0.039
Threonine, g	0.17	0.192	0.183	0.531	0.122
Isoleucine, g	0.172	0.219	0.218	0.49	0.181
Leucine, g	0.306	0.373	0.369	0.9	0.248
Lycine, g	0.323	0.389	0.407	1.02	0.286
Methionine, g	0.105	0.118	0.103	0.326	0.078
Cystine, g	0.046	0.065	0.058	0.135	0.064
Phenylalanine, g	0.153	0.183	0.162	0.449	0.142
Tyrosine, g	0.126	0.166	0.141	0.387	0.139
Valine, g	0.191	0.223	0.212	0.539	0.181
Arginine, g	0.268	0.314	0.382	0.792	0.267
Histidine, g	0.124	0.162	0.158	0.387	0.089
Alanine, g	0.262	0.365	0.346	0.751	0.240
Aspartic acid, g	0.366	0.497	0.502	1.11	0.345
Glutamic acid, g	0.598	0.827	0.833	1.85	0.459
Glycine, g	0.291	0.424	0.371	0.813	0.295
Proline, g	0.21	0.365	0.244	0.624	0.195
Serine, g	0.167	0.205	0.208	0.519	0.15

Luncheon and Sausage

	Knockwurst	Liver cheese	Liverwurst	Mortadella	Pepperoni
Measure	1 link	1 oz	1 oz	1 oz	1 slice
Weight, g	68	28	28	28	5.5[1]
Calories	209	86	93	88	27
Protein, g	8.08	4.3	4.01	4.64	1.15
Carbohydrate, g	1.2	0.59	0.63	0.87	0.16
Fiber, g	0	—	—	—	0
Vitamin A, IU	—	4958	—	—	—
Vitamin B$_1$, mg	0.233	0.06	0.077	0.034	0.018
Vitamin B$_2$, mg	0.095	0.631	0.292	0.043	0.014
Vitamin B$_6$, mg	0.11	0.13	—	0.035	0.01
Vitamin B$_{12}$, mcg	0.8	6.96	24.2	0.42	0.14
Niacin, mg	1.86	3.33	—	0.758	0.273
Pantothenic acid, mg	0.22	1	0.84	—	0.1
Folic acid, mcg	—	—	8	—	—
Vitamin C, mg	t	1	—	t	0.018
Vitamin E, IU	—	—	—	—	—
Calcium, mg	7	2	7	5	1
Copper, mg	0.04	0.11	—	0.02	0
Iron, mg	0.62	3.07	1.81	0.4	0.08
Magnesium, mg	8	3	—	3	1
Manganese, mg	—	0.057	—	0.008	—
Phosphorus, mg	67	59	65	27	7
Potassium, mg	136	64	—	46	19
Selenium, mcg	—	—	—	—	—
Sodium, mg	687	347	—	353	112
Zinc, mg	1.13	1.05	—	0.6	0.14
Total lipid, g	18.8	7.25	8.09	7.2	2.42
Total saturated, g	6.94	2.54	3	2.7	0.89
Total unsaturated, g	—	—	—	—	—
Total monounsaturated, g	—	—	—	—	—
Cholesterol, mg	39	49	45	16	—
Tryptophan, g	0.073	0.058	0.043	0.043	0.011
Threonine, g	0.326	0.185	0.192	0.179	0.047
Isoleucine, g	0.317	0.179	0.187	0.201	0.05
Leucine, g	0.558	0.377	0.326	0.344	0.087
Lycine, g	0.634	0.334	0.331	0.358	0.09
Methionine, g	0.195	0.097	0.081	0.112	0.029
Cystine, g	0.1	0.093	0.043	0.058	0.014
Phenylalanine, g	0.277	0.203	0.177	0.17	0.043
Tyrosine, g	0.245	0.132	0.104	0.15	0.037
Valine, g	0.35	0.229	0.246	0.208	0.054
Arginine, g	0.482	0.237	0.232	0.291	0.074
Histidine, g	0.245	0.111	0.128	0.147	0.037
Alanine, g	0.459	0.264	0.237	0.326	0.077
Aspartic acid, g	0.687	0.383	0.333	0.448	0.108
Glutamic acid, g	1.1	0.52	0.628	0.742	0.178
Glycine, g	0.478	0.265	0.314	0.374	0.087
Proline, g	0.367	0.203	0.244	0.312	0.067
Serine, g	0.324	0.196	0.199	0.188	0.047

[1] ⅛" thick.

Meats

Luncheon and Sausage

	Polish sausage	Pork and beef sausage	Pork sausage	Salami, hard	Summer sausage	Vienna sausage
Measure	1 oz	1 link	1 link	1 slice	1 slice	1
Weight, g	28	13	28	10[1]	23[2]	16
Calories	92	52	118	42	80	45
Protein, g	4	1.79	3.31	2.29	3.69	1.65
Carbohydrate, g	0.46	0.35	0.29	0.26	0.53	0.33
Fiber, g	0	0	0	0	0	0
Vitamin A, IU	—	—	—	—	—	—
Vitamin B_1, mg	0.142	0.096	0.155	0.06	0.039	0.014
Vitamin B_2, mg	0.042	0.019	0.046	0.029	0.069	0.017
Vitamin B_6, mg	0.05	0.01	0.07	0.05	0.07	0.02
Vitamin B_{12}, mcg	0.28	0.06	0.32	0.19	1.06	0.16
Niacin, mg	0.976	0.438	0.804	0.487	0.94	0.258
Pantothenic acid, mg	0.13	0.06	0.11	0.11	0.13	—
Folic acid, mcg	—	—	1	—	—	—
Vitamin C, mg	0	—	—	t	t	0
Vitamin E, IU	—	—	—	—	—	—
Calcium, mg	3	—	5	1	2	2
Copper, mg	0.03	0	0.02	0.01	0.02	0
Iron, mg	0.41	0.15	0.26	0.15	0.47	0.14
Magnesium, mg	4	1	3	2	3	1
Manganese, mg	0.014	—	—	0.004	0.007	0.005
Phosphorus, mg	39	14	34	14	23	8
Potassium, mg	67	—	58	38	53	16
Selenium, mcg	—	—	—	—	—	—
Sodium, mg	248	105	228	186	334	152
Zinc, mg	0.55	0.24	0.45	0.32	0.47	0.26
Total lipid, g	8.14	4.71	11.4	3.44	6.88	4.03
Total saturated, g	2.93	1.68	4.1	1.22	2.77	1.48
Total unsaturated, g	—	—	—	—	—	—
Total monounsaturated, g	—	—	—	—	—	—
Cholesterol, mg	20	—	19	8	16	8
Tryptophan, g	0.039	0.017	0.027	0.021	0.035	0.017
Threonine, g	0.168	0.072	0.131	0.096	0.158	0.057
Isoleucine, g	0.173	0.069	0.121	0.097	0.177	0.089
Leucine, g	0.305	0.127	0.222	0.173	0.241	0.128
Lycine, g	0.315	0.141	0.252	0.182	0.318	0.127
Methionine, g	0.107	0.043	0.081	0.059	0.081	0.042
Cystine, g	0.045	0.018	0.033	0.026	0.045	0.028
Phenylalanine, g	0.153	0.062	0.111	0.087	0.133	0.068
Tyrosine, g	0.126	0.053	0.096	0.071	0.125	0.055
Valine, g	0.192	0.077	0.133	0.108	0.185	0.092
Arginine, g	0.262	0.111	0.196	0.152	0.228	0.113
Histidine, g	0.126	0.054	0.096	0.07	0.108	0.044
Alanine, g	0.256	0.106	0.186	0.148	0.233	0.104
Aspartic acid, g	0.367	0.154	0.276	0.207	0.331	0.161
Glutamic acid, g	0.6	0.259	0.458	0.338	0.507	0.209
Glycine, g	0.281	0.117	0.201	0.164	0.254	0.162
Proline, g	0.202	0.085	0.154	0.119	0.198	0.097
Serine, g	0.166	0.069	0.128	0.094	0.156	0.069

[1] 1⁄16″ thick.
[2] 1⁄8″ thick.

Meats

Nuts and Seeds

	Almonds	Brazil nuts	Cashews, dry roasted	Chestnuts, raw, peeled	Coconut, shredded
Measure	1 C	1 C	1 C	1 oz	1 C
Weight, g	142	140	140	28	80
Calories	849	916	785	56	277
Protein, g	26.4	20	24.1	0.46	2.8
Carbohydrate, g	27.7	15.3	41	13	7.5
Fiber, g	17	7.5	4	—	7.2
Vitamin A, IU	14	0	0	7.4	0
Vitamin B$_1$, mg	0.34	1.34	0.6	0.04	0.04
Vitamin B$_2$, mg	1.31	0.17	0.35	0.005	0.02
Vitamin B$_6$, mg	0.142	0.238	0.325	0.1	0.035
Vitamin B$_{12}$, mcg	0	0	0	0	0
Niacin, mg	5	2.2	2.5	0.3	0.4
Pantothenic acid, mg	0.668	0.323	1.82	0.135	0.16
Folic acid, mcg	41	5.6	94	16	21
Vitamin C, mg	0	0.98	0	12	2
Vitamin E, IU	55	15.9	1.2	—	0.86
Calcium, mg	332	260	53	5.4	10
Copper, mg	1.18	2.14	2.82	0.12	0.368
Iron, mg	6.7	4.8	5.3	0.27	1.4
Magnesium, mg	386	351	374	8.5	37
Manganese, mg	2.7	3.9	—	0.095	1.05
Phosphorus, mg	716	970	522	11	76
Potassium, mg	1098	1001	650	137	205
Selenium, mcg	11	4144	16	—	8
Sodium, mg	6	1	21	0.57	18
Zinc, mg	4.14	7.1	6.1	0.14	0.88
Total lipid, g	77	93.7	64	0.35	28.2
Total saturated, g	6.2	18.7	10.9	0.067	24.3
Total unsaturated, g	17	34	37	0.14	0.29
Total monounsaturated, g	45	32	11	0.122	1.1
Cholesterol, mg	0	0	0	0	0
Tryptophan, g	0.508	0.364	0.325	0.005	0.001
Threonine, g	1.05	0.644	0.813	0.016	0.097
Isoleucine, g	1.23	0.841	1	0.018	0.105
Leucine, g	2.2	1.66	1.76	0.027	0.198
Lycine, g	0.946	0.757	1.12	0.027	0.118
Methionine, g	0.322	1.42	0.376	0.011	0.05
Cystine, g	0.508	0.489	0.389	0.015	0.053
Phenylalanine, g	1.58	1.04	1.09	0.02	0.135
Tyrosine, g	1	0.64	0.673	0.013	0.082
Valine, g	1.46	1.28	1.43	0.026	0.162
Arginine, g	3.54	3.35	2.39	0.033	0.437
Histidine, g	0.792	0.563	0.546	0.013	0.062
Alanine, g	1.34	0.798	0.962	0.03	0.136
Aspartic acid, g	3.33	1.89	2.06	0.08	0.26
Glutamic acid, g	8.43	4.4	4.97	0.06	0.609
Glycine, g	1.75	0.92	1.1	0.024	0.126
Proline, g	1.78	1.07	0.946	0.024	0.11
Serine, g	1.28	1.04	1.17	0.023	0.138

Nuts and Seeds

	Coconut liquid	Hazelnuts	Hickory nuts, dried	Macadamia nuts	Pecans
Measure	1 C	1 C	5	1 C	1 C
Weight, g	240	135	15	134	108
Calories	792	856	101	940	742
Protein, g	8.7	17	2.1	11	9.9
Carbohydrate, g	16	22.5	2	18.4	15.8
Fiber, g	5.3	13	0.95	11	10
Vitamin A, IU	0	144	20	0	83
Vitamin B_1, mg	0.07	0.62	0.08	0.469	0.93
Vitamin B_2, mg	0	0.738	0.02	0.147	0.14
Vitamin B_6, mg	0.045	0.735	0.03	0.368	0.183
Vitamin B_{12}, mcg	0	0	0	0	0
Niacin, mg	0.2	1.2	0.135	2.87	1
Pantothenic acid, mg	0.63	1.54	0.26	1	1.7
Folic acid, mcg	55	152	6	15	24
Vitamin C, mg	7	8	0.3	1.6	2
Vitamin E, IU	2.6	29.8	1.16	1	5.9
Calcium, mg	26	282	9	94	79
Copper, mg	0.9	1.72	0.214	0.397	1.14
Iron, mg	5.4	4.6	0.4	3.23	2.6
Magnesium, mg	67	313	24	155	142
Manganese, mg	3	5.67	0.69	5.5	1.54
Phosphorus, mg	292	455	49	183	312
Potassium, mg	780	950	64	493	651
Selenium, mcg	—	5.4	1.2	4.8	6.48
Sodium, mg	9	3	0.15	6	t
Zinc, mg	2.3	4	0.61	2.29	5.91
Total lipid, g	83	84.2	10.1	98.8	76.9
Total saturated, g	73	4.2	0.9	14.8	5.4
Total unsaturated, g	0.9	11	3.3	2	23
Total monounsaturated, g	3.5	62	4.89	79	44
Cholesterol, mg	0	0	0	0	0
Tryptophan, g	0.1	0.248	0.2	0.09	0.215
Threonine, g	0.32	0.515	0.06	0.352	0.273
Isoleucine, g	0.34	0.653	0.082	0.327	0.348
Leucine, g	0.65	1.27	0.146	0.619	0.562
Lycine, g	0.38	0.459	0.07	0.434	0.315
Methionine, g	0.16	0.189	0.042	0.123	0.201
Cystine, g	0.17	0.263	0.038	0.129	0.226
Phenylalanine, g	0.44	0.789	0.1	0.348	0.442
Tyrosine, g	0.27	0.521	0.064	0.452	0.307
Valine, g	0.53	0.761	0.1	0.43	0.417
Arginine, g	1.43	2.48	0.298	1.2	1.19
Histidine, g	0.2	0.376	0.05	0.225	0.245
Alanine, g	0.44	0.814	0.094	0.441	0.365
Aspartic acid, g	0.85	1.85	0.194	1.1	0.765
Glutamic acid, g	2	4.07	0.409	2.39	1.67
Glycine, g	0.4	0.81	0.1	0.497	0.407
Proline, g	0.36	0.585	0.081	0.531	0.389
Serine, g	0.45	0.769	0.115	0.47	0.406

Nuts and Seeds

	Pine nuts	Pistachios	Pumpkin and squash seeds	Sesame seeds	Sunflower seeds
Measure	1 oz	1 C	1 C	1 C	1 C
Weight, g	28	128	140	150	145
Calories	180	739	774	873	812
Protein, g	3.7	26	40.6	27.3	34.8
Carbohydrate, g	5.8	31.7	21	26.4	28.9
Fiber, g	1.3	13	5.4	17	15
Vitamin A, IU	10	707	100	99	70
Vitamin B_1, mg	0.36	1.05	0.34	0.27	2.84
Vitamin B_2, mg	0.07	0.223	0.442	0.2	0.33
Vitamin B_6, mg	0.031	2	0.31	0.126	1.8
Vitamin B_{12}, mcg	0	0	0	0	0
Niacin, mg	1.3	1.38	3.4	8.1	7.8
Pantothenic acid, mg	0.06	0.67	0.47	1.02	2
Folic acid, mcg	16	74	79	140	327
Vitamin C, mg	0.54	6	2.6	0	2
Vitamin E, IU	1.48	8.8	2	4.87	107
Calcium, mg	3	173	71	1404	174
Copper, mg	0.29	1.52	1.9	2.39	2.57
Iron, mg	1.5	8.67	15.7	3.6	10.3
Magnesium, mg	66	203	738	270	57
Manganese, mg	1.2	0.419	4	3.5	2.9
Phosphorus, mg	171	644	1620	888	1214
Potassium, mg	170	1399	1113	610	1334
Selenium, mcg	4.7	8.8	7.7	8.2	86
Sodium, mg	1	7	24	59	4
Zinc, mg	1.21	1.71	10.3	15.4	7.3
Total lipid, g	14.3	61.9	65.4	80	68.6
Total saturated, g	1.7	7.84	11.8	11.2	8.2
Total unsaturated, g	6	16.7	29	31	13
Total monounsaturated, g	5.4	29	19.6	27	47
Cholesterol, mg	0	0	0	0	0
Tryptophan, g	0.086	0.362	0.595	0.71	0.5
Threonine, g	0.216	0.924	1.25	1.77	1.34
Isoleucine, g	0.265	1.25	1.74	1.93	1.64
Leucine, g	0.491	2.15	2.87	3.22	2.39
Lycine, g	0.256	1.64	2.53	1.24	1.35
Methionine, g	0.122	0.488	0.76	1.34	0.711
Cystine, g	0.124	0.657	0.415	0.785	0.649
Phenylalanine, g	0.261	1.52	1.69	2.28	1.69
Tyrosine, g	0.249	0.914	1.41	1.69	0.959
Valine, g	0.352	1.8	2.72	2.22	1.9
Arginine, g	1.33	2.79	5.57	4.99	3.46
Histidine, g	0.163	0.686	0.94	1.02	0.91
Alanine, g	0.356	1.28	1.6	2.11	1.6
Aspartic acid, g	0.621	2.7	3.42	3.4	3.5
Glutamic acid, g	1.16	6.3	6	7.42	8.03
Glycine, g	0.347	1.4	2.48	2.84	2.1
Proline, g	0.366	1.2	1.4	2.04	1.7
Serine, g	0.289	1.73	1.58	1.97	1.55

Nuts and Seeds

	Nuts and Seeds		Chicken[1]
	Tahini	Walnuts, shelled	Light meat, from a 1-lb bird
Measure	1 T	1 C	4 oz
Weight, g	15	100	116
Calories	89	651	216
Protein, g	2.55	14.8	23.5
Carbohydrate, g	3.18	15.8	0
Fiber, g	1.4	6.7	0
Vitamin A, IU	10	30	115
Vitamin B$_1$, mg	0.183	0.33	0.068
Vitamin B$_2$, mg	0.071	0.13	0.1
Vitamin B$_6$, mg	0.022	0.73	0.56
Vitamin B$_{12}$, mcg	0	0	0.39
Niacin, mg	0.818	0.9	10.3
Pantothenic acid, mg	0.1	0.9	0.921
Folic acid, mcg	15	98	5
Vitamin C, mg	0	2	1.1
Vitamin E, IU	0.5	4.4	0.51
Calcium, mg	64	99	13
Copper, mg	0.242	1.39	0.046
Iron, mg	1.34	3.1	0.92
Magnesium, mg	14	131	27
Manganese, mg	0.22	1.8	0.021
Phosphorus, mg	110	380	189
Potassium, mg	62	450	237
Selenium, mcg	0.25	4.6	19
Sodium, mg	17	2	76
Zinc, mg	0.69	2.26	1.08
Total lipid, g	8.06	64	12.8
Total saturated, g	1.13	4.5	3.66
Total unsaturated, g	3.5	47	2.7
Total monounsaturated, g	3	8.9	5.24
Cholesterol, mg	0	0	78
Tryptophan, g	0.056	0.227	0.263
Threonine, g	0.106	0.538	0.973
Isoleucine, g	0.11	0.679	1.17
Leucine, g	0.195	1.19	1.71
Lycine, g	0.082	0.466	1.92
Methionine, g	0.084	0.336	0.628
Cystine, g	0.051	0.414	0.313
Phenylalanine, g	0.135	0.754	0.914
Tyrosine, g	0.107	0.527	0.760
Valine, g	0.143	0.868	1.14
Arginine, g	0.378	2.52	1.47
Histidine, g	0.075	0.431	0.693
Alanine, g	0.133	0.731	1.36
Aspartic acid, g	0.237	1.77	2.09
Glutamic acid, g	0.569	3.37	3.44
Glycine, g	0.175	0.906	1.49
Proline, g	0.116	0.664	1.12
Serine, g	0.139	0.938	0.828

[1]Chicken contains approx. .25 mg vitamin E/100 g; 4.54 mcg biotin/lb.

Chicken

	Dark meat, from a 1-lb bird	Light meat, w/o skin, from a 1-lb bird	Dark meat, w/o skin, from a 1-lb bird	Back, bone removed
Measure	5.6 oz	3 oz	3.8 oz	½
Weight, g	160	88	109	99
Calories	379	100	136	316
Protein, g	26.7	20.4	21.9	13.9
Carbohydrate, g	0	0	0	0
Fiber, g	0	0	0	0
Vitamin A, IU	273	25	78	248
Vitamin B_1, mg	0.98	0.06	0.084	0.05
Vitamin B_2, mg	0.234	0.081	0.201	0.115
Vitamin B_6, mg	0.39	0.48	0.36	0.19
Vitamin B_{12}, mcg	0.47	0.34	0.39	0.24
Niacin, mg	8.33	9.33	6.8	4.78
Pantothenic acid, mg	1.59	0.723	1.36	0.811
Folic acid, mcg	11	4	11	6
Vitamin C, mg	3.4	1.1	3.4	1.6
Vitamin E, IU	—	—	—	—
Calcium, mg	18	10	13	13
Copper, mg	0.086	0.035	0.069	0.047
Iron, mg	1.57	0.64	1.12	0.93
Magnesium, mg	30	24	25	15
Manganese, mg	0.03	0.016	0.023	0.018
Phosphorus, mg	217	164	177	112
Potassium, mg	285	210	241	142
Selenium, mcg	20	15.7	14.7	12
Sodium, mg	117	60	93	63
Zinc, mg	2.53	0.85	2.18	1.25
Total lipid, g	29.3	1.45	4.7	28.4
Total saturated, g	8.41	0.38	1.2	8.25
Total unsaturated, g	6.4	0.326	1.17	6
Total monounsaturated, g	12	0.34	1.46	12
Cholesterol, mg	130	51	87	79
Tryptophan, g	0.296	0.238	0.256	0.149
Threonine, g	1.09	0.862	0.924	0.564
Isoleucine, g	1.31	1.07	1.15	0.66
Leucine, g	1.93	1.53	1.64	0.985
Lycine, g	2.15	1.73	1.86	1.09
Methionine, g	0.706	0.565	0.606	0.357
Cystine, g	0.358	0.261	0.28	0.192
Phenylalanine, g	1.03	0.81	0.869	0.531
Tyrosine, g	0.85	0.689	0.739	0.43
Valine, g	1.29	1.01	1.08	0.663
Arginine, g	1.68	1.23	1.32	0.9
Histidine, g	0.776	0.634	0.679	0.389
Alanine, g	1.57	1.11	1.19	0.854
Aspartic acid, g	2.38	1.82	1.95	1.24
Glutamic acid, g	3.88	3.05	3.27	2
Glycine, g	1.8	1	1.07	1.08
Proline, g	1.33	0.84	0.9	0.759
Serine, g	0.946	0.702	0.753	0.501

Poultry

Chicken

	Breast, bone removed	Drumstick, bone removed	Leg, bone removed	Neck, bone and skin removed	Thigh, bone removed
Measure	½	1	1	1	1
Weight, g	145	73	167	20	94
Calories	250	117	312	31	199
Protein, g	30.2	14	30.3	3.5	16.2
Carbohydrate, g	0	0	0	0	0
Fiber, g	0	0	0	0	0
Vitamin A, IU	121	69	206	29	136
Vitamin B_1, mg	0.091	0.054	0.112	0.011	0.058
Vitamin B_2, mg	0.123	0.13	0.274	0.046	0.144
Vitamin B_6, mg	0.77	0.22	0.48	0.06	0.24
Vitamin B_{12}, mcg	0.5	0.25	0.54	0.06	0.28
Niacin, mg	14.3	3.97	9.07	0.824	5.1
Pantothenic acid, mg	1.16	0.863	1.85	0.218	0.97
Folic acid, mcg	6	6	19	2	7
Vitamin C, mg	1.5	2	4.1	0.5	2.1
Vitamin E, IU	—	0.32	—	—	—
Calcium, mg	16	8	17	5	9
Copper, mg	0.057	0.043	0.097	0.022	0.055
Iron, mg	1.07	0.75	1.68	0.41	0.93
Magnesium, mg	36	16	34	3	19
Manganese, mg	0.026	0.015	0.033	0.007	0.018
Phosphorus, mg	252	113	249	23	136
Potassium, mg	319	151	331	35	181
Selenium, mcg	19.2	10	21	2.7	12
Sodium, mg	91	61	132	16	71
Zinc, mg	1.16	1.46	2.96	0.54	1.5
Total lipid, g	13.4	6.34	20.2	1.76	14.3
Total saturated, g	3.86	1.75	5.7	0.45	4.08
Total unsaturated, g	2.8	1.4	4.4	0.44	3.1
Total monounsaturated, g	5.54	2.46	8.2	0.54	5.9
Cholesterol, mg	92	59	138	17	79
Tryptophan, g	0.344	0.159	0.341	0.041	0.18
Threonine, g	1.26	0.585	1.25	0.148	0.67
Isoleucine, g	1.54	0.715	1.52	0.185	0.807
Leucine, g	2.22	1.03	2.21	0.263	1.17
Lycine, g	2.5	1.16	2.47	0.298	1.31
Methionine, g	0.816	0.379	0.81	0.097	0.431
Cystine, g	0.397	0.185	0.402	0.045	0.217
Phenylalanine, g	1.18	0.55	1.18	0.139	0.630
Tyrosine, g	0.992	0.46	0.982	0.118	0.521
Valine, g	1.48	0.688	1.47	0.174	0.787
Arginine, g	1.87	0.872	1.89	0.212	1.02
Histidine, g	0.906	0.42	0.895	0.109	0.475
Alanine, g	1.72	0.804	1.75	0.191	0.951
Aspartic acid, g	2.7	1.25	2.7	0.313	1.44
Glutamic acid, g	4.46	2.07	4.44	0.525	2.37
Glycine, g	1.78	0.842	1.91	0.172	1.07
Proline, g	1.38	0.65	1.44	0.144	0.796
Serine, g	1.05	0.493	1.06	0.121	0.574

Chicken

	Wing, bone removed	Gizzard	Heart	Liver	Canned, boned
Measure	1	1	1	1	5 oz
Weight, g	49	37	6.1	32	142
Calories	109	44	9	40	234
Protein, g	8.98	6.73	0.95	5.75	30.9
Carbohydrate, g	0	0.21	0.04	1.09	0
Fiber, g	0	0	0	0	0
Vitamin A, IU	72	80	2	6576	166
Vitamin B$_1$, mg	0.024	0.013	0.009	0.044	0.021
Vitamin B$_2$, mg	0.043	0.07	0.044	0.628	0.183
Vitamin B$_6$, mg	0.17	0.05	0.02	0.24	0.5
Vitamin B$_{12}$, mcg	0.15	0.78	0.44	7.35	0.42
Niacin, mg	2.9	1.74	0.298	2.96	8.98
Pantothenic acid, mg	0.375	0.278	0.156	1.98	1.2
Folic acid, mcg	2	19	4	236	5.7
Vitamin C, mg	0.3	1.2	0.2	10.8	2.8
Vitamin E, IU	0.22	0.66	—	0.69	0.45
Calcium, mg	6	3	1	3	20
Copper, mg	0.02	0.036	0.021	0.126	0.065
Iron, mg	0.47	1.3	0.36	2.74	2.25
Magnesium, mg	9	6	1	6	17
Manganese, mg	0.009	0.024	0.005	0.083	0.02
Phosphorus, mg	65	50	11	87	158
Potassium, mg	76	87	11	73	196
Selenium, mcg	7.5	20.6	0.26	20	22
Sodium, mg	36	28	5	25	714
Zinc, mg	0.65	1.11	0.4	0.98	—
Total lipid, g	7.82	1.55	0.57	1.23	11.3
Total saturated, g	2.19	0.44	0.16	0.42	3.12
Total unsaturated, g	1.6	0.45	0.165	0.2	2.48
Total monounsaturated, g	3	0.396	0.14	0.3	4.5
Cholesterol, mg	38	48	8	140	88
Tryptophan, g	0.096	0.06	0.012	0.081	0.345
Threonine, g	0.363	0.31	0.043	0.256	1.27
Isoleucine, g	0.421	0.317	0.051	0.305	1.54
Leucine, g	0.632	0.472	0.083	0.519	2.24
Lycine, g	0.698	0.465	0.079	0.435	2.5
Methionine, g	0.228	0.176	0.023	0.136	0.815
Cystine, g	0.125	0.088	0.013	0.077	0.422
Phenylalanine, g	0.341	0.28	0.042	0.286	1.19
Tyrosine, g	0.275	0.205	0.034	0.202	0.993
Valine, g	0.426	0.302	0.054	0.363	1.49
Arginine, g	0.585	0.484	0.061	0.352	1.92
Histidine, g	0.248	0.136	0.025	0.153	0.903
Alanine, g	0.558	0.265	0.06	0.334	1.78
Aspartic acid, g	0.801	0.619	0.092	0.547	2.73
Glutamic acid, g	1.28	1.15	0.141	0.745	4.5
Glycine, g	0.723	0.353	0.053	0.334	1.97
Proline, g	0.502	0.35	0.048	0.285	1.47
Serine, g	0.325	0.302	0.038	0.247	1.08

| | **Chicken** | | **Duck** | | **Goose** |
	Liver paté	Cornish game hen	Domesticated, from a 1-lb bird	Liver	Domesticated, from a 1-lb bird
Measure	1 T	½	10 oz	1	11.2 oz
Weight, g	13	168	287	44	320
Calories	26	336	1159	60	1187
Protein, g	175	29	33	8.24	50.7
Carbohydrate, g	0.85	0	0	1.55	0
Fiber, g	0	0	0	0	0
Vitamin A, IU	94	181	483	17559	176
Vitamin B$_1$, mg	0.007	0.12	0.565	0.247	0.272
Vitamin B$_2$, mg	0.182	0.29	0.603	0.39	0.784
Vitamin B$_6$, mg	0.034	0.5	0.55	0.334	1.24
Vitamin B$_{12}$, mcg	1.1	0.55	0.73	23.7	1.1
Niacin, mg	0.977	9.5	11.3	2.86	11.5
Pantothenic acid, mg	0.34	1	2.73	2.7	1.4
Folic acid, mcg	42	5	37	325	14
Vitamin C, mg	1.3	0.84	8	1.98	13
Vitamin E, IU	0.19	0.74	2.98	5	8.3
Calcium, mg	1	19	30	2.62	38
Copper, mg	0.023	0.08	0.677	13.4	0.864
Iron, mg	1.19	1.3	6.89	—	8
Magnesium, mg	1.7	30	42	10	59
Manganese, mg	0.02	0.027	0.049	0.11	0.06
Phosphorus, mg	23	235	398	118	748
Potassium, mg	12	397	600	101	985
Selenium, mcg	6	19.8	36	30	46
Sodium, mg	50	103	3.91	62	234
Zinc, mg	0.28	1.9	113	1.35	5.5
Total lipid, g	1.7	23.5	37.9	2.04	107
Total saturated, g	0.52	6.5	68.1	0.63	31.3
Total unsaturated, g	0.32	4.65	14.6	0.277	12
Total monounsaturated, g	0.68	10	54	0.312	57
Cholesterol, mg	50	170	218	227	256
Tryptophan, g	0.025	0.32	0.413	0.116	0.66
Threonine, g	0.078	1.18	1.35	0.367	2.26
Isoleucine, g	0.096	1.4	1.54	0.438	2.38
Leucine, g	0.155	2.1	2.58	0.744	4.25
Lysine, g	0.124	2.3	2.61	0.624	4.01
Methionine, g	0.044	0.76	0.835	0.195	1.22
Cystine, g	0.028	0.39	0.517	0.111	0.79
Phenylalanine, g	0.09	1.1	1.31	0.41	2.12
Tyrosine, g	0.064	0.9	1.13	0.29	1.62
Valine, g	0.112	1.4	1.64	0.52	2.48
Arginine, g	0.106	1.8	2.21	0.505	3.15
Histidine, g	0.045	0.84	0.812	0.219	1.41
Alanine, g	0.1	1.7	2.23	0.479	3.12
Aspartic acid, g	0.16	2.56	3.16	0.784	4.56
Glutamic acid, g	0.25	4.2	4.9	1.06	7.54
Glycine, g	0.09	1.9	2.66	0.479	3.21
Proline, g	0.09	1.4	1.97	0.409	2.45
Serine, g	0.089	1	1.4	0.355	2.02

Poultry

	Goose	**Turkey**			
	Liver	Light meat, from a 1-lb bird	Dark meat, from a 1-lb bird	Liver	Canned, boned
Measure	1	6.4 oz	5.3 oz	1	5 oz
Weight, g	94	180	152	102	142
Calories	125	286	243	140	231
Protein, g	15.3	39	28.7	20.4	33.6
Carbohydrate, g	5.94	0	0	4.21	0
Fiber, g	0	0	0	0	0
Vitamin A, IU	29138	12	8	18403	0
Vitamin B_1, mg	0.528	0.101	0.111	0.062	0.02
Vitamin B_2, mg	0.838	0.207	0.307	2.21	0.243
Vitamin B_6, mg	0.72	0.86	0.49	0.78	0.47
Vitamin B_{12}, mcg	51	0.37	0.58	64.6	0.4
Niacin, mg	6.11	9.24	4.34	10.35	9.4
Pantothenic acid, mg	5.8	1.1	1.57	7.81	0.97
Folic acid, mcg	694	13	15	752	8.5
Vitamin C, mg	4.2	0	0	4.6	2.8
Vitamin E, IU	—	—	—	—	0.574
Calcium, mg	40	23	26	7	17
Copper, mg	7.07	0.135	0.208	0.512	0.1
Iron, mg	29	2.18	2.57	11	2.64
Magnesium, mg	23	43	31	21	28
Manganese, mg	0	0.032	0.032	0.294	0.024
Phosphorus, mg	245	331	259	319	230
Potassium, mg	216	489	396	303	318
Selenium, mcg	64	40	40	74	0.37
Sodium, mg	132	106	108	98	663
Zinc, mg	2.9	2.82	4.49	2.53	3.4
Total lipid, g	4.03	13.2	13.3	4.05	9.74
Total saturated, g	1.49	3.59	3.92	1.28	2.84
Total unsaturated, g	0.24	3	3.46	0.7	2.5
Total monounsaturated, g	0.76	5	4.56	1	3.2
Cholesterol, mg	484	117	109	475	94
Tryptophan, g	0.216	0.43	0.318	0.288	0.371
Threonine, g	0.684	1.7	1.25	0.908	1.46
Isoleucine, g	0.818	1.95	1.44	1.08	1.68
Leucine, g	1.38	3.02	2.23	1.84	2.6
Lycine, g	1.16	3.54	2.62	1.54	3.04
Methionine, g	0.365	1.09	0.81	0.483	0.939
Cystine, g	0.207	0.428	0.316	0.274	0.378
Phenylalanine, g	0.766	1.52	1.12	1.01	1.3
Tyrosine, g	0.541	1.47	1.09	0.718	1.27
Valine, g	0.97	2.02	1.49	1.28	1.74
Arginine, g	0.943	2.74	2.02	1.25	2.36
Histidine, g	0.409	1.17	0.866	0.543	1
Alanine, g	0.894	2.48	1.83	1.18	2.13
Aspartic acid, g	1.46	3.75	2.77	1.94	3.22
Glutamic acid, g	1.99	6.2	4.59	2.64	5.34
Glycine, g	0.894	2.35	1.71	1.18	2.02
Proline, g	0.763	1.81	1.33	1.01	1.55
Serine, g	0.663	1.71	1.27	0.879	1.47

Poultry

	Wild Game		Seafood and Seaweed	
	Pheasant, from a 1-lb bird	Quail, from a 1-lb bird	Abalone	Agar-agar
Measure	13 oz	14 oz	3 oz	2 T
Weight, g	371	405	85	10
Calories	670	780	89	2.6
Protein, g	84.2	79.4	14.5	0.05
Carbohydrate, g	0	0	5	0.68
Fiber, g	0	0	0	0.05
Vitamin A, IU	655	985	4.25	0
Vitamin B$_1$, mg	0.267	0.988	0.16	t
Vitamin B$_2$, mg	0.531	1.05	0.12	t
Vitamin B$_6$, mg	2.46	2.43	0.128	t
Vitamin B$_{12}$, mcg	2.85	1.7	0.62	0
Niacin, mg	23.8	30.5	1.3	t
Pantothenic acid, mg	3.44	3	2.55	0.03
Folic acid, mcg	22	30	4.3	8.5
Vitamin C, mg	19.6	24.6	1.7	0
Vitamin E, IU	1.64	4	5	0.01
Calcium, mg	46	52	27	5.4
Copper, mg	0.241	2.05	0.167	t
Iron, mg	4.25	16	2.7	0.19
Magnesium, mg	72	93	41	6.7
Manganese, mg	0.063	0.08	0.034	0.04
Phosphorus, mg	794	1112	173	0.5
Potassium, mg	900	874	213	23
Selenium, mcg	58	67	38	0.07
Sodium, mg	150	215	255	0.9
Zinc, mg	3.57	9.8	0.69	0.06
Total lipid, g	34.4	48.8	0.64	0.00
Total saturated, g	10	13.7	0.127	0.001
Total unsaturated, g	4.4	2	0.088	0.001
Total monounsaturated, g	16	17	0.09	0
Cholesterol, mg	263	308	72	0
Tryptophan, g	1.12	1.16	0.163	—
Threonine, g	4.11	3.82	0.626	—
Isoleucine, g	4.55	4.1	0.632	—
Leucine, g	6.93	6.53	1.02	—
Lycine, g	7.47	6.66	1.09	—
Methionine, g	2.38	2.39	0.328	—
Cystine, g	1.13	1.37	0.19	—
Phenylalanine, g	3.25	3.34	0.521	—
Tyrosine, g	2.68	3.43	0.465	—
Valine, g	4.56	4.18	0.635	—
Arginine, g	5.24	5.18	1.06	—
Histidine, g	3.2	2.82	0.279	—
Alanine, g	5.23	5.1	0.879	—
Aspartic acid, g	8.11	6.69	1.4	—
Glutamic acid, g	12.2	10.2	1.97	—
Glycine, g	4.56	6.24	0.91	—
Proline, g	3.48	3.5	0.593	—
Serine, g	3.6	3.79	0.651	—

Poultry

Seafood and Seaweed

	Anchovy, in oil, drained	Bass, sea	Bluefish
Measure	5	3 oz	3 oz
Weight, g	20	85	85
Calories	42	82	105
Protein, g	5.78	15	17
Carbohydrate, g	0	0	0
Fiber, g	0	0	0
Vitamin A, IU	14	156	338
Vitamin B_1, mg	0.016	0.09	0.049
Vitamin B_2, mg	0.073	0.03	0.068
Vitamin B_6, mg	0.041	0.34	0.342
Vitamin B_{12}, mcg	0.176	3.25	4.58
Niacin, mg	3.98	1.9	5.06
Pantothenic acid, mg	0.18	0.46	0.704
Folic acid, mcg	2.5	4.3	1.4
Vitamin C, mg	0	0	0
Vitamin E, IU	1	0.64	0.63
Calcium, mg	46	8.5	6
Copper, mg	0.068	0.026	0.045
Iron, mg	0.93	0.71	0.41
Magnesium, mg	14	35	28
Manganese, mg	0.02	0.013	0.018
Phosphorus, mg	50	174	193
Potassium, mg	109	232	316
Selenium, mcg	13.6	31	31
Sodium, mg	734	59	51
Zinc, mg	0.49	0.34	0.69
Total lipid, g3	1.94	1.98	3.6
Total saturated, g	0.441	0.431	0.778
Total unsaturated, g	0.5	0.63	0.9
Total monounsaturated, g	0.75	0.36	1.5
Cholesterol, mg	17	68	50
Tryptophan, g	0.065	0.169	0.19
Threonine, g	0.253	0.66	0.746
Isoleucine, g	0.266	0.694	0.785
Leucine, g	0.470	1.23	1.39
Lycine, g	0.531	1.38	1.56
Methionine, g	0.171	0.446	0.504
Cystine, g	0.062	0.162	0.183
Phenylalanine, g	0.226	0.588	0.665
Tyrosine, g	0.195	0.509	0.575
Valine, g	0.298	0.777	0.877
Arginine, g	0.346	0.902	1.02
Histidine, g	0.17	0.444	0.502
Alanine, g	0.349	0.911	1.03
Aspartic acid, g	0.592	1.54	1.74
Glutamic acid, g	0.862	2.25	2.54
Glycine, g	0.277	0.723	0.818
Proline, g	0.204	0.533	0.603
Serine, g	0.236	0.615	0.695

Seafood and Seaweed

	Carp	Catfish	Caviar, black and red	Clams	Cod
Measure	3 oz	3 oz	1 T	9 lge	3 oz
Weight, g	85	85	16	180	85
Calories	108	99	40	133	70
Protein, g	15	15.5	3.9	23	15
Carbohydrate, g	0	0	0.64	4.62	0
Fiber, g	0	0	0	0	0
Vitamin A, IU	25	43	299	540	34
Vitamin B$_1$, mg	0.008	0.038	0.03	0.18	0.065
Vitamin B$_2$, mg	0.036	0.09	0.1	0.38	0.055
Vitamin B$_6$, mg	0.162	0.1	0.05	0.14	0.208
Vitamin B$_{12}$, mcg	1.3	0.002	3.2	89	0.772
Niacin, mg	1.34	1.82	0.02	3.17	1.75
Pantothenic acid, mg	0.136	0.424	0.56	0.65	0.13
Folic acid, mcg	13	8.5	8	4.5	5.9
Vitamin C, mg	1.4	0.6	0	23	0.9
Vitamin E, IU	0.8	0.5	1.5	2.68	0.29
Calcium, mg	35	34	42	83	13
Copper, mg	0.048	0.08	0.02	0.619	0.024
Iron, mg	1.05	0.83	1.7	25	0.32
Magnesium, mg	25	21	48	17	27
Manganese, mg	0.036	0.013	t	0.9	0.013
Phosphorus, mg	352	181	54	304	173
Potassium, mg	283	296	27	564	351
Selenium, mcg	10.7	10.7	10.5	43	28
Sodium, mg	42	54	240	100	46
Zinc, mg	1.26	0.61	0.15	2.46	0.38
Total lipid, g	4.76	3.62	2.86	1.75	0.57
Total saturated, g	0.921	0.836	0.65	0.169	0.111
Total unsaturated, g	1.2	1.2	1.18	0.51	0.196
Total monounsaturated, g	1.98	1	0.74	0.14	0.08
Cholesterol, mg	56	49	94	60	37
Tryptophan, g	0.17	0.173	0.052	0.257	0.169
Threonine, g	0.665	0.677	0.202	0.99	0.664
Isoleucine, g	0.699	0.712	0.166	1	0.698
Leucine, g	1.23	1.25	0.341	1.62	1.23
Lycine, g	1.39	1.42	0.293	1.72	1.39
Methionine, g	0.449	0.457	0.103	0.518	0.448
Cystine, g	0.162	0.166	0.072	0.302	0.162
Phenylalanine, g	0.592	0.604	0.171	0.824	0.591
Tyrosine, g	0.512	0.522	0.155	0.736	0.511
Valine, g	0.781	0.796	0.202	1	0.779
Arginine, g	0.907	0.925	0.254	1.68	0.906
Histidine, g	0.446	0.455	0.104	0.441	0.445
Alanine, g	0.916	0.934	0.264	1.4	0.915
Aspartic acid, g	1.55	1.58	0.382	2.22	1.55
Glutamic acid, g	2.26	2.31	0.581	3.13	2.26
Glycine, g	0.728	0.741	0.118	1.44	0.727
Proline, g	0.536	0.547	0.192	0.938	0.536
Serine, g	0.619	0.631	0.304	1.03	0.617

Seafood and Seaweed

	Crab	Eel	Flat fish, flounder and sole species	Haddock	Halibut
Measure	3 oz	3 oz	3 oz	3 oz	3 oz
Weight, g	85	85	85	85	85
Calories	71	156	78	74	93
Protein, g	15.6	15.7	16	16	17.7
Carbohydrate, g	0	0	0	0	0
Fiber, g	0	0	0	0	0
Vitamin A, IU	20	2954	28	47	132
Vitamin B$_1$, mg	0.037	0.128	0.076	0.03	0.051
Vitamin B$_2$, mg	0.037	0.034	0.065	0.031	0.064
Vitamin B$_6$, mg	0.272	0.057	0.177	0.255	0.292
Vitamin B$_{12}$, mcg	9.08	2.55	1.29	1.02	1
Niacin, mg	0.934	2.98	2.46	3.23	11.97
Pantothenic acid, mg	0.54	0.204	0.428	0.108	0.28
Folic acid, mcg	3.6	12.8	6.8	1	1.8
Vitamin C, mg	1.8	1.3	1.45	0	0
Vitamin E, IU	—	5	2.4	0.49	1
Calcium, mg	39	17	15	28	40
Copper, mg	0.784	0.02	0.027	0.022	0.023
Iron, mg	0.5	0.43	0.3	0.89	0.71
Magnesium, mg	30.8	16.3	27	33	71
Manganese, mg	0.03	0.03	0.014	0.021	0.013
Phosphorus, mg	186	183	156	160	189
Potassium, mg	173	232	307	264	382
Selenium, mcg	31	5.5	30.4	26	31
Sodium, mg	711	43	69	58	46
Zinc, mg	5.05	1.38	0.39	0.32	0.35
Total lipid, g	0.51	9.9	1	0.61	1.95
Total saturated, g	0.076	2	0.241	0.111	0.267
Total unsaturated, g	0.11	0.805	0.28	0.2	0.62
Total monounsaturated, g	0.068	6.1	0.198	0.1	0.64
Cholesterol, mg	35	107	41	49	27
Tryptophan, g	0.217	0.176	0.179	0.18	0.198
Threonine, g	0.63	0.688	0.702	0.705	0.775
Isoleucine, g	0.754	0.723	0.738	0.74	0.815
Leucine, g	1.23	1.27	1.3	1.3	1.44
Lycine, g	1.35	1.44	1.47	1.48	1.62
Methionine, g	0.438	0.464	0.474	0.476	0.524
Cystine, g	0.174	0.168	0.172	0.173	0.19
Phenylalanine, g	0.657	0.612	0.626	0.627	0.691
Tyrosine, g	0.518	0.53	0.541	0.542	0.598
Valine, g	0.732	0.808	0.825	0.828	0.911
Arginine, g	1.36	0.938	0.959	0.961	1.06
Histidine, g	0.316	0.462	0.472	0.473	0.521
Alanine, g	0.881	0.948	0.969	0.972	1.07
Aspartic acid, g	1.6	1.6	1.64	1.65	1.81
Glutamic acid, g	2.65	2.34	2.39	2.4	2.64
Glycine, g	0.938	0.752	0.769	0.772	0.849
Proline, g	0.513	0.554	0.566	0.569	0.626
Serine, g	0.612	0.640	0.654	0.655	0.722

Seafood and Seaweed

	Kelp	Lobster	Mackerel	Oysters	Perch
Measure	2 T	3 oz	3 oz	6 med	3 oz
Weight, g	10	85	85	84	85
Calories	4.3	77	174	58	80
Protein, g	0.168	16	15.8	5.9	15.8
Carbohydrate, g	0.957	0.43	0	3.29	0
Fiber, g	0.13	0	0	0	0
Vitamin A, IU	12	60	140	282	34
Vitamin B_1, mg	t	0.368	0.15	0.128	0.08
Vitamin B_2, mg	0.015	0.041	0.265	0.139	0.094
Vitamin B_6, mg	0	0.05	0.339	0.042	0.2
Vitamin B_{12}, mcg	0	0.786	7.4	16	0.85
Niacin, mg	0.047	1.23	7.72	1.1	1.7
Pantothenic acid, mg	18	1.39	0.728	0.155	0.306
Folic acid, mcg	0.3	7.7	1	8.3	7.7
Vitamin C, mg	0.087	0	0.3	3	2.72
Vitamin E, IU	—	1.86	1.9	1.06	1.57
Calcium, mg	17	26	10	38	91
Copper, mg	0.013	1.41	0.062	3.74	0.022
Iron, mg	0.285	0.54	1.38	5.63	0.78
Magnesium, mg	12	15.6	64	46	26
Manganese, mg	0.02	0.047	0.013	0.378	0.013
Phosphorus, mg	42	166	184	117	184
Potassium, mg	8.9	236	267	192	232
Selenium, mcg	0.07	35	37.5	44.4	37
Sodium, mg	429	272	76	94	64
Zinc, mg	0.123	2.57	0.53	76.4	0.41
Total lipid, g	0.056	0.76	11.8	2.08	1.39
Total saturated, g	0.025	0.15	2.77	0.53	0.207
Total unsaturated, g	0.005	0.128	2.85	0.8	0.36
Total monounsaturated, g	0.01	0.22	4.64	0.26	0.53
Cholesterol, mg	0	81	60	46	36
Tryptophan, g	0.005	0.223	0.177	0.066	0.178
Threonine, g	0.006	0.647	0.693	0.255	0.694
Isoleucine, g	0.008	0.774	0.728	0.258	0.729
Leucine, g	0.008	1.29	1.28	0.417	1.29
Lysine, g	0.008	1.1	1.15	0.444	1.45
Methionine, g	0.003	0.45	0.468	0.134	0.468
Cystine, g	0.01	0.179	0.169	0.078	0.17
Phenylalanine, g	0.004	0.675	0.617	0.213	0.618
Tyrosine, g	0.003	0.532	0.534	0.19	0.535
Valine, g	0.007	0.751	0.814	0.259	0.816
Arginine, g	0.007	1.4	0.946	0.433	0.948
Histidine, g	0.002	0.325	0.466	0.114	0.466
Alanine, g	0.012	0.905	0.956	0.359	0.957
Aspartic acid, g	0.013	1.65	1.62	0.572	1.62
Glutamic acid, g	0.027	2.73	2.36	0.807	2.36
Glycine, g	0.01	0.964	0.759	0.371	0.76
Proline, g	0.007	0.527	0.559	0.242	0.56
Serine, g	0.01	0.629	0.645	0.265	0.646

Seafood and Seaweed

	Pike	Pollock	Salmon	Sardines, in oil, drained	Scallops
Measure	3 oz	3 oz	3 oz	2	3 oz
Weight, g	85	85	85	24	85
Calories	75	78	121	50	75
Protein, g	16.4	16.5	16.9	5.9	14.3
Carbohydrate, g	0	0	0	0	2
Fiber, g	0	0	0	0	0
Vitamin A, IU	60	30	34	54	43
Vitamin B_1, mg	0.049	0.04	0.19	0.019	0.01
Vitamin B_2, mg	0.054	0.157	0.32	0.054	0.055
Vitamin B_6, mg	0.099	0.244	0.695	0.04	0.13
Vitamin B_{12}, mcg	1.7	2.7	2.7	2.15	1.3
Niacin, mg	2.16	2.78	6.68	1.26	0.978
Pantothenic acid, mg	0.64	0.3	1.4	0.154	0.122
Folic acid, mcg	13	2.55	1.8	2.8	13.6
Vitamin C, mg	3.2	0	8.2	0	2.55
Vitamin E, IU	0.25	0.29	—	0.1	1.3
Calcium, mg	48	51	10	92	21
Copper, mg	0.043	0.043	0.18	0.045	0.045
Iron, mg	0.47	0.39	0.68	0.7	0.25
Magnesium, mg	27.2	57	26.2	9	48
Manganese, mg	0.018	0.013	0.009	0.026	0.077
Phosphorus, mg	187	188	170	118	186
Potassium, mg	220	302	417	95	274
Selenium, mcg	11	31	31	12.6	19
Sodium, mg	33	73	37	121	137
Zinc, mg	0.57	0.4	0.54	0.31	0.81
Total lipid, g	0.58	0.83	5.39	2.75	0.64
Total saturated, g	0.1	0.115	0.834	0.367	0.067
Total unsaturated, g	0.17	0.41	2.16	1.24	0.22
Total monounsaturated, g	0.133	0.095	1.79	0.93	0.03
Cholesterol, mg	33	60	47	34	28
Tryptophan, g	0.184	0.185	0.189	0.066	0.16
Threonine, g	0.717	0.724	0.74	0.259	0.614
Isoleucine, g	0.754	0.762	0.777	0.272	0.621
Leucine, g	1.33	1.34	1.37	0.48	1
Lycine, g	1.5	1.52	1.55	0.542	1.06
Methionine, g	0.485	0.49	0.499	0.175	0.322
Cystine, g	0.175	0.177	0.181	0.063	0.187
Phenylalanine, g	0.639	0.645	0.659	0.231	0.511
Tyrosine, g	0.553	0.558	0.57	0.199	0.456
Valine, g	0.843	0.852	0.869	0.304	0.623
Arginine, g	0.979	0.989	1	0.354	1.04
Histidine, g	0.482	0.486	0.496	0.174	0.274
Alanine, g	0.99	1	1.02	0.357	0.863
Aspartic acid, g	1.67	1.69	1.72	0.605	1.38
Glutamic acid, g	2.44	2.47	2.52	0.882	1.94
Glycine, g	0.785	0.793	0.81	0.283	0.893
Proline, g	0.579	0.585	0.597	0.209	0.582
Serine, g	0.668	0.674	0.689	0.241	0.639

Seafood/Seaweed

Seafood and Seaweed

	Shark	Shrimp	Smelt	Snails	Snapper
Measure	3 oz	3 oz	3 oz	3 oz	3 oz
Weight, g	85	85	85	85	85
Calories	111	90	83	117	85
Protein, g	17.8	17.3	15	20	17.4
Carbohydrate, g	0	0.77	0	6.6	0
Fiber, g	0	0	0	0	0
Vitamin A, IU	198	8.26	43	72	85
Vitamin B_1, mg	0.036	0.024	t	0.022	0.039
Vitamin B_2, mg	0.053	0.029	0.102	0.091	0.003
Vitamin B_6, mg	0.3	0.088	0.13	0.291	0.34
Vitamin B_{12}, mcg	1.27	0.987	2.92	7.7	2.6
Niacin, mg	2.5	2.17	1.23	0.893	0.241
Pantothenic acid, mg	0.59	0.235	0.542	0.177	0.64
Folic acid, mcg	3	2.6	3.4	5.4	4.3
Vitamin C, mg	0	1.7	0	—	1.4
Vitamin E, IU	1.2	1	0.6	—	0.64
Calcium, mg	29	44	51	48	27
Copper, mg	0.028	0.224	0.118	0.876	0.024
Iron, mg	0.71	2.05	0.77	4.28	0.15
Magnesium, mg	42	31	26	73	27
Manganese, mg	0.013	0.043	0.595	0.38	0.011
Phosphorus, mg	179	175	196	120	169
Potassium, mg	136	157	247	295	355
Selenium, mcg	32	32	31	—	33
Sodium, mg	67	126	51	175	54
Zinc, mg	0.36	0.94	1.4	1.39	0.3
Total lipid, g	3.83	1.47	2.06	0.34	1.14
Total saturated, g	0.786	0.279	0.384	0.026	0.242
Total unsaturated, g	1	0.569	0.75	—	0.39
Total monounsaturated, g	1.5	0.215	0.545	—	0.2
Cholesterol, mg	43	130	60	55	31
Tryptophan, g	0.2	0.241	0.167	0.263	0.196
Threonine, g	0.782	0.699	0.657	0.908	0.764
Isoleucine, g	0.822	0.837	0.69	0.704	0.803
Leucine, g	1.45	1.37	1.22	1.62	1.42
Lycine, g	1.64	1.5	1.38	1.25	1.6
Methionine, g	0.528	0.486	0.444	0.513	0.516
Cystine, g	0.191	0.194	0.161	0.159	0.187
Phenylalanine, g	0.696	0.729	0.585	0.7	0.681
Tyrosine, g	0.602	0.575	0.506	0.645	0.588
Valine, g	0.919	0.813	0.772	0.881	0.898
Arginine, g	1.07	1.51	0.897	2.1	1.04
Histidine, g	0.525	0.351	0.441	0.415	0.513
Alanine, g	1.08	0.978	0.906	1.32	1.05
Aspartic acid, g	1.83	1.78	1.53	2.18	1.79
Glutamic acid, g	2.66	2.95	2.24	3.12	2.6
Glycine, g	0.856	1.04	0.719	1.27	0.836
Proline, g	0.631	0.57	0.53	1	0.616
Serine, g	0.728	0.68	0.611	0.944	0.711

Seafood and Seaweed

	Spirulina	Swordfish	Trout	Tuna, bluefin	Tuna, light, in water
Measure	1 C	3 oz	3 oz	3 oz	1 can
Weight, g	15	85	85	85	165
Calories	44	103	126	123	191
Protein, g	8.6	16.8	17.7	20	42
Carbohydrate, g	3.6	0	0	0	0
Fiber, g	0.54	0	0	0	0
Vitamin A, IU	85.5	101	49	1856	92
Vitamin B_1, mg	0.357	0.031	0.277	0.21	0.05
Vitamin B_2, mg	0.55	0.081	0.261	0.21	0.122
Vitamin B_6, mg	0.055	0.281	1.43	0.387	0.58
Vitamin B_{12}, mcg	0	1.49	6.6	8	4.9
Niacin, mg	1.9	8.23	7.6	7.4	22
Pantothenic acid, mg	0.5	0.35	1.65	0.9	0.35
Folic acid, mcg	15	1.7	11.3	1.6	6.6
Vitamin C, mg	1.5	0.9	0.4	0	0
Vitamin E, IU	1.12	0.6	0.25	1.3	1.3
Calcium, mg	18	4	36	6.8	18
Copper, mg	0.9	0.107	0.16	0.07	0.08
Iron, mg	4.3	0.69	1.27	0.867	2.5
Magnesium, mg	29	23	19	43	45
Manganese, mg	0.285	0.016	0.723	0.013	0.02
Phosphorus, mg	18	224	208	216	268
Potassium, mg	205	245	307	214	391
Selenium, mcg	1.1	41	11	31	133
Sodium, mg	157	76	44	33	558
Zinc, mg	0.3	0.97	0.56	0.5	1.3
Total lipid, g	1.16	3.41	5.62	4.17	1.35
Total saturated, g	0.398	0.932	0.98	1.07	0.386
Total unsaturated, g	0.3	0.78	1.27	1.22	0.556
Total monounsaturated, g	0.1	1.3	2.77	1.36	0.26
Cholesterol, mg	0	33	49	32	50
Tryptophan, g	0.139	0.189	0.198	0.22	0.472
Threonine, g	0.446	0.738	0.774	0.87	1.85
Isoleucine, g	0.48	0.775	0.813	0.9	1.94
Leucine, g	0.74	1.37	1.44	1.6	3.4
Lycine, g	0.45	1.55	1.62	1.8	3.9
Methionine, g	0.17	0.498	0.523	0.59	1.25
Cystine, g	0.1	0.18	0.19	0.2	0.45
Phenylalanine, g	—	0.657	0.689	0.77	1.6
Tyrosine, g	—	0.568	0.596	0.7	1.4
Valine, g	—	0.867	0.91	0.1	2.17
Arginine, g	—	1	1.06	1.2	2.5
Histidine, g	—	0.496	0.519	0.58	1.24
Alanine, g	—	1.02	1.07	1.2	2.55
Aspartic acid, g	—	1.72	1.8	2	4.3
Glutamic acid, g	—	2.51	2.63	2.96	6.3
Glycine, g	—	0.808	0.847	0.95	2
Proline, g	—	0.595	0.624	0.7	1.5
Serine, g	—	0.687	0.72	0.81	1.7

Seafood and Seaweed

	Tuna, white, in water	Wakame	Whitefish
Measure	1 can	2 T	3 oz
Weight, g	172	10	85
Calories	220	0.5	114
Protein, g	41	0.3	16
Carbohydrate, g	0	0.9	0
Fiber, g	0	0.05	0
Vitamin A, IU	33	36	2050
Vitamin B_1, mg	0.014	t	0.128
Vitamin B_2, mg	0.076	0.023	0.108
Vitamin B_6, mg	0.37	0	0.255
Vitamin B_{12}, mcg	2	0	0.85
Niacin, mg	9.97	0.16	2.72
Pantothenic acid, mg	0.2	0.07	0.637
Folic acid, mcg	3.4	20	12.8
Vitamin C, mg	0	0.3	0
Vitamin E, IU	4	0.15	0.25
Calcium, mg	24	15	22
Copper, mg	0.067	0.03	0.061
Iron, mg	1.67	0.22	0.31
Magnesium, mg	57	11	28
Manganese, mg	0.03	0.14	0.057
Phosphorus, mg	373	8	230
Potassium, mg	408	5	269
Selenium, mcg	113	0.07	11
Sodium, mg	648	87	43
Zinc, mg	0.826	0.038	0.84
Total lipid, g	5.1	0.06	4.98
Total saturated, g	1.36	0.013	0.77
Total unsaturated, g	1.9	0.022	1.83
Total monounsaturated, g	1.35	0.006	1.7
Cholesterol, mg	72	0	51
Tryptophan, g	0.456	0.004	0.182
Threonine, g	1.78	0.017	0.711
Isoleucine, g	1.87	0.009	0.748
Leucine, g	3.3	0.026	1.32
Lycine, g	3.73	0.011	1.49
Methionine, g	1.2	0.006	0.48
Cystine, g	0.44	0.003	0.174
Phenylalanine, g	1.59	0.011	0.633
Tyrosine, g	1.37	0.005	0.547
Valine, g	2.1	0.021	0.836
Arginine, g	2.43	0.009	0.971
Histidine, g	1.2	0.002	0.478
Alanine, g	2.46	0.014	0.981
Aspartic acid, g	4.2	0.018	1.66
Glutamic acid, g	6.1	0.02	2.42
Glycine, g	1.95	0.01	0.779
Proline, g	1.44	0.009	0.574
Serine, g	1.66	0.008	0.662

Vegetables and Vegetable Juices

	Alfalfa sprouts	Artichoke, globe	Artichoke, Jerusalem	Arugula	Asparagus
Measure	1 C	1 med	1 C	½ C	1 C
Weight, g	33	128	150	10	134
Calories	10	65	114	2.5	30
Protein, g	1.32	3.4	3	0.258	4.1
Carbohydrate, g	1.25	15.3	26	0.365	4.94
Fiber, g	0.83	1.36	1.2	0.16	1.1
Vitamin A, IU	51	237	30	237	1202
Vitamin B_1, mg	0.025	0.1	0.3	T	0.15
Vitamin B_2, mg	0.042	0.077	0.09	T	0.166
Vitamin B_6, mg	0.011	0.143	0.116	T	0.2
Vitamin B_{12}, mcg	0	0	0	0	0
Niacin, mg	0.159	0.973	1.95	0.03	1.5
Pantothenic acid, mg	0.186	0.329	0.6	0.044	0.234
Folic acid, mcg	12.2	94.2	20	9.7	160
Vitamin C, mg	2.7	13.8	6	1.5	44
Vitamin E, IU	0.01	0.36	0.42	0.06	4
Calcium, mg	10	61	21	16	28
Copper, mg	0.052	0.095	0.2	t	0.2
Iron, mg	0.32	2.1	5.1	0.146	0.9
Magnesium, mg	9	60	26	4.7	24
Manganese, mg	0.062	0.426	0.09	0.032	0.286
Phosphorus, mg	23	99	117	5.2	70
Potassium, mg	26	434	644	37	404
Selenium, mcg	0.2	0.256	1.05	0.03	3
Sodium, mg	2	102	6	2.7	2
Zinc, mg	0.3	0.56	0.18	0.047	0.94
Total lipid, g	0.23	0.19	0.02	0.066	0.3
Total saturated, g	0.023	0.045	0	0.009	0.068
Total unsaturated, g	0.135	0.081	0.002	0.032	0.118
Total monounsaturated, g	0.018	0.006	0.006	0.005	0.008
Cholesterol, mg	0	0	0	0	0
Tryptophan, g	—	—	—	—	0.04
Threonine, g	0.044	—	—	—	0.114
Isoleucine, g	0.047	—	—	—	1.5
Leucine, g	0.088	—	—	—	0.178
Lycine, g	0.071	—	—	—	0.194
Methionine, g	—	—	—	—	0.038
Cystine, g	—	—	—	—	0.048
Phenylalanine, g	—	—	—	—	0.096
Tyrosine, g	—	—	—	—	0.064
Valine, g	0.048	—	—	—	0.158
Arginine, g	—	—	—	—	0.192
Histidine, g	—	—	—	—	0.062
Alanine, g	—	—	—	—	0.192
Aspartic acid, g	—	—	—	—	0.476
Glutamic acid, g	—	—	—	—	0.672
Glycine, g	—	—	—	—	0.132
Proline, g	—	—	—	—	0.218
Serine, g	—	—	—	—	0.156

Vegetables/Juices

Vegetables and Vegetable Juices

	Beets	Beet green	Broccoli	Brussels sprouts	Cabbage, common
Measure	1 C	1 C	1 C	1 C	1 C
Weight, g	136	38	88	88	70
Calories	60	0.8	24	38	16
Protein, g	2	0.7	2.6	3.3	0.84
Carbohydrate, g	13.6	1.5	4.6	7.88	2.76
Fiber, g	3.8	1.4	2.6	3.3	1.6
Vitamin A, IU	28	2308	1356	778	88
Vitamin B_1, mg	0.068	0.038	0.058	0.12	0.03
Vitamin B_2, mg	0.028	0.08	0.1	0.08	0.02
Vitamin B_6, mg	0.06	0.04	0.14	0.19	0.066
Vitamin B_{12}, mcg	0	0	0	0	0
Niacin, mg	0.54	0.152	0.56	0.65	0.2
Pantothenic acid, mg	0.2	0.096	0.47	0.27	0.098
Folic acid, mcg	126	5.6	62	54	39
Vitamin C, mg	15	11	82	74	33
Vitamin E, IU	0.6	0.85	2	1	0.1
Calcium, mg	22	46	42	36	32
Copper, mg	0.1	0.07	0.04	0.06	0.016
Iron, mg	1.24	1.2	0.78	1.2	0.4
Magnesium, mg	28	28	22	20	10
Manganese, mg	0.47	0.15	0.2	0.29	0.11
Phosphorus, mg	66	16	58	60	16
Potassium, mg	440	208	286	342	172
Selenium, mcg	0.95	0.34	2.6	1.4	0.63
Sodium, mg	98	76	24	22	12
Zinc, mg	0.5	0.14	0.36	0.36	0.12
Total lipid, g	0.2	0.02	0.3	0.26	0.189
Total saturated, g	0.02	0.004	0.048	0.05	0.023
Total unsaturated, g	0.083	0.008	0.147	0.135	0.085
Total monounsaturated, g	0.045	0.005	0.021	0.02	0.013
Cholesterol, mg	0	0	0	0	0
Tryptophan, g	0.024	0.012	0.026	0.03	0.008
Threonine, g	0.06	0.02	0.08	0.1	0.03
Isoleucine, g	0.06	0.014	0.096	0.1	0.04
Leucine, g	0.08	0.03	0.116	0.13	0.044
Lycine, g	0.072	0.02	0.124	0.13	0.04
Methionine, g	0.024	0.006	0.03	0.028	0.008
Cystine, g	0.024	0.006	0.018	0.02	0.008
Phenylalanine, g	0.05	0.018	0.074	0.086	0.028
Tyrosine, g	0.05	0.016	0.056	—	0.014
Valine, g	0.07	0.02	0.112	0.136	0.026
Arginine, g	0.03	0.02	0.128	0.178	0.048
Histidine, g	0.028	0.01	0.044	0.066	0.018
Alanine, g	0.07	0.026	0.104	—	0.03
Aspartic acid, g	0.14	0.04	0.188	—	0.084
Glutamic acid, g	0.74	0.084	0.33	—	0.19
Glycine, g	0.04	0.026	0.084	—	0.018
Proline, g	0.05	0.016	0.1	—	0.166
Serine, g	0.07	0.022	0.088	—	0.05

Vegetables and Vegetable Juices

	Cabbage, Chinese	Carrots	Carrot juice	Cauliflower	Celery
Measure	1 C	1 C	1 C	1 C	1 C
Weight, g	70	110	227	100	120
Calories	9	48	96	24	18
Protein, g	1.05	1	2.47	1.98	0.8
Carbohydrate, g	1.53	11	22	4.9	4.36
Fiber, g	0.7	3	1.9	2.5	2
Vitamin A, IU	2100	30942	24750	16	152
Vitamin B_1, mg	0.028	0.1	0.13	0.076	0.036
Vitamin B_2, mg	0.049	0.064	0.12	0.058	0.036
Vitamin B_6, mg	—	0.16	0.534	0.23	0.036
Vitamin B_{12}, mcg	0	0	0	0	0
Niacin, mg	0.35	1	1.35	0.634	0.36
Pantothenic acid, mg	0.06	0.216	0.54	0.14	0.2
Folic acid, mcg	46	15	9	66	10.6
Vitamin C, mg	31.5	10	20	71	7.6
Vitamin E, IU	0.13	0.75	0.035	0.06	0.64
Calcium, mg	74	30	8.3	28	44
Copper, mg	0.015	0.05	0.11	0.032	0.042
Iron, mg	0.56	0.54	1.5	0.58	0.58
Magnesium, mg	13	16	51	14	14
Manganese, mg	0.11	0.156	0.31	0.2	0.164
Phosphorus, mg	26	48	81	46	32
Potassium, mg	176	356	767	356	340
Selenium, mcg	0.35	2.2	1.4	0.7	1.1
Sodium, mg	45	38	105	14	106
Zinc, mg	0.133	0.22	0.43	0.18	0.2
Total lipid, g	0.14	0.2	0.35	0.18	0.168
Total saturated, g	0.018	0.034	0.066	0.028	0.044
Total unsaturated, g	0.067	0.085	0.192	0.099	0.083
Total monounsaturated, g	0.011	0.009	0.017	0.014	0.032
Cholesterol, mg	0	0	0	0	0
Tryptophan, g	0.011	0.012	—	0.026	0.01
Threonine, g	0.034	0.042	—	0.072	0.022
Isoleucine, g	0.06	0.046	—	0.076	0.024
Leucine, g	0.062	0.048	—	0.116	0.038
Lycine, g	0.062	0.044	—	0.108	0.032
Methionine, g	0.006	0.008	—	0.028	0.006
Cystine, g	0.012	0.008	—	0.024	0.004
Phenylalanine, g	0.031	0.036	—	0.072	0.022
Tyrosine, g	0.02	0.022	—	0.044	0.01
Valine, g	0.046	0.048	—	0.1	0.032
Arginine, g	0.059	0.048	—	0.096	0.024
Histidine, g	0.018	0.018	—	0.04	0.014
Alanine, g	0.06	0.064	—	0.106	0.026
Aspartic acid, g	0.076	0.15	—	0.234	0.136
Glutamic acid, g	0.252	0.222	—	0.266	0.1
Glycine, g	0.03	0.034	—	0.064	0.026
Proline, g	0.022	0.032	—	0.086	0.02
Serine, g	0.034	0.038	—	0.104	0.024

Vegetables/Juices

Vegetables and Vegetable Juices

	Celeriac	Chard, Swiss	Chapote	Chicory greens	Chives
Measure	1 C	1 C	1 C	1 C	1 T
Weight, g	156	36	132	180	3
Calories	65	6	25	41	1
Protein, g	2.3	0.64	1.08	3	0.08
Carbohydrate, g	14	1.34	5.9	8.5	0.11
Fiber, g	2.8	0.58	2	7	0.075
Vitamin A, IU	0	1188	74	7200	192
Vitamin B$_1$, mg	0.078	0.014	0.03	0.11	0.003
Vitamin B$_2$, mg	0.094	0.032	0.038	0.18	0.005
Vitamin B$_6$, mg	0.257	0.036	0.1	0.189	0.005
Vitamin B$_{12}$, mcg	0	0	0	0	0
Niacin, mg	1.1	0.144	0.62	0.9	0.021
Pantothenic acid, mg	0.549	0.062	0.33	2	0.005
Folic acid, mcg	13	5	123	197	3
Vitamin C, mg	—	10.8	10	43	2.4
Vitamin E, IU	0.8	1	0.24	6	0.008
Calcium, mg	67	18	22	180	2
Copper, mg	0.1	0.16	0.16	0.53	0.011
Iron, mg	1.1	0.64	0.45	1.6	0.05
Magnesium, mg	31	30	16	54	2
Manganese, mg	0.25	0.45	0.25	0.77	0.011
Phosphorus, mg	179	16	24	85	2
Potassium, mg	468	136	165	756	8
Selenium, mcg	1.1	0.32	0.26	0.54	0.027
Sodium, mg	156	76	2.6	81	0
Zinc, mg	0.52	0.13	0.98	0.756	0.017
Total lipid, g	0.468	0.08	0.17	0.54	0.02
Total saturated, g	0.123	0.011	0.037	0.13	0.003
Total unsaturated, g	0.23	0.025	0.075	0.236	0.008
Total monounsaturated, g	0.09	0.014	0.013	0.011	0.003
Cholesterol, mg	0	0	0	0	0
Tryptophan, g	—	0.006	0.015	0.056	0.001
Threonine, g	—	0.03	0.053	0.085	0.003
Isoleucine, g	—	0.052	0.058	0.182	0.004
Leucine, g	—	0.046	0.1	0.133	0.005
Lycine, g	—	0.036	0.05	0.12	0.004
Methionine, g	—	0.006	0.001	0.018	0.001
Cystine, g	—	—	—	—	—
Phenylalanine, g	—	0.04	0.06	0.074	0.003
Tyrosine, g	—	—	0.04	—	0.002
Valine, g	—	0.04	0.08	0.14	0.004
Arginine, g	—	0.042	0.05	0.223	0.006
Histidine, g	—	0.012	0.02	0.05	0.001
Alanine, g	—	—	0.067	—	0.004
Aspartic acid, g	—	—	0.121	—	0.008
Glutamic acid, g	—	—	0.165	—	0.017
Glycine, g	—	—	0.054	—	0.004
Proline, g	—	—	0.058	—	0.006
Serine, g	—	—	0.06	—	0.004

Vegetables and Vegetable Juices

	Collards	Corn	Cucumber	Dandelion greens	Eggplant
Measure	1 C	1 C	1 C	1 C	1 C
Weight, g	36	154	104	55	82
Calories	11	132	14	25	22
Protein, g	0.8	4.96	0.56	1.5	0.9
Carbohydrate, g	2	29	3	5	5
Fiber, g	1	4	0.8	1.9	2
Vitamin A, IU	1376	432	46	7700	58
Vitamin B$_1$, mg	0.019	0.208	0.032	0.1	0.074
Vitamin B$_2$, mg	0.047	0.09	0.02	0.14	0.016
Vitamin B$_6$, mg	0.059	0.084	0.054	0.138	0.078
Vitamin B$_{12}$, mcg	0	0	0	0	0
Niacin, mg	0.267	2.6	0.321	0.44	0.492
Pantothenic acid, mg	0.096	1.17	0.26	0.046	0.066
Folic acid, mcg	60	70.6	14.4	15	14.4
Vitamin C, mg	13	10.6	4.8	19	0.14
Vitamin E, IU	1.2	0.2	0.12	2	0.04
Calcium, mg	52	4	14	103	30
Copper, mg	0.014	0.084	0.042	0.09	0.092
Iron, mg	0.068	0.8	0.28	1.7	0.44
Magnesium, mg	3.2	58	12	20	10
Manganese, mg	0.1	0.248	0.064	0.19	0.1
Phosphorus, mg	3.6	138	18	36	26
Potassium, mg	61	416	156	218	180
Selenium, mcg	0.41	0.9	0	0.275	0.246
Sodium, mg	7	23	2	42	2
Zinc, mg	0.047	0.7	0.24	0.225	0.12
Total lipid, g	0.15	1.8	0.14	0.385	0.08
Total saturated, g	0.02	0.28	0.034	0.094	0.016
Total unsaturated, g	0.07	0.86	0.028	0.168	0.06
Total monounsaturated, g	0.01	0.53	0.104	0.008	0.013
Cholesterol, mg	0	0	0	0	0
Tryptophan, g	0.011	0.036	0.004	—	0.008
Threonine, g	0.03	0.102	0.198	—	0.032
Isoleucine, g	0.036	0.198	0.018	—	0.04
Leucine, g	0.05	0.536	0.024	—	0.056
Lycine, g	0.04	0.21	0.022	—	0.042
Methionine, g	0.012	0.1	0.004	—	0.01
Cystine, g	0.009	0.04	0.004	—	0.004
Phenylalanine, g	0.03	0.232	0.016	—	0.038
Tyrosine, g	0.024	0.19	0.01	—	0.024
Valine, g	0.043	0.28	0.018	—	0.046
Arginine, g	0.045	0.2	0.036	—	0.05
Histidine, g	0.017	0.138	0.008	—	0.02
Alanine, g	0.038	0.454	0.018	—	0.046
Aspartic acid, g	0.067	0.366	0.034	—	0.146
Glutamic acid, g	0.073	0.98	0.16	—	0.164
Glycine, g	0.034	0.196	0.02	—	0.036
Proline, g	0.038	0.45	0.012	—	0.038
Serine, g	0.028	0.236	0.016	—	0.036

Vegetables/Juices

Vegetables and Vegetable Juices

	Endive	Garlic	Green beans	Jicama	Kale
Measure	1 C	1 clove	1 C	1 C	1 C
Weight, g	50	3	110	120	67
Calories	8	4	34	46	33
Protein, g	0.62	0.2	2	0.86	2.21
Carbohydrate, g	1.68	0.9	7.85	11	6.7
Fiber, g	1.4	0.05	3.7	5.9	1
Vitamin A, IU	1026	0	735	25	5963
Vitamin B_1, mg	0.04	0.006	0.092	0.024	0.074
Vitamin B_2, mg	0.038	t	0.116	0.035	0.087
Vitamin B_6, mg	0.1	0.037	0.081	0.05	0.182
Vitamin B_{12}, mcg	0	0	0	0	0
Niacin, mg	0.2	0.02	0.827	0.24	0.67
Pantothenic acid, mg	0.45	0.02	0.103	0.16	0.061
Folic acid, mcg	71	0.1	40	14	19.6
Vitamin C, mg	3.2	0.9	17.9	24	80.4
Vitamin E, IU	0.3	0	0.67	0.8	0.8
Calcium, mg	26	5	41	14	90
Copper, mg	0.05	0.008	0.076	0.058	0.194
Iron, mg	0.42	0.05	1.14	0.72	1.14
Magnesium, mg	8	1	27	14	23
Manganese, mg	0.21	0.05	0.235	0.07	0.519
Phosphorus, mg	14	6	42	22	38
Potassium, mg	158	16	230	180	299
Selenium, mcg	0.1	0.42	0.66	0.84	0.6
Sodium, mg	12	1	6	4.8	29
Zinc, mg	0.4	0.038	0.26	0.19	0.29
Total lipid, g	0.1	0.015	0.013	0.108	0.47
Total saturated, g	0.024	0.003	0.029	0.025	0.06
Total unsaturated, g	0.04	0.007	0.065	0.052	0.226
Total monounsaturated, g	0.002	0	0.006	0.006	0.035
Cholesterol, mg	0	0	0	0	0
Tryptophan, g	0.002	0.002	0.021	—	0.027
Threonine, g	0.026	0.005	0.087	0.022	0.098
Isoleucine, g	0.036	0.007	0.073	0.02	0.132
Leucine, g	0.05	0.009	0.123	0.03	0.155
Lycine, g	0.032	0.008	0.097	0.03	0.132
Methionine, g	0.008	0.002	0.024	0.008	0.021
Cystine, g	0.006	0.002	0.02	0.007	0.029
Phenylalanine, g	0.026	0.005	0.074	0.02	0.113
Tyrosine, g	0.02	0.002	0.046	0.014	0.078
Valine, g	0.032	0.009	0.099	0.03	0.121
Arginine, g	0.032	0.019	0.08	0.04	0.123
Histidine, g	0.012	0.003	0.037	0.023	0.046
Alanine, g	0.032	0.004	0.092	0.024	0.111
Aspartic acid, g	0.066	0.015	0.281	0.24	0.198
Glutamic acid, g	0.084	0.024	0.206	0.05	0.251
Glycine, g	0.03	0.006	0.072	0.02	0.107
Proline, g	0.03	0.003	0.075	0.03	0.131
Serine, g	0.024	0.006	0.109	0.03	0.093

Vegetables/Juices

Vegetables and Vegetable Juices

	Kohlrabi	Leeks	Lettuce, iceberg	Lettuce, Romaine	Mushrooms
Measure	1 C	1 C	1 C	1 C	1 C
Weight, g	140	124	75	56	70
Calories	38	54	10	8	18
Protein, g	2.38	1.3	0.7	0.9	1.46
Carbohydrate, g	8.68	13	2.2	1.3	3
Fiber, g	4.9	1.6	0.77	0.9	0.84
Vitamin A, IU	50	85	250	1456	0
Vitamin B$_1$, mg	0.07	0.05	0.05	0.056	0.072
Vitamin B$_2$, mg	0.028	0.037	0.05	0.056	0.3
Vitamin B$_6$, mg	0.21	0.2	0.028	0.02	0.068
Vitamin B$_{12}$, mcg	0	0	0	0	0
Niacin, mg	0.56	0.496	0.148	0.28	2.88
Pantothenic acid, mg	0.231	0.12	0.1	0.09	1.54
Folic acid, mcg	22	0.015	31	76	8.4
Vitamin C, mg	86.8	14.9	5	13.4	2.4
Vitamin E, IU	0.96	1	0.23	0.37	0.12
Calcium, mg	34	73	15	20	4
Copper, mg	0.21	0.09	0.035	0.02	0.34
Iron, mg	0.56	2.6	0.4	0.62	0.86
Magnesium, mg	27	35	5	4	8
Manganese, mg	0.16	0.43	0.12	0.36	0.078
Phosphorus, mg	64	43	17	26	72
Potassium, mg	490	223	131	162	260
Selenium, mcg	0.95	0.89	0.1	0.1	8.54
Sodium, mg	28	25	7	4	2
Zinc, mg	0.04	0.1	0.1	0.14	0.344
Total lipid, g	0.14	0.267	0.12	0.12	0.3
Total saturated, g	0.018	0.036	0.02	0.007	0.08
Total unsaturated, g	0.065	0.148	0.055	0.06	0.097
Total monounsaturated, g	0.009	0.004	0.004	0.004	0.004
Cholesterol, mg	0	0	0	0	0
Tryptophan, g	0.014	0.015	0.008	0.006	0.032
Threonine, g	0.069	0.078	0.044	0.042	0.066
Isoleucine, g	0.1	0.064	0.06	0.058	0.058
Leucine, g	0.094	0.119	0.056	0.054	0.09
Lycine, g	0.078	0.097	0.06	0.058	0.048
Methionine, g	0.018	0.022	0.012	0.012	0.028
Cystine, g	0.01	0.031	0.012	0.01	0.004
Phenylalanine, g	0.055	0.068	0.04	0.038	0.056
Tyrosine, g	—	0.051	0.024	0.022	0.032
Valine, g	0.07	0.069	0.048	0.048	0.068
Arginine, g	0.147	0.097	0.052	0.05	0.072
Histidine, g	0.027	0.031	0.016	0.016	0.04
Alanine, g	—	0.092	0.04	0.04	0.11
Aspartic acid, g	—	0.174	0.1	0.1	0.134
Glutamic acid, g	—	0.28	0.128	0.128	0.25
Glycine, g	—	0.086	0.04	0.04	0.066
Proline, g	—	0.082	0.036	0.034	0.1
Serine, g	—	0.114	0.028	0.028	0.066

Vegetables and Vegetable Juices

	Mushrooms, enoki	Mushrooms, portabello	Mushrooms, shiitake, dried	Mustard greens	Okra
Measure	1 med.		4	1 C	1 C
Weight, g	3	100	15	56	100
Calories	1	26	44	15	38
Protein, g	0.07	2.5	1.4	1.5	2
Carbohydrate, g	0.2	5	11	2.7	7.6
Fiber, g	0.078	1.5	1.7	1.8	3.2
Vitamin A, IU	0.2	0	0	2968	660
Vitamin B$_1$, mg	t	0.077	0.045	0.045	0.2
Vitamin B$_2$, mg	t	0.48	0.19	0.06	0.06
Vitamin B$_6$, mg	t	0.1	0.145	0.1	0.2
Vitamin B$_{12}$, mcg	0	0.05	0	0	0
Niacin, mg	0.11	4.5	2	0.448	1
Pantothenic acid, mg	0.028	1.5	3.3	0.12	0.246
Folic acid, mcg	0.9	22	25	105	88
Vitamin C, mg	0.36	0	0.525	39	21
Vitamin E, IU	—	0.19	0.03	1.68	1
Calcium, mg	0.03	8	1.65	58	82
Copper, mg	t	0.4	0.775	0.08	0.94
Iron, mg	0.03	0.6	0.258	0.82	0.8
Magnesium, mg	0.48	11	20	18	56
Manganese, mg	t	0.14	0.176	0.27	0.99
Phosphorus, mg	3.4	130	44	24	64
Potassium, mg	11	484	230	198	302
Selenium, mcg	0.48	11	20	0.5	0.7
Sodium, mg	0.09	6	1.95	14	8
Zinc, mg	0.017	0.6	1.15	0.11	0.6
Total lipid, g	0.012	0.2	0.148	0.112	0.1
Total saturated, g	0.001	0.026	0.037	0.006	0.026
Total unsaturated, g	0.005	0.078	0.02	0.021	0.027
Total monounsaturated, g	0	0.003	0.046	0.052	0.017
Cholesterol, mg	0	0	0	0	0
Tryptophan, g	0.002	0.056	0.005	0.017	0.018
Threonine, g	0.003	0.113	0.075	0.04	0.066
Isoleucine, g	0.001	0.099	0.06	0.055	0.07
Leucine, g	0.004	0.153	0.1	0.046	0.1
Lycine, g	0.005	0.252	0.05	0.069	0.082
Methionine, g	0.001	0.048	0.03	0.014	0.022
Cystine, g	—	0.006	0.03	0.022	0.02
Phenylalanine, g	0.004	0.097	0.07	0.04	0.066
Tyrosine, g	0.003	0.054	0.048	0.08	0.088
Valine, g	0.002	0.115	0.07	0.059	0.092
Arginine, g	0.006	0.123	0.097	0.1	0.084
Histidine, g	0.002	0.067	0.024	0.27	0.032
Alanine, g	0.005	0.187	0.085	—	0.074
Aspartic acid, g	0.008	0.228	0.114	—	0.146
Glutamic acid, g	0.01	0.43	0.387	—	0.272
Glycine, g	0.003	0.11	0.06	—	0.044
Proline, g	0.006	0.176	0.06	—	0.046
Serine, g	0.003	0.13	0.076	—	0.044

Vegetables and Vegetable Juices

	Onions, green	Onions, mature	Parsley	Parsnips	Peppers, sweet
Measure	1 C	1 C	1 C	1 C	1 C
Weight, g	100	160	60	133	93
Calories	26	54	26	102	24
Protein, g	1.7	1.88	2.2	2.3	0.86
Carbohydrate, g	5.5	11.7	5.1	23	5.3
Fiber, g	2.6	2.9	1.98	6.5	1.2
Vitamin A, IU	385	0	3120	0	530
Vitamin B_1, mg	0.07	0.096	0.07	0.11	0.086
Vitamin B_2, mg	0.14	0.016	0.16	0.12	0.05
Vitamin B_6, mg	0.06	0.25	0.098	0.13	0.164
Vitamin B_{12}, mcg	0	0	0	0	0
Niacin, mg	0.2	0.16	0.7	0.2	0.54
Pantothenic acid, mg	0.144	0.2	0.18	0.9	0.036
Folic acid, mcg	64	31.8	91	89	16.8
Vitamin C, mg	18	13.4	80	16	82
Vitamin E, IU	0.19	0.3	1.5	—	0.9
Calcium, mg	60	40	122	50	6
Copper, mg	0.06	0.064	0.293	0.17	0.1
Iron, mg	1.88	0.58	3.7	0.9	1.2
Magnesium, mg	20	16	24.5	40	14
Manganese, mg	0.16	0.2	0.563	0.75	0.14
Phosphorus, mg	32	46	38	96	22
Potassium, mg	256	248	436	587	196
Selenium, mcg	0.6	9.6	0.06	2.4	0.276
Sodium, mg	4	4	27	12	4
Zinc, mg	0.44	0.28	0.44	0.8	0.18
Total lipid, g	0.19	0.25	0.4	0.4	0.175
Total saturated, g	0.032	0.07	0.079	0.067	0.026
Total unsaturated, g	0.074	0.09	0.07	0.06	0.09
Total monounsaturated, g	0.027	0.037	0.177	0.149	0.012
Cholesterol, mg	0	0	0	0	0
Tryptophan, g	0.02	0.028	0.022	—	0.012
Threonine, g	0.068	0.044	—	—	0.03
Isoleucine, g	0.074	0.068	—	—	0.028
Leucine, g	0.1	0.066	—	—	0.044
Lycine, g	0.088	0.09	0.132	—	0.038
Methionine, g	0.02	0.016	0.01	—	0.01
Cystine, g	—	0.34	—	—	0.016
Phenylalanine, g	0.056	0.048	—	—	0.026
Tyrosine, g	0.05	0.046	—	—	0.018
Valine, g	0.078	0.044	—	—	0.036
Arginine, g	0.126	0.262	—	—	0.042
Histidine, g	0.03	0.03	—	—	0.018
Alanine, g	0.078	0.052	—	—	0.036
Aspartic acid, g	0.162	0.1	—	—	0.124
Glutamic acid, g	0.36	0.3	—	—	0.1
Glycine, g	0.086	0.078	—	—	0.032
Proline, g	0.1	0.06	—	—	0.038
Serine, g	0.078	0.056	—	—	0.034

Vegetables/Juices

Vegetables and Vegetable Juices

	Peppers, hot	Pickles, dill	Potato	Pumpkin	Purslane
Measure	½ C	1 sm	1 C	1 C	1 C
Weight, g	75	37	150	116	43
Calories	30	6	114	30	7
Protein, g	1.5	0.3	3.2	1.16	0.6
Carbohydrate, g	7	1.5	25.7	7.5	1.48
Fiber, g	1.35	0.4	2.4	0.58	—
Vitamin A, IU	8062	121	0	1856	568
Vitamin B$_1$, mg	0.068	t	0.15	0.058	0.02
Vitamin B$_2$, mg	0.068	0.01	0.06	0.13	0.048
Vitamin B$_6$, mg	0.21	0.005	0.4	0.07	0.03
Vitamin B$_{12}$, mcg	0	0	0	0	0
Niacin, mg	0.713	0.022	2.3	0.7	0.21
Pantothenic acid, mg	0.046	0.02	0.57	0.35	0.015
Folic acid, mcg	17.5	0.37	19.2	19	5
Vitamin C, mg	182	0.7	30	10	9
Vitamin E, IU	0.77	0.09	0.13	1.8	—
Calcium, mg	13	3	11	24	28
Copper, mg	0.13	0.03	0.388	0.147	0.05
Iron, mg	0.9	0.2	0.9	0.93	0.86
Magnesium, mg	19	4	51	14	29
Manganese, mg	0.178	t	0.394	0.145	0.13
Phosphorus, mg	34	8	80	51	19
Potassium, mg	255	43	611	394	212
Selenium, mcg	0.38	0	0.45	0.348	0.39
Sodium, mg	5	474	5	1.2	19
Zinc, mg	0.23	0.05	0.58	0.37	0.07
Total lipid, g	0.15	0.07	0.2	0.015	0.043
Total saturated, g	0.016	0.018	0.04	0.116	—
Total unsaturated, g	0.082	0.028	0.032	0.06	—
Total monounsaturated, g	0.008	0.001	0.002	0.006	—
Cholesterol, mg	0	0	0	0	0
Tryptophan, g	0.02	0.002	0.048	0.014	0.006
Threonine, g	0.056	0.006	0.1	0.034	0.019
Isoleucine, g	0.049	0.007	0.12	0.036	0.02
Leucine, g	0.079	0.01	0.186	0.053	0.034
Lycine, g	0.067	0.01	0.19	0.063	0.026
Methionine, g	0.018	0.002	0.05	0.013	0.005
Cystine, g	0.029	0.001	0.04	0.003	0.004
Phenylalanine, g	0.047	0.006	0.138	0.037	0.02
Tyrosine, g	0.032	0.004	0.1	0.049	0.009
Valine, g	0.063	0.007	0.176	0.04	0.027
Arginine, g	0.072	0.015	0.14	0.06	0.021
Histidine, g	0.031	0.003	0.068	0.02	0.009
Alanine, g	0.062	0.008	0.096	0.032	0.02
Aspartic acid, g	0.215	0.014	0.76	0.12	0.03
Glutamic acid, g	0.198	0.065	0.52	0.213	0.08
Glycine, g	0.056	0.008	0.094	0.03	0.017
Proline, g	0.065	0.005	0.1	0.03	0.03
Serine, g	0.06	0.007	0.136	0.05	0.017

Vegetables and Vegetable Juices

	Radish	Rutabaga	Sauerkraut	Spinach	Squash, summer
Measure	10	1 C	1 C	1 C	1 C
Weight, g	45	140	235	30	130
Calories	7	64	42	6	25
Protein, g	0.27	1.5	2.4	0.86	1.4
Carbohydrate, g	1.6	15.4	9.4	1	5.5
Fiber, g	0.7	3.5	5.9	0.8	2.5
Vitamin A, IU	3	810	120	2014	530
Vitamin B$_1$, mg	0.002	0.1	0.07	0.023	0.07
Vitamin B$_2$, mg	0.02	0.1	0.09	0.057	0.12
Vitamin B$_6$, mg	0.032	0.14	0.31	0.059	0.186
Vitamin B$_{12}$, mcg	0	0	0	0	0
Niacin, mg	0.135	1.5	0.5	0.22	1.3
Pantothenic acid, mg	0.04	0.22	0.22	0.02	0.468
Folic acid, mcg	12.2	29	56	58	30
Vitamin C, mg	10.3	60	33	8	29
Vitamin E. IU	0	0.6	0.35	0.85	—
Calcium, mg	9	92	85	30	36
Copper, mg	0.018	0.11	0.235	0.04	0.22
Iron, mg	0.13	0.6	1.2	0.8	0.5
Magnesium, mg	4	20	31	24	21
Manganese, mg	0.032	0.056	0.356	0.27	0.185
Phosphorus, mg	8	55	42	15	38
Potassium, mg	104	335	329	167	263
Selenium, mcg	0.3	0.98	1.4	0.3	0.26
Sodium, mg	11	7	1755	24	1
Zinc, mg	0.13	0.48	0.448	0.16	0.33
Total lipid, g	0.24	0.28	0.33	0.105	0.28
Total saturated, g	0.014	0.038	0.083	0.017	0.057
Total unsaturated, g	0.02	0.123	0.144	0.044	0.13
Total monounsaturated, g	0.01	0.035	0.031	0.003	0.023
Cholesterol, mg	0	0	0	0	0
Tryptophan, g	0.002	0.018	—	0.012	0.014
Threonine, g	0.013	0.064	—	0.037	0.036
Isoleucine, g	0.014	0.07	—	0.044	0.055
Leucine, g	0.017	0.053	—	0.067	0.09
Lycine, g	0.016	0.055	—	0.05	0.085
Methionine, g	0.003	0.014	—	0.016	0.022
Cystine, g	0.002	0.015	—	0.01	0.016
Phenylalanine, g	0.01	0.043	—	0.04	0.053
Tyrosine, g	0.006	0.032	—	0.03	0.04
Valine, g	0.014	0.067	—	0.05	0.069
Arginine, g	0.018	0.207	—	0.05	0.065
Histidine, g	0.006	0.042	—	0.02	0.033
Alanine, g	0.01	0.046	—	0.043	0.081
Aspartic acid, g	0.022	0.122	—	0.07	0.187
Glutamic acid, g	0.059	0.199	—	0.1	0.164
Glycine, g	0.01	0.038	—	0.04	0.057
Proline, g	0.008	—	—	0.034	0.048
Serine, g	0.009	0.049	—	0.03	0.062

Vegetables/Juices

Vegetables and Vegetable Juices

	Squash, winter	Sweet potato	Taro	Tomato, med	Tomato juice
Measure	1 C	1	1 C	1	1 C
Weight, g	205	130	104	123	243
Calories	129	136	116	24	46
Protein, g	3.7	2	1.5	1.1	2.2
Carbohydrate, g	31.6	32	28	5.3	10.4
Fiber, g	2.6	3.9	4	1.35	0.97
Vitamin A, IU	8610	26082	0	766	1351
Vitamin B$_1$, mg	0.1	0.086	0.1	0.074	0.12
Vitamin B$_2$, mg	0.27	0.191	0.03	0.062	0.07
Vitamin B$_6$, mg	0.18	0.334	0.3	0.059	0.366
Vitamin B$_{12}$, mcg	0	0	0	0	0
Niacin, mg	1.4	0.876	0.6	0.738	1.9
Pantothenic acid, mg	0.56	0.768	0.32	0.304	0.607
Folic acid, mcg	25	18	23	11.5	48
Vitamin C, mg	27	30	4.7	21.6	39
Vitamin E, IU	0.21	0.54	3.7	0.7	3.3
Calcium, mg	57	29	45	8	17
Copper, mg	0.1	0.22	0.18	0.095	0.246
Iron, mg	1.6	0.76	0.57	0.59	2.2
Magnesium, mg	45	14	34	14	20
Manganese, mg	0.2	0.46	0.4	0.15	0.188
Phosphorus, mg	98	37	87	29	44
Potassium, mg	945	265	614	254	552
Selenium, mcg	0.46	0.78	0.73	0.8	1.2
Sodium, mg	2	17	11	10	486
Zinc, mg	0.28	0.36	0.24	0.13	0.1
Total lipid, g	0.26	0.38	0.208	0.4	0.2
Total saturated, g	0.05	0.083	0.043	0.055	0.02
Total unsaturated, g	0.1	0.172	0.086	0.166	0.058
Total monounsaturated, g	0.02	0.014	0.017	0.06	0.02
Cholesterol, mg	0	0	0	0	0
Tryptophan, g	0.041	0.026	0.024	0.009	0.012
Threonine, g	0.082	0.107	0.07	0.027	0.042
Isoleucine, g	0.112	0.107	0.056	0.026	0.036
Leucine, g	0.125	0.157	0.1	0.041	0.052
Lycine, g	0.09	0.105	0.07	0.041	0.054
Methionine, g	0.031	0.053	0.02	0.01	0.01
Cystine, g	0.02	0.017	0.03	0.015	0.01
Phenylalanine, g	0.112	0.129	0.085	0.028	0.04
Tyrosine, g	0.089	0.088	0.057	0.018	0.024
Valine, g	0.122	0.14	0.085	0.028	0.036
Arginine, g	0.158	0.1	0.1	0.027	0.036
Histidine, g	0.041	0.04	0.035	0.016	0.03
Alanine, g	0.121	0.117	0.076	0.031	0.058
Aspartic acid, g	0.302	0.367	0.2	0.151	0.232
Glutamic acid, g	0.522	0.209	0.18	0.402	0.74
Glycine, g	0.1	0.096	0.077	0.027	0.03
Proline, g	0.1	0.094	0.006	0.021	0.042
Serine, g	0.103	0.111	0.096	0.03	0.044

Vegetables and Vegetable Juices

	Tomato paste	Turnips	Turnip greens	Vegetable juice cocktail	Water chestnuts
Measure	1 C	1 C	1 C	1 C	4 avg
Weight, g	262	130	55	242	36
Calories	215	39	15	41	35
Protein, g	8.9	1.3	0.83	2.2	0.5
Carbohydrate, g	48.7	8.6	3	8.7	8.6
Fiber, g	10	2.3	1.7	1.9	1
Vitamin A, IU	8650	0	4180	2831	0
Vitamin B_1, mg	0.52	0.05	0.039	0.12	0.04
Vitamin B_2, mg	0.31	0.09	0.055	0.07	0.05
Vitamin B_6, mg	0.996	0.117	0.145	0.338	0.118
Vitamin B_{12}, mcg	0	0	0	0	0
Niacin, mg	8.1	0.8	0.33	1.9	0.2
Pantothenic acid, mg	1.97	0.26	0.21	0.6	0.17
Folic acid, mcg	60	19	107	51	6
Vitamin C, mg	128	27	33	22	1
Vitamin E, IU	16	0.06	0.88	1.15	0.64
Calcium, mg	71	51	105	29	1
Copper, mg	1.4	0.09	0.193	0.484	0.117
Iron, mg	9.2	0.7	0.61	1.2	0.2
Magnesium, mg	50	25	17	26	2.4
Manganese, mg	1.3	0.052	0.256	0.242	0.12
Phosphorus, mg	183	39	23	53	16
Potassium, mg	2237	348	163	535	125
Selenium, mcg	3.6	0.78	0.66	1.2	0.25
Sodium, mg	100	64	22	484	5
Zinc, mg	2	0.35	0.1	0.48	0.18
Total lipid, g	2	0.13	0.17	0.2	0.036
Total saturated, g	0.332	0.014	0.039	0.03	0.009
Total unsaturated, g	0.6	0.069	0.066	0.09	0.015
Total monounsaturated, g	0.2	0.008	0.01	0.034	0.001
Cholesterol, mg	0	0	0	0	0
Tryptophan, g	0.068	0.012	0.014	—	—
Threonine, g	0.226	0.033	0.045	—	—
Isoleucine, g	0.192	0.047	0.043	—	—
Leucine, g	0.276	0.043	0.075	—	—
Lycine, g	0.282	0.047	0.054	—	—
Methionine, g	0.05	0.014	0.019	—	—
Cystine, g	0.058	0.007	0.009	—	—
Phenylalanine, g	0.2	0.022	0.051	—	—
Tyrosine, g	0.134	0.017	0.032	—	—
Valine, g	0.2	0.039	0.056	—	—
Arginine, g	0.2	0.031	0.052	—	—
Histidine, g	0.158	0.018	0.02	—	—
Alanine, g	0.3	0.046	0.057	—	—
Aspartic acid, g	1.24	0.082	0.087	—	—
Glutamic acid, g	3.95	0.169	0.112	—	—
Glycine, g	0.16	0.033	0.05	—	—
Proline, g	0.218	0.034	0.039	—	—
Serine, g	0.236	0.038	0.034	—	—

Vegetables and Vegetable Juices

	Watercress	Yams
Measure	1 C	1 C
Weight, g	35	150
Calories	7	177
Protein, g	0.8	3
Carbohydrate, g	1.1	41
Fiber, g	0.5	6
Vitamin A, IU	1720	0
Vitamin B$_1$, mg	0.03	0.18
Vitamin B$_2$, mg	0.06	0.05
Vitamin B$_6$, mg	0.045	0.51
Vitamin B$_{12}$, mcg	0	0
Niacin, mg	0.3	1.2
Pantothenic acid, mg	108	0.5
Folic acid, mcg	3	42
Vitamin C, mg	28	18
Vitamin E, IU	0.5	0.36
Calcium, mg	53	8
Copper, mg	0.032	0.44
Iron, mg	0.6	1.2
Magnesium, mg	6.5	62
Manganese, mg	0.189	0.6
Phosphorus, mg	19	100
Potassium, mg	99	1508
Selenium, mcg	0.31	1
Sodium, mg	18	17
Zinc, mg	0.037	0.43
Total lipid, g	0.04	0.255
Total saturated, g	0.01	0.056
Total unsaturated, g	0.012	0.114
Total monounsaturated, g	0.003	0.009
Cholesterol, mg	0	0
Tryptophan, g	0.01	0.018
Threonine, g	0.046	0.081
Isoleucine, g	0.032	0.078
Leucine, g	0.056	0.144
Lycine, g	0.046	0.089
Methionine, g	0.006	0.032
Cystine, g	0.002	0.079
Phenylalanine, g	0.038	0.107
Tyrosine, g	0.022	0.06
Valine, g	0.046	0.093
Arginine, g	0.052	0.191
Histidine, g	0.014	0.051
Alanine, g	0.046	0.095
Aspartic acid, g	0.064	0.233
Glutamic acid, g	0.064	0.272
Glycine, g	0.038	0.08
Proline, g	0.032	0.081
Serine, g	0.02	0.122

REFERENCES

1. Williams, M.J.A., et al. "Impaired endothelial function following a meal rich in used cooking fat," *J. Am. Coll. of Cardio.* **33**(4): 1050 (1999).

2. Taddei, S., et al. "Vitamin C improves endotheoium-dependent vasodilation by restoring nitric oxide activity in essential hypertension," *Circulation* **97**: 2222–29 (1998).

3. Stampfer, M.J., et al. "Vitamin E consumption and the risk of coronary heart disease in men," *N. Engl. J. Med.* **328**: 1450–56; in women, 1444–49, 1993.

4. Stephens, N.G., et al. "Randomised controlled trial of vitamin E in patients with coronary disease," *Lancet* **347**: 781–86 (1996).

5. Schnaubelt, K. *Advanced Aromatherapy.* Rochester, Vermont: Healing Arts Press, 1998, p. 31.

6. Ibid. p. 40.

7. Ibid. p. 40.

8. Verma, S.K., et al. "Effect of Commiphora mukul (gum guggulu) in patients of hyperlipidemia with special reference to HDL-cholesterol," *Indian J. Med. Res.* **87**: 356–60 (1988).

9. Singh, K., et al. "Guggulsterone, a potent hypolipidaemic, prevents oxidation of low density lipoprotein," *Phytother. Res.* **11**: 291–94 (1997).

10. Carper, J. *Food: Your Miracle Medicine.* New York: Harper Collins, 1994, p. 428.

11. Weil, A. *Natural Health Natural Medicine.* New York: Houghton Mifflin Co., 1998, p. 241.

12. Zhang, Z.C. "Preliminary report on the use of Momordica charantia extract by HIV patients," *J. of Naturo. Med.* **3**(1): 65–69 (1992).

13. Durant, J., et al. "Efficacy and safety of Buxus sempervirens L. preparations in HIV-infected asymptomatic patients: A multicentre, randomized, double-blind, placebo-controlled trial," *Phytomedicine* **5**(1): 1–10 (1998).

14. Pelletier, K. *The Best Alternative Medicine.* New York: Simon and Schuster, 2000, p. 146.

15. Schmidt, R., et al. "Plasma antioxidants and cognitive performance in middle-aged and older adults: Results of the Austrian Stroke Prevention Study," *J. Am. Geriatr. Soc.* **46**: 1407–10 (1998).

16. Crook, T., et al. "Effects of phosphatidylserine in Alzheimer's disease," *Psychopharmacol. Bull.* **28**: 61–66 (1992).

17. Pettegrew, J.W., et al. "Clinical and neurochemical effects of acetyl-L-carnitine in Alzheimer's disease," *Neurobio. Aging* **16**: 1–4 (1995).

18. Drovanti, A., et al. "Therapeutic activity of oral glucosamine sulfate in osteoarthritis: A

placebo-controlled double-blind investigation," *Clin. Ther.* **3**(4): 260–72 (1980).

19. Bucsi, L., et al. "Efficacy and tolerability of oral chondroitin sulfate as a symptomatic slow-acting drug for osteoarthritis in the treatment of knee osteoarthritis," *Osteoarthr. Cartilage,* **6**(A): 31–6 (1998).

20. Carper. *Food: Your Miracle Medicine.* p. 383.

21. Weil. *Natural Health and Natural Medicine.* p. 258.

22. Ibid. p. 258.

23. Denke, M.A., et al. "Comparison of effects of lauric acid and palmitic acid on plasma lipids and lipoproteins," *Am. J. Clin. Nutr.* **56**: 895–98 (1992).

24. Brevetti, G., et al. "Increases in walking distance in patients with peripheral vascular disease treated with L-carnitine: A double-blind, cross-over study," *Circulation* **77**: 767–73 (1988).

25. Braquet, P. et al. "Perspectives in platelet activating factor research," *Pharmacol. Rev.* **39**: 97–210 (1987).

26. Kiesewetter, H., et al. "Effect of garlic on thrombocyte aggregation, microcirculation and other risk factors," *Int. J. Pharm. Ther. Toxicol.* **29**(4): 151–54 (1991).

27. Araghiniknam, M., et al. "Antioxidant activity of dioscorea and dehydroepiandrosterone in older humans," *Life Sci.* **11**: 147–57 (1996).

28. Singh, K. "Guggulsterone a potent hypolipidaemic, prevents oxidation of low density lipoprotein," *Phytother. Res.* **11**: 291–94 (1997).

29. Shealy, C.N. *Alternative Healing Therapies.* Boston, MA: Element Books Ltd., 1999, p. 344.

30. Weil. *Natural Health and Natural Medicine.* p. 265.

31. Berstein A.L., et al. "Effect of pharmacologic doses of vitamin B_6 on carpal tunnel syndrome, electronencephalographic results, and pain," *J. Am. Coll. Nutri.* **12**: 73–76 1993.

32. Melchart, D., et al. "Immunomodulation with echinacea—a systematic review of controlled clinical trials," *Phytomedicine* **1**: 245–54 (1994).

33. Belluzzi, A., et al. "Effect of an enteric-coated fish oil preparation on relapses in Crohn's disease," *N. Engl. J. Med.* **334**: 1557–60 (1996).

34. Sobota, A.E. "Inhibition of bacterial adherence by cranberry juice: Potential use for the treatment of urinary tract infections," *J. Urol.* **131**: 1013–16 (1984).

35. Weil. *Natural Health and Natural Medicine.* p. 282.

36. Harrer, G., et al. "Treatment of mild/moderate depression with Hypericum," *Phytomedicine* **1**: 3–8 (1994).

37. Paolisso, G., et al. "Pharmacologic doses of vitamin E improve insulin action in healthy subjects and non-insulin dependent diabetic patients," *Am. J. Clin. Nutri.* **57**: 650–56 (1993).

38. Zhang, T., et al. "Ginseng root: Evidence for numerous regulatory peptides and insulinotropic activity," *Biomed. Res.* **11**: 49–54 (1990).

39. Sotaniemi, E.A., et al. "Ginseng therapy in non-insulin-dependent diabetic patients," *Diabetes Care* **18**: 1373–75 (1995).

40. Bleichner, G., et al. "Saccharomyces boulardii prevents diarrhea in critically ill tube-fed patients. A multicenter, randomized, double-blind placebo-controlled trial," *Intensive Care Med.* **23**: 517–23, 1997.

41. Duncan, B., et al. "Exclusive breast feeding for at least four months protects against otitis media," *Pediatraics* **91**(5): 867–72, 1993.

42. Weil. *Natural Health and Natural Medicine.* p. 290.

43. Mian, E., et al. "Anthocyanosides and the walls of microvessels: Further aspects of the mechanism of action of their protective in syndromes due to abnormal capillary fragility," *Minerva Med.* **68**: 3565–81 (1977).

44. Duke, J. *The Green Pharmacy.* Emmaus, PA: Rodale Press, 1997, p. 208.

45. Ibid. p. 223.

46. Palevitch, D. "Feverfew as a prophylactic treatment for migraine: A double-blind placebo-controlled study," *Phytother. Res.* **11**: 508–11 (1997).

47. Carper. *Food: Your Miracle Medicine.* p. 321.

48. Kamikawa, T., et al. "Effects of coenzyme Q10 on exercise tolerance in chronic stable angina pectoris," *Am. J. Cardiol.* **56**: 247 (1985).

49. Cacciatore, L. "The therapeutic effect of L-carnitine in patients with exercise-induced stable angina: A controlled study," *Drugs Exp. Clin. Res.* **17**: 225–35 (1991).

50. Wolf, A., et al. "Dietary L-arginine supplementation normalizes platelet aggregation in hypercholesterolemic humans," *J. Am. Coll. Cardiol.* **29**: 479–85 (1997).

51. Tauchert, M., et al. "Effectiveness of hawthorn extract LI 132 compared with the ACE inhibitor Captopril: Multicenter double-blind study with 132 patients NYHA stage II," *Munch. Med. Wochenschr.* **132**: S27–33 (1994).

52. Duke. *The Green Pharmacy.* p. 239.

53. Jenkins, P.J., et al. "Use of polyunsaturated phosphatidyl choline in HBsAg negative chronic active hepatitis: Results of prospective double-blind controlled trial," *Liver* **2**: 77–81 (1982).

54. Galli, M., et al. "Attempt to treat acute type B hepatitis with an orally administered thymic extract: Preliminary results," *Drugs Exp. Clin. Res.* **11**: 665–69 (1985).

55. Buzzelli, G., et al. "A pilot study on the liver protective effect of silybinphosphatidylcholine complex in chronic active hepatitis," *Int. J. Clin. Pharmacol. Ther. Toxicol.* **31**: 456–60 (1993).

56. Digiesi, V., et al. "Effect of coenzyme Q10 on essential arterial hypertension," *Curr. Ther. Res.* **47**: 841–45 (1990).

57. Leathwood, P.D., et al. "Aqueous extract of valerian root improves sleep quality in man," *Pharmacol. Biochem. Behav.* **17**: 65–71 (1982).

58. Pittler, M.H. "Peppermint oil for irritable bowel syndrome: A critical review and meta-analysis," *Am. J. Gastroenterol.* **93**: 1131–35 (1998).

59. Lindberg, J., et al. "Effect of magnesium citrate and magnesium oxide on the crystallization of calcium salts in urine: Changes produced by food-magnesium interaction," *J. Urol.* **143**: 248–51 (1990).

60. Cangiano, C., et al. "Eating behavior and adherence to dietary prescriptions in obese adult subjects treated with 5-hydroxytryptophan," *Am. J. Clin. Nutr.* **56**: 863–67 (1992).

61. Cracium, A.M., et al. "Improved bone metabolism in female elite athletes after vitamin K supplementation," *Int. J. Sports Med.* **19**: 479–84 (1998).

62. Lauritzen, C., et al. "Treatment of premenstrual tension syndrome with Vitex agnus castus: Controlled, double-blind study versus pyridoxine," *Phytomedicine* **4**: 183–89 (1997).

63. Berges, R.R., et al. "Randomized, placebo-controlled, double-blind clinical trial of beta-sitosterol in patients with benign prostatic hyperplasia," *Lancet* **345**: 1529–32 (1995).

64. Wilt, T.J., et al. "Saw palmetto extracts for treatment of benign prostatic hyperplasia: A systematic review," *JAMA* **280**: 1604–1609 (1998).

65. Andro, M.C., et al. "Pygeum africanum extract for the treatment of patients with benign prostatic hyperplasia: A review of 25 years of published experience," *Curr. Ther. Res.* **56**: 796–817 (1995).

66. Carper. *Food: Your Miracle Medicine.* p. 445.

67. Duke. *The Green Pharmacy.* p. 414.

68. Smith, B.L. "Organic foods versus supermarket foods: Element levels," *J. Appl. Nutr.* **45**(1): 35–37 (1993).

69. Pelletier. *The Best Alternative Medicine.* p. 97.

70. Wood, R. *The New Whole Foods Encyclopedia.* New York: Penguin Books, 1999, p. 22.

SELECTED BIBLIOGRAPHY

Barlow, Wilfred. *The Alexander Technique.* New York: Alfred A. Knopf, 1991.

Beinfield, Harriet. *Between Heaven and Earth: A Guide to Chinese Medicine.* New York: Ballantine Books, 1991.

Blumenthal, Mark (senior ed.). *The Complete German Commission E Monographs.* Boston, MA: Integrative Medicine Communications, 1998.

Borysenko, Joan. *Minding the Body, Mending the Mind.* Reading, MA: Bantam, 1988.

Brand-Miller, Jennie; Wolever, Thomas M.S.; Colagiuri, Stephen; Foster-Powell, Kaye. *The Glucose Revolution: The Authoritative Guide to the Glycemic Index.* New York: Marlowe & Company, 1999.

Carper, Jean. *Food Your Miracle Medicine.* New York: Harper Collins, 1994.

Coplan-Griffiths, Michael. *Dynamic Chiropractic Today: The Complete and Authoritiative Guide to This Major Therapy.* San Francisco, CA: Harper Collins, 1991.

Dong, Paul; Esser, Aristide H. *Chi Kung, The Ancient Chinese Way to Health.* New York: Paragon House, 1990.

Elman, Dave. *Hypnotherapy.* Glendale, CA: Westwood Publishing Co., 1984.

Duke, James. *The Green Pharmacy.* Emmaus, PA: Rodale Press, 1997.

Feldenkrais, Moshe. *The Potent Self: A Guide to Spontaneity.* San Francisco, CA: Harper & Row, 1992.

Gach, Michael, R. *Acupressure's Potent Points.* New York: Bantam Books, 1990.

Jenkins, Nancy Harmon; Trichopoulou, Antonia. *The Mediterranean Diet Cookbook: A Delicious Alternative for Lifelong Health.* New York: Bantam Doubleday Dell, 1994.

Kaptchuk, Ted. *The Web That Has No Weaver: Understanding Chinese Medicine.* Chicago, IL: Contemporary Books, 1985.

Kunz, Kevin, Barbara. *Hand and Foot Reflexology: A Self-Help Guide.* New York: Simon & Schuster, 1987.

Lawless, Julia. *The Complete Illustrated Guide to Aromatherapy.* Boston, MA: Element Books, 1997.

Lininger, Schuyler W., ed. *The Natural Pharmacy.* Roseville, CA: Prima Publ., 1999.

Locke, Steven; Colligan, Douglas. *The Healer Within: The New Medicine of Mind and Body.* New York: E.P. Dutton, 1986.

Lockie, Andrew; Geddes, Nicola. *The Complete Guide to Homeopathy.* New York: DK Publishing Inc., 1995.

Lundberg, Paul. *The Book of Shiatsu.* New York: Fireside, 1992.

McCabe, Vinton. *Practical Homeopathy.* New York: St. Martins Press, 2000.

McGill, Leonard. *The Chiropractic's Health Book.* New York: Three Rivers Press, 1997.

Murray, Michael; Pizzorno, Joseph. *Encyclopedia of Natural Medicine.* Revised 2nd ed. Rocklin, CA: Prima Publ, 1998.

Peirce, Andrea. *The American Pharmaceutical Association's Practical Guide to Natural Medicines.* New York: William Morrow & Co, 1999.

Pelletier, Kenneth R. *The Best Alternative Medicine.* New York: Simon & Schuster, 2000.

Pitchford, Paul. *Healing with Whole Foods: Oriental Traditions and Modern Nutrition.* Berkeley: North Atlantic Books, 1996.

Rolf, Ida P. *Rolfing: The Integration of Human Structures.* New York: Harper & Row, 1977.

Schnaubelt, Kurt. *Advanced Aromatherapy.* Translated from the German by J. Michael Beasley. Rochester, VT: Healing Arts Press, 1998.

Shealy, Norman C. *Alternative Healing Therapies.* Boston, MA: Element Books Inc., 1999.

Shealy, Norman C. *Illustrated Encyclopedia of Healing Remedies.* Boston, MA: Element Books, Inc., 1998.

Thomas, Sara. *Massage for Common Ailments.* New York: Fireside, 1989.

Tiwari, Maya. *Ayurveda—A Life of Balance: The Complete Guide to Ayurvedic Nutrition and Body Types.* Rochester, VT: Healing Arts Press, 1994.

Tyler, Varro E. *Herbs of Choice, The Therapeutic Use of Phyto Medicinals.* New York: Pharmaceutical Products Press, 1994.

Ullman, Dana. *Discovering Homeopathy: Your Introduction to the Science and Art of Homeopathic Medicine.* Berkeley, CA: North Atlantic Books, 1991.

Vishnudevananda, Swami. *The Complete Illustrated Book of Yoga.* New York: Harmony Books, 1980.

Weil, Andrew. *Health and Healing.* New York: Houghton Mifflin Co., 1983.

Weil, Andrew. *Natural Health, Natural Medicine.* New York: Houghton Mifflin Co., 1998.

Weil, Andrew. *Eating Well for Optimum Health.* New York: Alfred A. Knopf, 2000.

Wood, Rebecca. *The New Whole Foods Encyclopedia.* New York: Penguin, 1999.

Xiangcai, Xu. *Qigong for Treating Common Ailments.* Boston, MA: YMAA Publications, 2000.

INDEX

A

Abalone, nutrients in, 234
Abbreviations (in tables), 158
Abdominal pain, essential oils to avoid with, 23
Abscesses, 37–38
Absorption, 4
Acetate fragments, 8
Acetylcholine, 12, 44
Acid reflux, 95
Acidic foods, glycemic index and, 151
Acidophilus, 136
Acne, 38–40
Acupressure, 26
Adenosine triphosphate (ATP), 11, 15
Adequate intakes (AIs), 160–161
Adrenal glands, 12, 22
Aduki beans, 138, 208
Agar, 140
Agar-agar, nutrients in, 234
Aging process, 8, 14, 137
AIDS, 40–42
AIs (see Adequate Intakes)
Alexander technique, 26
Alfalfa sprouts, 138, 243
Allergies, 10, 42–44
    and arthritis, 47
    and asthma, 47
    and bronchitis, 56
    and canker sores, 64

Allergies (Cont.)
    and chronic fatigue syndrome, 66
    and Crohn's disease, 71
    and ear infections, 81
    and eczema, 81
    and epileptic seizures, 83
    food intolerances vs., 136
    and gallbladder disease, 87
    and glaucoma, 84
    herbs to avoid with, 29, 30, 32
    and insomnia, 104
    and migraines, 91
    and reaction to essential oils, 22
Allopathic medicine, 21
Almond oil, nutrients in, 178
Almonds, nutrients in, 225
Aloe vera, 29
Alpha carotene, 11
Alpha tocopherol, 136
Alternative medicine and therapies, 21–33
    aromatherapy, 21–23
    Ayurvedic medicine, 23–25
    biofeedback, 32–33
    bodywork, 25–27
    Chinese medicine, 27–28
    chiropractic, 28
    deep tissue manipulation, 25–26
    energy balancing, 26–27
    herbal therapy, 28–31
    homeopathy, 32–32

Alternative medicine and therapies (*Cont.*)
  hypnotherapy, 33
  imagery, 33
  massage, 25–26
  meditation, 32
  mindbody therapy, 32–33
  movement therapies, 26
  reflexology, 27
  therapeutic massage, 25
Alzheimer's disease, 12, 44–45
Amaranth, 138, 139, 197
Amasake, 141
Amenorrhea, 112
American cheese, nutrients in, 171
American ginseng, 30
Amino acids, 4, 5, 9, 10
  homocysteine, 12
  neuropeptides/peptides, 32
Ammonia, 10
Amylase, 3
Amylopectic starches, 151
Amylopectin, 6
Amylose, 6
Amylose starches, 151
Analgesic foods, 142
Anaphylactic shock, 42
Anasazi beans, 138
Anchovies, nutrients in, 235
Anemia, 12, 15, 45–47
Angina, 52, 93
Anthocyanins, 10, 13
Antibacterial agents:
  essential oils as, 22
  foods as, 142
Antibiotic activity of yogurt, 140
Antibiotics, 37–38
Antibodies, 42
Anticancer foods, 142–143
Anticoagulants:
  foods as, 143
  herbs to avoid with, 30
Anticonvulsant drugs, 83
Antidepressant drugs, herbs to avoid with, 32
Anti-inflammatory agents, essential oils
    as, 22
Antioxidants, 10, 11, 13, 15
  and color of foods, 137
  foods high in, 143
  and macular degeneration, 84
  selenium, 16

Antiviral agents:
  essential oils as, 142
  foods as, 143
Anxiety disorders, 30, 32
Apithery, 114
Appetite, loss of, 22
Apple cider vinegar, 141
Apple juice, nutrients in, 183
Apples, nutrients in, 183
Applesauce, nutrients in, 183
Apricot kernel, nutrients in, 178
Apricot nectar, nutrients in, 184
Apricots, nutrients in, 183–184
Arame, 140
Aromatherapy, 21–23
  for abscess, 38
  for acne, 40
  for AIDS, 42
  for allergy, 44
  for Alzheimer's disease, 45
  for anemia, 46
  for arthritis, 49
  for asthma, 51
  for atherosclerosis, 54
  for back pain, 56
  for bronchitis, 58
  for bruises, 59
  for burns, 60
  for bursitis, 62
  for cancer, 64
  for carpal tunnel syndrome, 66
  for chronic fatigue syndrome, 67
  for colds and flu, 69
  for constipation, 70
  for Crohn's disease, 72
  for cystitis, 73
  for depression, 75
  for diabetes, 78
  for diarrhea, 79
  for ear infection, 81
  for eczema, 82
  for epilepsy, 83
  for fibromyalgia, 86
  for gallbladder disease, 88
  for gingivitis, 89
  for gout, 90
  for headache, 92
  for heart attack, 94–95
  for hemorrhoids, 97
  for hepatitis, 98

Aromatherapy (*Cont.*)
    for herpes, 100
    for hypertension, 101
    for infection, 104
    for insomnia, 105
    for irritable bowel syndrome, 107
    for kidney stones, 108
    for menopause, 111
    for menstrual problems, 113
    for multiple sclerosis, 114
    for overweight, 117
    for pregnancy, 120
    for premenstrual syndrome, 121
    for psoriasis, 124
    for Raynaud's disease, 125
    for stress, 127
    for stroke, 129
    for ulcers, 130
    for vaginitis, 132
Arrythmias, 93
Arteries:
    disease, arterial, 8
    spasms of, 93
    stroke, 128
Arthritis, 47–50
Artichokes, nutrients in, 243
Arugula, 137, 243
Ascorbic acid (vitamin C), 13, 146
Asparagus, nutrients in, 243
Aspartame, 141–142
Aspirin, 13, 30, 32
Asthma, 23, 50–52
Aston-Patterning, 25
Atherosclerosis, 8, 9, 12, 15, 52–54
Athlete's foot, 54
Atopic dermatitis, 81
ATP (*see* Adenosine triphosphate)
Attention deficit disorder, 8
Attention problems, 44
Autism, 8
Autoimmune diseases, 10
    (*See also* specific diseases)
Autonomic nervous system, 28
Avocado oil, nutrients in, 178
Avocados, nutrients in, 184
Ayurvedic medicine, 23–25
    for abscess, 38
    for acne, 40
    for AIDS, 42
    for allergy, 44

Ayurvedic medicine (*Cont.*)
    for Alzheimer's disease, 45
    for anemia, 47
    for arthritis, 49
    for asthma, 51
    for atherosclerosis, 54
    for back pain, 56
    for bronchitis, 58
    for burns, 60
    for bursitis, 62
    for cancer, 64
    for chronic fatigue syndrome, 67
    for colds and flu, 69
    for constipation, 70
    for Crohn's disease, 72
    for cystitis, 73
    for depression, 75
    for diabetes, 78
    for diarrhea, 79
    for ear infection, 81
    for eczema, 82
    for epilepsy, 83
    for fibromyalgia, 86
    for gallbladder disease, 88
    for gingivitis, 89
    for gout, 90
    for headache, 92
    for heart attack, 95
    for hemorrhoids, 97
    for hepatitis, 98
    for herpes, 100
    for hypertension, 101
    for infection, 104
    for insomnia, 105
    for irritable bowel syndrome, 107
    for kidney stones, 108
    for lupus, 109
    for menopause, 111
    for menstrual problems, 113
    for multiple sclerosis, 114
    for osteoporosis, 116
    for overweight, 117
    for pregnancy, 120
    for premenstrual syndrome, 121
    for prostate problems, 123
    for psoriasis, 124
    for Raynaud's disease, 125
    for stress, 127
    for stroke, 129
    for ulcers, 130

B

B complex vitamins, 11–13, 39, 145
Back pain, 54–56
Bacon, nutrients in, 217
Bacteria, 5
Bagels, nutrients in, 201
Bananas, nutrients in, 184
Barberry, 29
Barley, 138, 139, 197
Barley malt, 141
Basmati rice, 139
Bass, sea, nutrients in, 235
Beans, 137–138
    cooking process for, 138
    nutrients in, 208–211
Beef, nutrients in, 213–215
Beef sausage, nutrients in, 224
Beer, nutrients in, 163
Beet greens, 137, 244
Beets, nutrients in, 244
Benign prostatic hyperplasia (BPH), 122
Beta carotene, 11
Beverages, composition of, 163–164
Bile, 4
Bile salts, 4
Biofeedback, 32–33
Bioflavonoids, 13, 147
Biotin, 12, 140, 146
Birth abnormalities, 12
Birth control pills, 11–13, 15
    and acne, 39
    and depression, 74
Bismuth, herbs to avoid with, 30
Bitter melon, 29
Black beans, 138, 208
Black cohosh, 29
Blackberries, nutrients in, 184
Blackeyed peas, nutrients in, 208
Blackstrap molasses, 141
Bladder, cystitis in, 72
Blepharitis, 84
Blood circulation, 8
Blood fat abnormalities, 6
Blood pressure, 13, 15, 16, 100
    (See also Hypertension)
Blood sugar levels, 6
    (See also Glycemic index)
Bloodroot, 29
Blue cheese, nutrients in, 165

Blue cohosh, 29
Blue corn, 139
Blueberries, nutrients in, 185
Bluefish, nutrients in, 235
Bodywork, 25–27
    for abscess, 38
    for acne, 40
    for AIDS, 42
    for allergy, 44
    for Alzheimer's disease, 45
    for anemia, 47
    for arthritis, 49–50
    for asthma, 51–52
    for atherosclerosis, 54
    for back pain, 56
    for bronchitis, 58
    for bursitis, 62
    for cancer, 64
    for carpal tunnel syndrome, 66
    for chronic fatigue syndrome, 67
    for colds and flu, 69
    for constipation, 70–71
    for Crohn's disease, 72
    for cystitis, 73
    for depression, 75
    for diabetes, 78
    for diarrhea, 80
    for diverticulitis, 80
    for ear infection, 81
    for eczema, 83
    for epilepsy, 83
    for fibromyalgia, 87
    for gout, 91
    for headache, 92
    for heart attack, 95
    for heartburn, 96
    for hemorrhoids, 97
    for hepatitis, 99
    for hypertension, 102
    for infection, 104
    for insomnia, 106
    for irritable bowel syndrome, 107
    for kidney stones, 108
    for lupus, 109
    for menopause, 111
    for menstrual problems, 113
    for multiple sclerosis, 115
    for osteoporosis, 116
    for overweight, 117
    for pregnancy, 120

Bodywork (*Cont.*)
  for premenstrual syndrome, 121
  for prostate problems, 123
  for psoriasis, 124
  for Raynaud's disease, 126
  for stress, 127
  for stroke, 129
  for ulcers, 131
Boericke, William, 37
Boils, 37
Bologna, nutrients in, 221
Bones:
  broken, 48
  and osteoporosis, 115
Boneset, 29
Bottled water, 17
Boysenberries, nutrients in, 185
BPH (benign prostatic hyperplasia), 122
Brain, 6
  essential oils' effects on, 22
  imagination and, 33
Bratwurst, nutrients in, 221
Braunschweiger, nutrients in, 221
Brazil nuts, nutrients in, 225
Breads:
  glycemic indexes of, 6, 151
  nutritional composition of, 201–206
Breast cancer, 62
  essential oils to avoid with, 23
  herbs to avoid with, 30
Breast disease, fibrocystic, 85–86
Breathing, 16, 126
Brick cheese, nutrients in, 165
Brie cheese, nutrients in, 165
Broccoli, 137, 244
Broken bones, 48
Bronchi, 47
Bronchitis, 56–58
Brotwurst, nutrients in, 222
Brown rice, nutrients in, 200
Brown rice syrup, 141
Brown rice vinegar, 141
Brown sugar, 141
Bruises, 58–59
Brussels sprouts, 137, 244
Buchu, 29
Buckwheat, 138, 139
Buckwheat flour, nutrients in, 206
Buckwheat groats, nutrients in, 197
Bulgur, 138, 139, 197

Burns, 59–60
Bursitis, 61–62
Butter, nutrients in, 178
Buttermilk, 140, 174

C

Cabbage, 137, 244–245
Calcium, 13, 14
  and atherosclerosis, 52
  in kidney stones, 107
  and osteoporosis, 115
  rich food sources of, 147
Calmati rice, 139
Camembert cheese, nutrients in, 165
Canadian bacon, nutrients in, 217
Cancer, 8, 62–64
  essential oils to avoid with, 23
  and selenium, 16
  and vitamin A, 10–11
  and vitamin C, 13
Cane juices/sugars, 141
Canker sores, 64–65
Canola oil, 8, 179
Cantaloupe, nutrients in, 190
Capacity measurements, 158
Carbohydrates, 5–7
  cholesterol and high-GI, 8, 9
  digestion of, 4
  rich food sources of, 144
  simple, 5
  (*See also* Glycemic index)
Cardiovascular disease, 6
Carob, 137, 208
Carotenoids, 10, 11, 136, 147
Carp, nutrients in, 236
Carpal tunnel syndrome, 11, 65–66
Carrot juice, nutrients in, 245
Carrots, nutrients in, 245
Casaba melons, nutrients in, 190
Cashews, nutrients in, 225
Cataracts, 84
Catfish, nutrients in, 236
Cat's claw, 29
Cauliflower, nutrients in, 245
Caviar, nutrients in, 236
Celeriac, nutrients in, 246
Celery, 29, 137, 245
Cell metabolism, free radical activity and, 137

Cellulose, 6
Central nervous system, 28
Cerebral arteries, 52
Cervical dysplasia, 63
Chamomile, 29
Chaparral, 29
Chapote, nutrients in, 246
Chard, 137
Cheddar cheese, nutrients in, 165
Cheese spread, nutrients in, 171
Cheeses, 140, 165–171
Cherimoya, nutrients in, 185
Cherries, nutrients in, 185
Cheshire cheese, nutrients in, 166
Chestnuts, nutrients in, 225
Chewing, 3
Chicken, 139, 228–232
Chicken fat, nutrients in, 179
Chicorygreens, nutrients in, 246
Children:
    DRIs for, 159–161
    RDAs for, 159–161
Chinese cabbage, nutrients in, 245
Chinese ginseng, 30
Chinese medicine, 27–28
    for abscess, 38
    for acne, 40
    for AIDS, 42
    for allergy, 44
    for Alzheimer's disease, 45
    for anemia, 47
    for arthritis, 49
    for asthma, 51
    for atherosclerosis, 54
    for back pain, 56
    for bronchitis, 58
    for bruises, 59
    for burns, 60
    for bursitis, 62
    for cancer, 64
    for canker sores, 65
    for carpal tunnel syndrome, 66
    for chronic fatigue syndrome, 67
    for colds and flu, 69
    for constipation, 70
    for Crohn's disease, 72
    for cystitis, 73
    for depression, 75
    for diabetes, 78
    for diarrhea, 79

Chinese medicine (*Cont.*)
    for diverticulitis, 80
    for ear infection, 81
    for eczema, 83
    for epilepsy, 83
    for fibromyalgia, 86
    for gallbladder disease, 88
    for gingivitis, 89
    for gout, 90
    for headache, 92
    for heart attack, 95
    for heartburn, 96
    for hemorrhoids, 97
    for hepatitis, 98–99
    for herpes, 100
    for hypertension, 102
    for infection, 104
    for insomnia, 105
    for irritable bowel syndrome, 107
    for kidney stones, 108
    for lupus, 109
    for menopause, 111
    for menstrual problems, 113
    for multiple sclerosis, 114
    for osteoporosis, 116
    for overweight, 117
    for pregnancy, 120
    for premenstrual syndrome, 121
    for prostate problems, 123
    for psoriasis, 124
    for Raynaud's disease, 125
    for stress, 127
    for stroke, 129
    for ulcers, 130
Chiropractic, 28
    for arthritis, 49
    for asthma, 51
    for back pain, 56
    for carpal tunnel syndrome, 66
    for chronic fatigue syndrome, 67
    for depression, 75
    for diverticulitis, 80
    for ear infection, 81
    for epilepsy, 83
    for fibromyalgia, 87
    for headache, 92
    for heart attack, 95
    for heartburn, 96
    for hypertension, 102
    for insomnia, 105

Chiropractic (*Cont.*)
    for menstrual problems, 113
    for osteoporosis, 116
    for pregnancy, 120
    for premenstrual syndrome, 121
    for Raynaud's disease, 126
Chives, nutrients in, 246
Chocolate, glycemic index of, 153
Chocolate milk, nutrients in, 175
Cholesterol, 4, 8–9, 13
    and atherosclerosis, 52
    foods that lower, 144
    guggul for lowering, 24
    in meats, poultry, 139
    and soluble fibers, 6
Choline, 12, 146
Chromium, 14–15, 147
Chromium GTF, 6
Chronic fatigue syndrome, 15, 66–67
Chyme, 4
Cinnamon, 29
Cirrhosis, 97
Clams, nutrients in, 236
Claudication, intermittent, 52
Clove, 29
Coca Cola, glycemic index of, 153
Coconut, nutrients in, 225
Coconut liquid, nutrients in, 226
Coconut oil, nutrients in, 179
Cod, nutrients in, 236
Cod liver oil, nutrients in, 179
Coenzymes:
    biotin, 12
    niacin, 11
    vitamins as, 10
Coffee, 81, 163
Coffee cream, nutrients in, 172
Colas:
    glycemic index of, 153
    nutrients in, 163
Colby cheese, nutrients in, 166
Colds, 67–69
Colitis, 71
Collards, 137, 247
Colon, 5
    and Crohn's disease, 71
    fiber and cancer of, 6
Color of foods, antioxidant activity and, 137
Comfrey, 29
Commission E (Germany), 29

Complex carbohydrates, 7
Compresses, herb, 29
Condensed milk, nutrients in, 175
Conjunctivitis, 84
Constipation, 69–71
Contraceptives (*see* Birth control pills)
Conventional medicine, 21
Copper, 13, 15
    and PMS (premenstrual syndrome), 15
    rich food sources of, 147–148
Corn, 139, 247
Corn flour, nutrients in, 206
Corn oil, nutrients in, 179
Corn pasta, nutrients in, 198
Corn syrup, 141
Corned beef, nutrients in, 213
Cornish game hens, nutrients in, 232
Cornmeal, nutrients in, 198
Coronary arteries, 52, 93
Coronary heart disease, 10
Cortisone, 8
Cottage cheese, nutrients in, 166
Cottonseed oil, nutrients in, 180
Couscous, 138, 139, 199
Crabapples, nutrients in, 186, 237
Cracked wheat bread, nutrients in, 201
Crackers:
    glycemic index of, 153
    nutrients in, 205–206
Cranberries, nutrients in, 186
Cream, nutrients in, 172
Cream cheese, nutrients in, 166
Crohn's disease, 71–72
Cruciferous vegetables, 137
Cryptococcal meningitis (*see* Human immuno-
    deficiency virus)
Cryptoxanthin, 11
Cucumber, nutrients in, 247
Currants, nutrients in, 186
Cystitis, 72–73

D

Daikon, 137
Dairy products, 140
    glycemic indexes of, 151–152
    nutritional composition of, 165–177
Dandelion, 29
Dandelion greens, 137, 247

Date sugar, 141
Dates, nutrients in, 186
Decoctions, herb, 29
Deep breathing, 126
Deep tissue manipulation, 25–26
Degenerative diseases, 10
Demineralization of bones, 13
Depression, 8, 11, 12, 22, 73–76
Dermatitis, 12, 81
Detoxification, 5
Devil's claw, 30
DHA, 136
DHEA, 136
Diabetes, 6, 11, 12, 76–78, 150
   and glycemic index of foods, 151
   herbs to avoid with, 30
Diagnosis:
   in Ayurvedic medicine, 23–24
   in Chinese medicine, 27
Diarrhea, 78–80
Diet:
   and cancer, 63
   and heart disease, 93
   high protein intake, 9–10
   and immune system strength, 102
Dietary intake charts, 158–161
Dietary Reference Intakes (DRIs), 158–161
Digestion, 3–5, 9
Digestive tract, 3
Digitalis, herbs to avoid with, 30
Dill pickles, nutrients in, 252
Disaccharides, 5
Discoid lupus erythermatosus, 109
Diverticulitis, 7, 80
Dizziness, herbs causing, 32
DNA, 9, 62, 63, 137
Dong quai, 30
Doshas (Ayurvedic medicine), 23–24
Dried beef, nutrients in, 213
Dried fruits, 141
Drugs:
   anticonvulsant, 83
   antidepressant, 32
   and constipation, 69
   herbal interactions with, 29
   monoamine oxidase inhibitor, 30
   prescription, 28
   selective serotonin reuptake inhibitor, 30
Duck, 139, 232
Dulse, 140

Duodenum, 4, 129
Dysmenorrhea, 111

E

Ear infection, 80
Echinacea, 30
Eczema, 81–83
Edam cheese, nutrients in, 167
Eel, nutrients in, 237
EFAs (*see* Essential fatty acids)
Effleurage, 25
Eggnog, nutrients in, 176
Eggplant, nutrients in, 247
Eggs, 140, 177
Eicosanoids, 47, 135
Elderberries, nutrients in, 186
Emotions, immune system and, 32
Endive, nutrients in, 248
Endocrine system, mindbody therapy and, 32
Endogenous depression, 73
Endometriosis, 111
Energy:
   DRIs for, 159–161
   and fats/fatty acids, 7
   and glycemic index of foods, 151
   levels of, 6
   RDAs for, 159–161
Energy balancing, 26–27
English muffins, nutrients in, 202
Enoki mushrooms, nutrients in, 250
Enzymes, 3–4, 9
   intrinsic factor, 12
   and manganese, 15
   superoxide dismutase, 14–15
   and zinc, 16
   (*See also* specific enzymes)
EPA, 136
Ephedra, 30
Epilepsy, 23, 83–84
Equal (sweetener), 142
Equivalents, table of, 158
Eriodictyol, 13
Esophagus, 3
Essential amino acids, 10
Essential fatty acids (EFAs), 7, 8
Essential oils, 21–23
Estrogen(s), 8, 109, 135
Eucalyptus, 30

Evaporated milk, nutrients in, 175
Extracts, herb, 29
Eye problems, 84–85
Eyelid, inflammation of, 84

F

Fatigue, 6, 12
    aromatherapy for, 22
    chronic fatigue syndrome, 15
    and fibromayalgia, 86
Fat(s), 7–9
    breakdown/metabolism of, 5
    digestion of, 4
    and glycemic index, 6, 151
    nutritional composition of, 178–182
    rich food sources of, 149–150
Fat-soluble vitamins, 10
Fatty acids, 7–9
    in foods, 135–136
    rich food sources of, 150
    (*See also* Omega-3 fatty acids; Omega-6 fatty
      acids)
Fava beans, nutrients in, 208
Feet, reflexology and, 27
Feldendrais method, 26
Females:
    DRIs for, 159–161
    RDAs for, 159–161
Fennel, 7
Fermented foods, 141
Fermented red clover, 30
Fertility, 16
Feta cheese, nutrients in, 167
Fever, herbs to avoid with, 30
Feverfew, 30
Fiber, 5–7, 69
    and diverticulitis, 80
    functions of, 6
    and glycemic index, 6
    suggested amounts of, 6
Fibrocystic breast disease, 85–86
Fibromyalgia, 86–87
Figs, nutrients in, 187
Fish, 140
    (*See also* specific types of fish)
Flat fish, nutrients in, 237
Flatulence, 7
Flavanones, 13

Flavans, 13
Flavones, 13
Flavonols, 13
Flaxseed, 109
Flaxseed oil, 8
Flounder, nutrients in, 237
Flour(s), 138, 206–207
Flu, 67–69
Fluid retention, 16
Folic acid, 12, 145
Fontina cheese, nutrients in, 167
Food additives, digestion and, 4
Food groups, 137–142
    beverages, 163–164
    dairy products, 140, 165–177
    eggs, 140, 177
    fats and oils, 178–182
    fruits and fruit juices, 137, 183–196
    grains, 138–139, 197–207
    legumes, 137–138, 208–212
    meats, 139–140, 213–224
    nuts and seeds, 139, 225–228
    poultry, 139–140, 228–234
    seafood and seaweed, 140, 234–243
    sweeteners, 141–142
    vegetables and vegetable juices, 137,
      243–256
Food intolerances, 5, 136, 140
Foods, 135–153
    for abscess, 38
    for acne, 39
    for AIDS, 41
    for allergy, 43
    for Alzheimer's disease, 45
    for anemia, 46
    for arthritis, 48
    for asthma, 50
    for atherosclerosis, 53
    Ayurvedic categorization of, 24
    for back pain, 55
    for bronchitis, 57
    for bruises, 59
    for burns, 60
    for bursitis, 61
    for cancer, 63
    for canker sores, 65
    for carpal tunnel syndrome, 65–66
    for chronic fatigue syndrome, 66–67
    for colds and flu, 68
    for constipation, 70

Foods (*Cont.*)
  for Crohn's disease, 71
  for cystitis, 72–73
  for depression, 74–75
  for diabetes, 77
  for diarrhea, 78–79
  for diverticulitis, 80
  for eczema, 82
  fatty acids in, 135–136
  fermented, 141
  for fibrocystic breast disease, 85
  for fibromyalgia, 86
  for gallbladder disease, 87
  for gingivitis, 89
  glycemic index of, 150–153
  for gout, 90
  groups, food (*see* Food groups)
  for headache, 91–92
  for heart attack, 93–94
  for heartburn, 95
  for hemorrhoids, 96
  for hepatitis, 98
  for herpes, 99
  for hypertension, 101
  for infection, 103
  for insomnia, 104–105
  intolerances of/sensitivities to, 136, 140
  for irritable bowel syndrome, 106
  for kidney stones, 107–108
  for lupus, 109
  for menopause, 110
  for menstrual problems, 112
  for multiple sclerosis, 114
  nutrient-rich, 144–150
  organically-grown, 136
  for osteoporosis, 115–116
  for overweight, 116–117
  pharmacological activity of, 142–144
  for pregnancy, 119
  for premenstrual syndrome, 120–121
  for prostate problems, 122
  for psoriasis, 123–124
  for Raynaud's disease, 125
  for stress, 126–127
  for stroke, 128
  supplements vs., 136–137
  for ulcers, 129
  for vaginitis, 131
  (*See also* specific foods)
Frankfurters, nutrients in, 222

Free radicals, 8, 62, 137
French bread, nutrients in, 202
Friction massage, 25
Frozen desserts, nutrients in, 173
Fructose, 5, 141
Fruits, 137
  glycemic indexes of, 152
  nutritional composition of, 183–196
  as source of sweeteners, 141
  (*See also* specific fruits)
Fungicides, 136
Fungus (in celery), 137

G

Galactose, 5
Gallbladder, 4, 11
Gallbladder disease, 87–88
Gallstones, 29, 30, 32, 87
Gamma tocopherol, 136
Garbanzo beans, 138
Garbanzo beans, nutrients in, 209
Garlic, 7, 30, 248
Gastric acids, 4
Gastritis, 29, 30, 32, 129
Genistein, 13
GI (*see* Glycemic index)
Ginger, 7, 30
Gingivitis, 88–89
Ginkgo biloba, 44
Ginseng, 30
Gjetost cheese, nutrients in, 167
Glands:
  adrenal, 12
  oil, 8
  in stomach, 3–4
  sweat, 16
  thyroid, 15
Glandulars, 136
Glaucoma, 15, 84
  essential oils to avoid with, 23
  herbs to avoid with, 29, 30
Glucose, 5–6, 9
  (*See also* Glycemic index)
Glucose tolerance factor (GTF), 14
Glycemic index (GI), 6, 150–153
  calculation of, 151
  and diabetes, 76
  and method of food processing, 151

Glycemic index (GI) (*Cont.*)
of processed grains, 138
Glycogen, 5, 6, 9
Goat's milk, 140, 176
Goldenrod, 29
Goldenseal, 30
Goose, 139, 232
Gooseberries, nutrients in, 187
Gouda cheese, nutrients in, 167
Gout, 11, 89–91
Graham crackers:
glycemic index of, 153
nutrients in, 205
Grains, 138–139
glycemic indexes of, 152
nutritional composition of, 197–207
(*See also* specific grains)
Grape juice, nutrients in, 188
Grapefruit, nutrients in, 187
Grapefruit juice, nutrients in, 187
Grapes, nutrients in, 188
Grapeseed oil, nutrients in, 180
Green beans, nutrients in, 248
Green onions, nutrients in, 251
Ground beef, nutrients in, 213–214
Gruyere cheese, nutrients in, 168
GTF (glucose tolerance factor), 14
Guavas, nutrients in, 188
Guggul, 24
Gums, 6
infection of, 102
inflammation of, 88

H

Haddock, nutrients in, 237
Hair loss, 12
Half and half, nutrients in, 172
Halibut, nutrients in, 237
Hallucinations, herbs causing, 32
Ham, nutrients in, 217
Hazelnut oil, nutrients in, 180
Hazelnuts, nutrients in, 226
HCl (*see* Hydrochloric acid)
HDL (*see* High-density lipoproteins)
Headaches, 13, 91–92
aromatherapy for, 22
herbs causing, 32
homeopathic treatment of, 31

Health conditions, 37, 135
(*See also* specific conditions)
Heart, chicken, nutrients in, 231
Heart attacks, 8, 9, 11, 13, 93–95
Heart disease, 8, 10, 12, 30, 150
Heartburn, 30, 95–96
Helicobacter pylori, 129
Hellerwork, 25
Hemicellulose, 6
Hemorrhaging, essential oils to avoid with, 23
Hemorrhoids, 96–97
Hepatitis, 97–99
Herb tea, nutrients in, 164
Herbal therapy, 28–31
for abscess, 38
for acne, 39
for AIDS, 41–42
for allergy, 43
for Alzheimer's disease, 45
for anemia, 46
for arthritis, 48–49
for asthma, 51
for atherosclerosis, 53
for athlete's foot, 54
for back pain, 55
for bronchitis, 57
for bruises, 59
for burns, 60
for bursitis, 61
for cancer, 64
for canker sores, 65
for carpal tunnel syndrome, 66
for chronic fatigue syndrome, 67
for colds and flu, 68
for constipation, 70
for Crohn's disease, 72
for cystitis, 73
for depression, 75
for diabetes, 77
for diarrhea, 79
for diverticulitis, 80
for ear infection, 81
for eczema, 82
for epilepsy, 83
for fibrocystic breast disease, 85–86
for fibromyalgia, 86
for gallbladder disease, 88
for gingivitis, 89
for gout, 90
for headache, 92

Herbal therapy (*Cont.*)
  for heart attack, 94
  for heartburn, 95–96
  for hemorrhoids, 96–97
  for hepatitis, 98
  for herpes, 99–100
  for hypertension, 101
  for infection, 103
  for insomnia, 105
  for irritable bowel syndrome, 106
  for kidney stones, 108
  for lupus, 109
  for menopause, 110–111
  for menstrual problems, 112–113
  for multiple sclerosis, 114
  for osteoporosis, 116
  for overweight, 117
  for pregnancy, 119
  for premenstrual syndrome, 121
  for prostate problems, 123
  for psoriasis, 124
  for Raynaud's disease, 125
  for stress, 127
  for stroke, 128
  for ulcers, 130
  for vaginitis, 131
Herpes, 99–100
Hesperetin, 13
Hesperidin, 13
Hiatal hernia, 95
Hickory nuts, nutrients in, 226
High blood pressure (*see* Hypertension)
High-density lipoproteins (HDL), 8, 9
Histamine, 13
Histamines, 47
HIV (*see* Human immunodeficiency virus)
Hives, 43
Hiziki, 140
Homeopathy, 32–32, 37
  for abscess, 38
  for acne, 39–40
  for AIDS, 42
  for allergy, 43–44
  for anemia, 46–47
  for arthritis, 49
  for asthma, 51
  for atherosclerosis, 54
  for back pain, 55–56
  for bronchitis, 57–58
  for bruises, 59

Homeopathy (*Cont.*)
  for burns, 60
  for bursitis, 62
  for cancer, 64
  for canker sores, 65
  for carpal tunnel syndrome, 66
  for chronic fatigue syndrome, 67
  for colds and flu, 68–69
  for constipation, 70
  for Crohn's disease, 72
  for cystitis, 73
  for depression, 75
  for diabetes, 77
  for diarrhea, 79
  for diverticulitis, 80
  for ear infection, 81
  for eczema, 82
  for epilepsy, 83
  for fibrocystic breast disease, 86
  for fibromyalgia, 86
  for gallbladder disease, 88
  for gingivitis, 89
  for gout, 90
  for headache, 92
  for heart attack, 94
  for heartburn, 96
  for hemorrhoids, 97
  for hepatitis, 98
  for herpes, 100
  for hypertension, 101
  for infection, 103–104
  for insomnia, 105
  for irritable bowel syndrome, 106–107
  for kidney stones, 108
  for menopause, 111
  for menstrual problems, 113
  for multiple sclerosis, 114
  for osteoporosis, 116
  for pregnancy, 119–120
  for premenstrual syndrome, 121
  for prostate problems, 122
  for psoriasis, 124
  for Raynaud's disease, 125
  for stress, 127
  for ulcers, 130
  for vaginitis, 131
Homocysteine, 12
Honey, 141
Honeydew melons, nutrients in, 190
Hormone replacements, 109

Hormones:
    and aromatherapy, 22
    and cholesterol, 8
    and protein, 9
    thyroid, 15
Horse chestnut, 30
Hot peppers, nutrients in, 252
Human immunodeficiency virus (HIV),
    30, 40
Human milk, nutrients in, 176
Hydrangea, 30
Hydrochloric acid (HCl), 4, 39, 95
Hydrogenated fats, 8
Hyperactivity, 15
Hypertension, 6, 15, 16, 100–102, 150
    essential oils to avoid with, 23
    and headaches, 91
    herbs to avoid with, 30, 32
Hypnotherapy, 33
Hypoglycemia, 6, 29
Hypothalamus, 16
Hypothyroidism, essential oils to avoid with, 23

I

Ice cream, nutrients in, 173
Iceberg lettuce, nutrients in, 249
IgE (immunoglobulin E), 42
Ileocccal valve, 5
Illness(es):
    causes of, 21, 24
    invisible, 27
    responding to aromatherapy, 22
Imagery, 33
Immune system, 10, 16
    emotional states and, 32
    and infection, 102
    memory of, 32
Immunoglobulin E (IgE), 42
Impotence, 122
Incontinence, 32
Infants:
    DRIs for, 159–161
    RDAs for, 159–161
Infection(s), 10, 102–104
    cystitis, 72
    ear, 80
    herbs to avoid with, 30
    of respiratory tract, 67–68

Infectious illnesses, 22
Infinitesimal Dose, Law of, 31
Inflammations, 87, 102
Infusions, herb, 29
Inositol, 12, 146
Inositol hexanicotinate, 11
Insoluble fibers, 6–7
Insomnia, 104–106
    aromatherapy for, 22
    essential oils to avoid with, 23
Insulin, 6, 9, 76, 150, 151
Intermittent claudication, 52
Intestinal tract, 4, 5
Intolerances, food, 136, 140
Intrinsic factor, 12
Iodine, 15
    and acne, 39
    rich food sources of, 148
Iron, 14, 15, 148
Irritable bowel syndrome, 7, 106–107
Isoflavones, 13, 109
Italian sausage, nutrients in, 222

J

Jam, glycemic index of, 153
Jaundice, 97
Jelly beans, glycemic index of, 153
Jicama, nutrients in, 248
Joints:
    and arthritis, 47–50
    and gout, 89
Juices:
    for abscess, 38
    for acne, 39
    for allergy, 43
    for anemia, 46
    for arthritis, 48
    for asthma, 50–51
    for atherosclerosis, 53
    for bronchitis, 57
    for bruises, 59
    for burns, 60
    for bursitis, 61
    for cancer, 63
    for canker sores, 65
    for chronic fatigue syndrome, 67
    for colds and flu, 68
    for constipation, 70

Juices (*Cont.*):
    for Crohn's disease, 71
    for cystitis, 73
    for diarrhea, 79
    for diverticulitis, 80
    for eczema, 82
    fruit, 141, 183–196
    for gallbladder disease, 88
    for gingivitis, 89
    for gout, 90
    for headache, 92
    for heart attack, 94
    for heartburn, 95
    for hemorrhoids, 96
    for hepatitis, 98
    for herpes, 99
    for hypertension, 101
    for infection, 103
    for insomnia, 105
    for irritable bowel syndrome, 106
    for kidney stones, 108
    for lupus, 109
    for menopause, 110
    for menstrual problems, 112
    for multiple sclerosis, 114
    for osteoporosis, 116
    for overweight, 117
    for prostate problems, 122
    for psoriasis, 124
    for Raynaud's disease, 125
    for stress, 127
    for stroke, 128
    for ulcers, 129–130
    vegetable, 243–256
Juniper, 30

K

Kale, 137, 248
Kamut, 138, 139
Kapha dosha, 24
Kava kava, 30
Kefir, 141
Kelp, 140, 238
Ketones (in essential oils), 23
Kidney beans, nutrients in, 209
Kidney disease, herbs to avoid with, 30, 32
Kidney stones, 13, 107–108
Kidneys, 10, 16, 23

Kielbasa, nutrients in, 222
Kiwis, nutrients in, 188
Knockwurst, nutrients in, 223
Kohlrabi, 137, 249
Kombu, 140
Kombucha, 141
Korean ginseng, 30
Kumquats, nutrients in, 189

L

LA (linoleic acid), 7
Lack of appetite, 12
Lactating women:
    DRIs for, 159–161
    herbs to avoid by, 29, 30, 32
    RDAs for, 159–161
Lactose, 5, 140
Lactose intolerances, 5, 140
Lamb, nutrients in, 216
Large intestine, 5
    and diarrhea, 78
    and diverticulitis, 80
Law of Infinitesimal Dose, 31
Law of Similars, 31
LDL (*see* Low-density lipoproteins)
Lecithin, 12
Leeks, nutrients in, 249
Leg pain, 52
Legumes, 137–138
    glycemic indexes of, 152
    nutritional composition of, 208–212
    (*See also* specific legumes)
Lemon juice, nutrients in, 189
Lentils and lentil sprouts, 137, 209
Lettuce, nutrients in, 249
Licorice, 30
Lignins, 6
Lima beans, nutrients in, 209
Limburger cheese, nutrients in, 168
Lime juice, nutrients in, 189
Linoleic acid (LA), 7
Linolenic acid (LNA), 7
Lipase, 4, 39
Lipoproteins, 8–9
Liquids, digestion of, 4
Liver (as food):
    beef, 214
    chicken, 231

Liver (as food) (*Cont.*):
　duck, 232
　goose, 233
　lamb, 216
　turkey, 233
　veal, 219
Liver cheese, nutrients in, 223
Liver diseases, 11, 29, 30
Liver (human organ), 4, 5, 10, 11
　dysfunction of, 5
　and hepatitis, 97
　herbs toxic to, 29
　vitamin A storage in, 10–11
Liver paté, chicken, 232
Liverwurst, nutrients in, 223
LNA (linolenic acid), 7
Lobelia, 30
Lobster, nutrients in, 238
Loganberries, nutrients in, 189
Loquats, nutrients in, 189
Low blood sugar (*see* Hypoglycemia)
Low-density lipoproteins (LDL), 8–9
Luncheon meats, nutrients in, 221–224
Lupus, 30, 108–109
Lutein, 10, 11
Lychee, nutrients in, 190
Lycopene, 10, 11, 136

M

Ma huang, 30
Macadamia nuts, nutrients in, 226
Macaroni, nutrients in, 199
Mackerel, nutrients in, 238
Macronutrients, 5–10
　carbohydrates, 5–7
　fats, 7–9
　proteins, 9–10
Macular degeneration, 84–85
Magnesium, 15, 148
Males:
　DRIs for, 159–161
　RDAs for, 159–161
Maltose, 5
Manganese, 15, 148
Mangoes, nutrients in, 190
MAO inhibitor drugs, herbs to avoid with, 30
Maple sugar, 141
Maple syrup, 141

Margarine, nutrients in, 180
Massage, 25–26
Materia Medica Repertory (William Boericke), 37
Meadowsweet, 30
Measures, 157, 158
Meats, 139–140
　and glycemic index, 151
　nutritional composition of, 213–224
Medications (*See* Drugs)
Medicine, conventional (allopathic), 21
　(*See also* Alternative medicine and therapies)
Meditation, 32
Melatonin, 136
Melons, nutrients in, 190
Memory (of immune system), 32
Memory problems, 44
Men (*See* Males)
Menopause, 14, 109–111
Menorrhagia, 112
Menstrual problems, 23, 111–113
Meridians, 26
Metric conversions, 157
Metropolitan Life height and weight chart, 117–118
Micronutrients, 10–17
　B complex vitamins, 11–12
　biotin, 12
　calcium, 14
　choline, 12
　chromium, 14–15
　copper, 15
　folic acid, 12
　inositol, 12
　iodine, 15
　iron, 15
　magnesium, 15
　manganese, 15
　PABA, 12–12
　pantothenic acid, 12
　para amino benzoic acid, 12
　potassium, 16
　selenium, 16
　sodium, 16
　vitamin A, 10–11
　vitamin C (ascorbic acid), 13
　vitamin D, 13
　vitamin E, 13–14
　vitamin K, 14
　zinc, 16

Microvilli, 4
Middle ear infections, 80–81
Migraines, 91
Milk, 140
    and diabetes, 76
    nutrients in, 173–176
Millet, 138, 198
Mindbody therapy, 32–33
    for acne, 40
    for AIDS, 42
    for allergy, 44
    for Alzheimer's disease, 45
    for anemia, 47
    for arthritis, 50
    for asthma, 52
    for atherosclerosis, 54
    for back pain, 56
    for bronchitis, 58
    for bruises, 59
    for burns, 60
    for cancer, 64
    for canker sores, 65
    for carpal tunnel syndrome, 66
    for chronic fatigue syndrome, 67
    for colds and flu, 69
    for constipation, 71
    for Crohn's disease, 72
    for cystitis, 73
    for depression, 76
    for diabetes, 78
    for diarrhea, 80
    for diverticulitis, 80
    for eczema, 83
    for epilepsy, 84
    for fibrocystic breast disease, 86
    for fibromyalgia, 87
    for gallbladder disease, 88
    for gout, 91
    for headache, 92
    for heart attack, 95
    for heartburn, 96
    for hemorrhoids, 97
    for hepatitis, 99
    for herpes, 100
    for hypertension, 102
    for infection, 104
    for insomnia, 106
    for irritable bowel syndrome, 107
    for lupus, 109
    for menopause, 111

Mindbody therapy (*Cont.*)
    for menstrual problems, 113
    for multiple sclerosis, 115
    for osteoporosis, 116
    for overweight, 117
    for pregnancy, 120
    for premenstrual syndrome, 121
    for prostate problems, 123
    for psoriasis, 124
    for Raynaud's disease, 126
    for stress, 127–128
    for stroke, 129
    for ulcers, 131
Minerals, 10, 14–16, 159–161
    calcium, 14
    chromium, 14–15
    copper, 15
    DRIs for, 159–161
    iodine, 15
    iron, 15
    magnesium, 15
    manganese, 15
    potassium, 16
    RDAs for, 159–161
    selenium, 16
    sodium, 16
    zinc, 16
Ministrokes, 128
Miso, 141, 210
Mixed-grain bread, nutrients in, 202
Molasses, 141
Molybdenum, rich food sources of, 148
Monoamine oxidase (MAO) inhibitor drugs,
        herbs to avoid with, 30
Monosaccharides, 5
Monounsaturated fats (MUFAs), 7–9
Monounsaturated fatty acids, rich food sources
        of, 149, 150
Monterey Jack cheese, nutrients in, 168
Mortadella, nutrients in, 223
Mouth, 3
Movement therapies, 26
Mozzarella cheese, nutrients in, 168
Mucus, 4
Muenster cheese, nutrients in, 169
MUFAs (*see* Monounsaturated fats)
Mulberries, nutrients in, 191
Multiple sclerosis, 30, 113–115
Mung bean sprouts, nutrients in, 210
Muscles, deep tissue massage of, 25–26

Mushrooms, 137, 249–250
Music therapy, 44
Mustard, 30
Mustard greens, 137, 250

N

Narcolepsy, 104
Natto, 141, 210
Nausea, 12
Navy beans, nutrients in, 210
Nectarines, nutrients in, 191
Nerve compression injuries, 11
Nervous conditions, aromatherapy for, 22
Nervous system, 28
Neufchatel cheese, nutrients in, 169
Neuropeptides, 32
Neurotransmitters, depression and, 74
Niacin (vitamin B_3), 11, 145
Niacinamide, 11
Night blindness, 85
Night vision, 10
Nitric oxide, 13
Nitrites, 139
Nonfat dry milk, nutrients in, 175
Nori, 140
Nutrasweet, 142
Nutrient-rich foods:
    lists of, 144–150
    organic foods as, 136
Nutrients, 3–16
    for abscess, 38
    for acne, 39
    for AIDS, 40–41
    for allergy, 43
    for Alzheimer's disease, 44–45
    for anemia, 46
    for arthritis, 47–48
    for asthma, 50
    for atherosclerosis, 52–53
    B complex vitamins, 11–12
    for back pain, 55
    biotin, 12
    for bronchitis, 56–57
    for bruises, 58–59
    for burns, 60
    for bursitis, 61
    calcium, 14
    for cancer, 63

Nutrients (*Cont.*)
    for canker sores, 64
    carbohydrates, 5–7
    for carpal tunnel syndrome, 65
    choline, 12
    chromium, 14–15
    for chronic fatigue syndrome, 66
    for colds and flu, 68
    for constipation, 69
    copper, 15
    for Crohn's disease, 71
    for cystitis, 72
    for depression, 74
    for diabetes, 76–77
    for diarrhea, 78
    digestion of, 3–5
    for ear infection, 81
    for eczema, 82
    for epilepsy, 83
    equilibrium of, 136
    fats, 7–9
    for fibrocystic breast disease, 85
    for fibromyalgia, 86
    folic acid, 12
    for gallbladder disease, 87
    for gingivitis, 88–89
    for gout, 90
    for headache, 91
    for heart attack, 93
    for hemorrhoids, 96
    for hepatitis, 97–98
    for herpes, 99
    for hypertension, 100–101
    for infection, 102–103
    inositol, 12
    for insomnia, 104
    iodine, 15
    iron, 15
    for irritable bowel syndrome, 106
    for kidney stones, 107
    for lupus, 109
    macronutrients, 5–10
    magnesium, 15
    manganese, 15
    for menopause, 110
    for menstrual problems, 112
    micronutrients, 10–17
    minerals, 14–16
    for multiple sclerosis, 114
    for osteoporosis, 115

Nutrients (*Cont.*)
    for overweight, 116
    PABA, 12–13
    pantothenic acid, 12
    para amino benzoic acid, 12
    potassium, 16
    for pregnancy, 118–119
    for premenstrual syndrome, 120
    in processed grains, 138
    for prostate problems, 122
    proteins, 9–10
    for psoriasis, 123
    for Raynaud's disease, 125
    selenium, 16
    sodium, 16
    for stress, 126
    for stroke, 128
    for ulcers, 129, 130
    for vaginitis, 131
    vitamin A, 10–11
    vitamin C (ascorbic acid), 13
    vitamin D, 13
    vitamin E, 13–14
    vitamin K, 14
    and water, 16–17
    zinc, 16
Nutritional yeast, 136
Nuts and seeds, 139
    and glycemic index, 151
    nutritional composition of, 225–228
    oxidation of, 8

O

Oak, 30
Oats, 138, 198
Obesity, 6
Oil glands, 8
Oils, 8
    essential, 21–23
    nutritional composition of, 178–182
Okra, nutrients in, 250
Olive oil, 8, 180
Omega-3 fatty acids, 7, 47, 135–136
    and atherosclerosis, 52
    fish as source of, 140
    rich food sources of, 150
Omega-6 fatty acids, 7, 52, 135, 136, 150
Onions, nutrients in, 251

Oral contraceptives (*see* Birth control pills)
Orange juice, nutrients in, 191
Oranges, nutrients in, 191
Oregon grape, 30
Organ meats, 139
Organically-grown foods, 136
Osteoarthritis, 47
Osteoporosis, 12, 14, 115–116
Otitis media, 80
Overweight, 116–118
    and arthritis, 47
    and diabetes, 76
    and glycemic index of foods, 151
Oxalates, 107
Oxidation:
    of fats, 8
    sources of, 137
    (*See also* Antioxidants)
Oysters, nutrients in, 238

P

PABA (*see* Para amino benzoic acid)
Palm kernel oil, nutrients in, 181
Palm oil, nutrients in, 181
Pancreas, 3, 4, 150
Pantothenic acid, 12, 145–146
Pap smears, 63
Papayas, nutrients in, 191
Para amino benzoic acid (PABA), 12, 146
Parmesan cheese, nutrients in, 169
Parsley, nutrients in, 251
Parsnips, nutrients in, 251
Partially hydrogenated fats, 8
Passion flower, 30
Passion fruit, nutrients in, 192
Pasta, nutrients in, 198–199
Pastrami, nutrients in, 214
Pau d'arco, 30
Peach nectar, nutrients in, 192
Peaches, nutrients in, 192
Peanut butter, nutrients in, 211
Peanut oil, nutrients in, 181
Peanuts, 137, 210
Pear nectar, nutrients in, 193
Pearl barley, 139
Pears, nutrients in, 192–193
Peas, 137, 211

Pecans, nutrients in, 226
Peppermint, 7, 30
Pepperoni, nutrients in, 223
Peppers, nutrients in, 251–252
Pepsin, 4, 95, 129
Peptic ulcers, 32, 129
Peptides, 32
Perch, nutrients in, 238
Periodentitis, 88
Peripheral nervous system, 28
Peristalsis, 3, 4
Pernicious anemia, 46
Persimmons, nutrients in, 193
Pesticides, 136
Pettrisage, 25
Pharmacological activity:
    of foods, 142–144
    of herbs, 28–29
Pharynx, 3
Pheasant, nutrients in, 234
Phosphorus, 13
Photomedicines, 29
Phytochemicals, 10, 11, 136, 137
Phytoestrogens, 10, 109
Pickles, nutrients in, 252
Pike, nutrients in, 239
Pine nuts, nutrients in, 227
Pineapple juice, nutrients in, 194
Pineapples, nutrients in, 193
Pinto beans, nutrients in, 211
Pistachios, nutrients in, 227
Pita bread, nutrients in, 203
Pitta dosha, 24
Plantains, nutrients in, 194
Plaque, arterial, 8
Plums, nutrients in, 194
PMS (*see* Premenstrual syndrome)
Polarity therapy, 26
Polish sausage, nutrients in, 224
Pollock, nutrients in, 239
Polyphenols, 10
Polysaccharides, 10
Polyunsaturated fats (PUFAs), 7–9, 149–150
Pomegranates, nutrients in, 194
Popcorn, nutrients in, 200
Pork, nutrients in, 217–218
Pork sausage, nutrients in, 224
Port du salut cheese, nutrients in, 169
Portabello mushrooms, nutrients in, 250
Portal vein, 5

Positron emission tomography, 33
Posture, 25
Potassium, 16, 148
Potatoes, 137, 252
Poultices , herb, 29
Poultry, 139–140, 228–234
Pregnancy, 11, 14, 15, 37, 118–120
    DRIs for women during, 159–161
    essential oils to avoid during, 23
    herbs to avoid during, 29–31
    RDAs for women during, 159–161
Premarin, 109
Premature aging, 8
Premenstrual syndrome (PMS), 11, 15, 120–121
Prescription drugs, herbs used in, 28
Prickly pears, nutrients in, 195
Primrose, 30
Proanthocyanidins, 10
Processed cheese, nutrients in, 171
Progesterone, 109
Prostate problems, 23, 122–123
Prostitis, 122
Protease, 4
Protein, 9–10
    and allergies, 42
    digestion of, 4
    DRIs for, 159–161
    in legumes, 137
    in meats, 139
    RDAs for, 159–161
    rich food sources of, 144
Protein supplements, 136
Proteolytic enzymes, 4
Prothrombin, 14
Provolone cheese, nutrients in, 170
Prozac, herbs to avoid with, 30
Prune juice, nutrients in, 195
Prunes, nutrients in, 195
Psoriasis, 123–124
Psychological disorders, 22, 32
Psychoneuroimmunology, 32
Ptyalin, 3
PUFAs (*see* Polyunsaturated fats)
Pumpernickel bread, nutrients in, 203
Pumpkin, nutrients in, 252
Pumpkin seeds, nutrients in, 227
Purslane, nutrients in, 252
Pyridoxine (vitamin B_6), 11–12, 145

Q

Qi, 27
Qigong, 26
Quail, nutrients in, 234
Quercetin, 13
Quercetrin, 13
Quince, nutrients in, 195
Quinoa, 138, 139, 201

R

Rabbit, nutrients in, 220
Radishes, 137, 253
Ragweed allergy, herbs to avoid with, 29
Raisins, nutrients in, 195
Rapadura, 141
Raspberries, nutrients in, 196
Raw sugar, 141
Raynaud's disease, 124–126
RDAs (*see* Recommended Dietary
    Allowances)
Receptors, 9
Recommended Dietary Allowances (RDAs),
    158–161
Rectal cancer, fiber and, 6
Red blood cells, 45
Red clover, 30
Refined foods, 5, 151
Reflexology, 27
Reproductive cancers, 62
Respiratory tract infections, 67–68
Restless leg syndrome, 104
Rheumatoid arthritis, 47
Rhubarb, 30, 196
Riboflavin (vitamin B_2), 11, 145
Ribosomes, 9
Rice, 138, 139, 200–201
Ricotta cheese, nutrients in, 170
Roasts, beef, 214
Rolf, Ida, 25
Rolfing, 25, 26
Rolls, nutrients in, 203–204
Romaine lettuce, nutrients in, 249
Romano cheese, nutrients in, 170
Roquefort cheese, nutrients in, 170
Rosacea, 39
Rutabaga, 137, 253
Rutin, 13

Rye, 138
Rye bread, nutrients in, 204
Rye flour, nutrients in, 207

S

s-adenosyl-L-methionine (SAMe), 12
Safflower oil, 8, 181
Sage, 30
Salami, nutrients in, 224
Salicylate activity in foods, 144
Salmon, nutrients in, 239
Salt, digestion and, 4
SAMe (s-adenosyl-L-methionine), 12
Sandalwood, 30
Sardines, nutrients in, 239
Sarsaparilla, 30
Saturated fats:
    and atherosclerosis, 52
    in means, poultry, 139
Saturated fatty acids (SFAs), 7–8, 149, 150
Sauerkraut, nutrients in, 253
Sausage, nutrients in, 221–224
Scallops, nutrients in, 239
Scar formation, 14
Schizophrenia, 15
Scullcap, 30
Sea bass, nutrients in, 235
Seafood, 140
Seafood and seaweed, composition of, 234–243
Seaweed, 140
Sedative foods, 144
Seeds (*see* Nuts and seeds)
Selective serotonin reuptake inhibitor drugs,
    herbs to avoid with, 30
Selenium, 16, 148
Sensitivities, food, 64, 136
Serotonin, 104
Serum cholesterol, 52
Sesame oil, nutrients in, 181
Sesame seeds, nutrients in, 227
SFAs (*see* Saturated fatty acids)
Shark, nutrients in, 240
Shellfish, 140
Sherbet, nutrients in, 173
Shiatsu, 26
Shiitake mushrooms, nutrients in, 250
Short ribs, nutrients in, 215
Shrimp, nutrients in, 240

Siberian ginseng, 30
Sickle cell anemia, 46
Silicon, rich food sources of, 149
Similars, Law of, 31
Simple carbohydrates, 5
Situational depression, 73
Skin cancer, 62
Skin irritation:
    eczema as cause of, 81
    herbs causing, 32
    herbs to avoid with, 30
    from psoriasis, 123
SLE (*see* Systemic lupus erythematosus)
Sleep apnea, 104
Sleep disorders, 104
    (*See also* Insomnia)
Small intestine, 4, 5, 10
Smelt, nutrients in, 240
Smoked beef, nutrients in, 215
Snails, nutrients in, 240
Snapper, nutrients in, 240
Snickers bars, glycemic index of, 153
Soba noodles, 139
SOD (superoxide dismutase), 14
Soda crackers, nutrients in, 205
Sodium, 16
Sole, nutrients in, 237
Sour cream, nutrients in, 173
Soy products, 137, 138
    fermented, 141
    milk, soy, 137, 138, 212
Soy sauce, 141
Soybean oil, nutrients in, 182
Soybean sprouts, nutrients in, 212
Soybeans, 109, 138, 211
Spaghetti, nutrients in, 199
Spareribs, nutrients in, 218
Spastic colon (*see* Irritable bowel syndrome)
Spelt, 138, 139
Spider bites, 42
Spinach, 137, 253
Spirulina, nutrients in, 241
Split peas, nutrients in, 211
Sprains, 48
Sprouts, 138
Squash, nutrients in, 253–254
Squash seeds, nutrients in, 227
St. John's wort, 29, 30
Starches, 6, 151
    (*See also* Carbohydrates)

Steaks, beef, nutrients in, 213, 214, 215
Stevia, 141
Stimulants, digestion and, 4
Stings, 42
Stomach, 3–4
Stomach ulcers, herbs to avoid with, 29
Strawberries, nutrients in, 196
Stress, 32, 126–128
Stroke, 8, 12, 128–129
Subluxation, 28
Substrate, 9
Sucrose, 5
Sugar(s), 6, 141
    and diabetes, 76
    and glycemic index, 151
    glycemic indexes of, 152
    (*See also* Carbohydrates; *specific types*)
Sulfur, rich food sources of, 149
Summer sausage, nutrients in, 224
Summer squash, nutrients in, 253
Sunflower oil, nutrients in, 182
Sunflower seeds, nutrients in, 227
Superoxide dismutase (SOD), 14
Supplements:
    and equilibrium of nutrients, 136
    foods vs., 136–137
Sweat glands, 16
Sweet peppers, nutrients in, 251
Sweet potatoes, nutrients in, 254
Sweetbreads, nutrients in, 220
Sweetened condensed milk, nutrients in, 175
Sweeteners, 141–142
Swiss chard, 137, 246
Swiss cheese, nutrients in, 171
Swordfish, nutrients in, 241
Sympathetic nervous system, 32, 126
Syrups, 141
Systemic lupus erythematosus (SLE), 108–109

T

Tabouli, 139
Tahini, nutrients in, 228
T'ai chi, 26
Tangerine juice, nutrients in, 196
Tangerines, nutrients in, 196
Tapotement massage, 25
Taro, nutrients in, 254
Taxmati rice, 139

Tea, nutrients in, 163–164
Tea tree, 30
Tearing, 16
Tef, 138, 139
Tempeh, 137, 141, 212
Temporomandibular joint syndrome (TMJ), 88
Tendonitis, 61
Tension, aromatherapy for, 22
Testosterone, 8
TFAs (trans fatty acids), 8
Therapeutic massage, 25
Therapy (*see* Alternative medicine and therapies)
Thiamine (vitamin B_1), 11, 145
Thirst, 16–17, 76
Thujone, 23
Thyroid gland, 15, 43
Thyroxine, 15
TIAs (*see* Transient ischemic attacks)
Tilsit cheese, nutrients in, 171
Tinctures, herb, 29
TMJ (temporomandibular joint syndrome), 88
Tocopherols, 14, 136
Tofu, 137, 138, 212
Tomato juice, nutrients in, 254
Tomato paste, nutrients in, 255
Tomatoes, nutrients in, 254
Tonsillitis, 102
Toothpaste, 64
Toxic effects:
    of herbs, 29, 30
    of ketones, 23
Toxins (in fish), 140
Trager approach (movement therapy), 26
Trans fatty acids (TFAs), 8
Transient ischemic attacks (TIAs), 52, 128
Treatments, 37
    (*See also* Alternative medicine and therapies)
Triglycerides, 7, 9
Trout, nutrients in, 241
Tuberculosis, herbs to avoid with, 30
Tumors:
    essential oils to avoid with, 23
    prostate, 122
Tuna, nutrients in, 241–242
Turbinado sugar, 141
Turkey, 139, 233
Turmeric, 31
Turnip greens, nutrients in, 255
Turnips, 137, 255

Tylenol, 97
Type I and II diabetes, 76

U

Ulcers, 11, 29, 30, 129–131
Umeboshi, 141
Urinary tract infection, essential oils to avoid with, 23
Uterine fibroids, 111
Uva ursi, 31

V

Vaginitis, 131–132
Vanadium, rich food sources of, 149
Varicose veins, 118
Vata dosha, 24
Veal, nutrients in, 219–220
Vegetable juice cocktail, nutrients in, 255
Vegetable shortening, nutrients in, 182
Vegetables, 137
    cruciferous, 137
    glycemic indexes of, 153
    nutritional composition of, 243–256
    (*See also* specific vegetables)
Vegetarians, 46
Veins, varicose veins, 118
Venison, nutrients in, 220
Ventricular fibrillation, 93
Vertebrae, 28
Vienna sausage, nutrients in, 224
Villi, 4
Vinegars, 141
Viruses, 68
Vision:
    glaucoma, 15
    night, 10
Vitamin(s), 10–14
    A, 10–11, 144–145
    B_1 (thiamine), 11, 145
    B_2 (riboflavin), 11, 145
    B_3 (niacin), 11
    B_6 (pyridoxine), 11–12, 145
    B_{12}, 12, 13, 145
    C (ascorbic acid), 13, 146
    D, 13, 146
    DRIs for, 159–161

Vitamin(s) (*Cont.*)
  E, 13–14, 44, 147
  K, 14, 147
  RDAs for, 159–161
  water-soluble vs. fat-soluble, 10
Vitex, 31

W

Wakame, 140, 242
Walnut oil, nutrients in, 182
Walnuts, nutrients in, 228
Water, 16–17
Water chestnuts, nutrients in, 255
Watercress, nutrients in, 256
Watermelon, nutrients in, 196
Water-soluble fibers, 6
Water-soluble vitamins, 10
Waxes, food, 136
Weakness, 6
Weight:
  Metropolitan Life height and weight chart,
    117–118
Weight loss, 13
Weights, 157
Wheat bread, nutrients in, 204
Wheat germ, 136, 138
Wheat germ oil, nutrients in, 182
Whipping/whipped cream, nutrients in, 172
White bread, nutrients in, 205
White flour, nutrients in, 207
White willow, 31

Whitefish, nutrients in, 242
Whole wheat bread, nutrients in, 205
Whole wheat crackers, nutrients in, 206
Whole wheat flour, nutrients in, 207
Wild game, nutrients in, 220
Wild indigo, 31
Wild rice, 138, 201
Wines, nutrients in, 164
Winter squash, nutrients in, 254
Women (*See* Females)
Wormwood, 31
Wounds, healing, 102

Y

Yams, nutrients in, 256
Yarrow, 31
Yin/yang, 26, 27
Yoga, 32
Yogurt, 138, 140, 141, 176–177
Yohimbe, 31
Yucca, 31

Z

Zeaxanthin, 10, 11
Zinc, 15, 16
  and acne, 39
  rich food sources of, 149
  and vitamin A use, 11

ABOUT THE AUTHOR

Lavon J. Dunne was the author of the highly successful Third Edition of McGraw-Hill's *Nutrition Almanac*.